HIGH-RISK PREGNANCY AND DELIVERY
NURSING PERSPECTIVES

HIGH-RISK PREGNANCY *and* DELIVERY

NURSING PERSPECTIVES

Elizabeth Stepp Gilbert, RN, MS

Assistant Professor,
Grand Canyon College,
Phoenix, Arizona

Judith Smith Harmon, RN, MS

Perinatal Clinical Nurse Specialist,
Good Samaritan Medical Center,
Phoenix, Arizona
Faculty, University of Phoenix, Phoenix, Arizona

with 66 illustrations

THE C. V. MOSBY COMPANY

St. Louis • Toronto • Princeton   1986

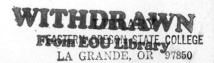

MOSBY

A TRADITION OF PUBLISHING EXCELLENCE

Editor: Barbara Ellen Norwitz
Developmental editor: Sally Adkisson
Editing supervisor: Lin Dempsey
Manuscript editor: Steve Ketterer
Book design: Nancy Steinmeyer
Production: Suzanne C. Glazer, Jeanne Gulledge

Printed in the United States of America

The C.V. Mosby Company
11830 Westline Industrial Drive, St. Louis, Missouri 63146

Library of Congress Cataloging in Publication Data

Gilbert, Elizabeth Stepp.
   High-risk pregnancy and delivery.

   Includes index.
      1. Obstetrical nursing.   2. Pregnancy, Complications
of.   3. Labor, Complicated.   I. Harmon, Judith Smith.
II. Title.   [DNLM: 1. Obstetrical Nursing.
2. Perinatology—nurses' instruction.   3. Pregnancy
Complications—nurses' instruction. WY 157 G464h]
RG951.G54   1986   610.73'678   85-3102
ISBN 0-8016-1896-7

C/VH/VH   9   8   7   6   5   4   3   2   1   01/D/043

Preface

The field of perinatal nursing is developing at a rapid pace. Out of this growth has come expanded knowledge leading to sophisticated care of the mother and fetus; the aim is to ensure an optimal outcome for the neonate and well-being of the mother while promoting the unity of the family. Not all high-risk pregnant women have ready access to a sophisticated perinatal obstetric service in a tertiary care center. Thus staff members in all obstetric care facilities, including primary care settings, must be prepared to screen for risk factors, render immediate stabilizing care in preparation for transport, and provide for preventive management. Nurses practicing in primary care settings must be able to assess and intervene rapidly and efficiently on the basis of scientific knowledge.

It is our conviction that thorough, sophisticated care of the maternal-fetal unit by all obstetric nurses can considerably decrease neonatal morbidity and mortality and lessen the incidence of later complications in children. Perinatal texts usually devote considerable attention to the care of the sick neonate; the intent of this text is to fill the void of nursing care knowledge of the high-risk maternal-fetal unit to improve the neonatal outcome.

This book is designed to provide obstetric nurses, practitioners, clinicians, and upper-division undergraduate and graduate students a text and reference for rendering high-risk maternal and fetal nursing care. The format was selected to provide for concise and systematic retrieval of information, focusing on knowledge beyond basic understanding. Additional references and resources are included for the reader who desires further information.

High-Risk Pregnancy and Delivery: Nursing Perspectives focuses on the physiologic and psychologic stressors of a high-risk pregnancy as they relate to the mother and the fetus. It is designed to provide the reader with a strong background in physiologic and pathophysiologic changes in pregnancy, their effects on the mother and fetus, and their potential effects on the neonate if optimal care is not implemented. Psychologic concepts are emphasized in one special unit and are interwoven throughout the text.

The text is organized into units and chapters based on physiologic adaptations to pregnancy, identification of high-risk pregnancy, antepartum and intrapartum assessment, psychologic implications of high-risk pregnancy, complicating conditions in pregnancy, and labor disorders. The content within the

v

chapters is organized according to the following format: incidence, etiology, and physiology, including pathophysiology and maternal and fetal/neonatal effects. The usual medical management is summarized so the nurse will be familiar with the possible plans of care and can thereby prepare and support the patient in considering her available options. A strong emphasis on the nursing process is a primary focus of each chapter. A major role of the nurse when caring for the expectant mother and her unborn child is one of prevention and early recognition; therefore patient education, assessment, intervention, and evaluation are heavily emphasized. Most chapters also include a suggested plan of nursing care, including potential patient problems, outcome criteria, and assessments and interventions. Other reference guides and tables are provided to consolidate critical information into a concise form.

ELIZABETH STEPP GILBERT
JUDITH SMITH HARMON

Contents

UNIT I PHYSIOLOGIC CONSIDERATIONS OF A HIGH-RISK PREGNANCY

1 Physiologic adaptations to pregnancy, *3*
2 Identification of a high-risk pregnancy, *22*
3 Antepartum and intrapartum assessment of fetal well-being, *31*

UNIT II PSYCHOLOGIC IMPLICATIONS OF A HIGH-RISK PREGNANCY

4 Psychologic adaptations to high-risk pregnancy, *71*

UNIT III HEALTH DISORDERS COMPLICATING PREGNANCY

5 Diabetes and pregnancy, *87*
6 Cardiac disease and pregnancy, *116*
7 Renal disease and pregnancy, *135*

UNIT IV COMPLICATIONS IN PREGNANCY

8 Spontaneous abortion, *157*
9 Ectopic pregnancy, *186*
10 Gestational trophoblastic disease, *208*
11 Third-trimester bleeding: abruptio placentae and placenta previa, *223*
12 Disseminated intravascular coagulopathy, *257*
13 Hypertensive disorders of pregnancy, *267*
14 Preterm labor, *306*
15 Premature rupture of membranes, *347*
16 Hemolytic incompatibility, *363*

UNIT V   ALTERATIONS IN THE MECHANISM OF LABOR

17   Dysfunctional labor, *383*
18   Postterm pregnancy, *419*
19   Labor stimulation, *432*

UNIT I

PHYSIOLOGIC CONSIDERATIONS OF A HIGH-RISK PREGNANCY

Significant changes occur in female physiology following impregnation. Within a very few weeks alterations are measurable in many body systems. The mother must acquire and circulate increased quantities of nutrients to herself and the conceptus. Her body must form and maintain a new organ, the placenta. Through this, her body must dispose of fetal waste products and provide for fetal nutrition and respiration. Throughout the pregnancy, homeostatic mechanisms must adapt to provide for protection of the fetus and to guard against its rejection as a foreign substance.

When caring for the high-risk pregnant woman, the nurse must consider numerous physiologic aspects of pregnancy, such as adaptations in maternal body functions and the development of the maternal-fetal unit. Through analysis of these, specific antenatal assessments can be made and high-risk pregnancies can be identified. Special antepartum and intrapartum assessments of fetal well-being, including fetal monitoring and other surveillance modes, can also be instituted.

CHAPTER 1

Physiologic adaptations to pregnancy

In the sections to follow, adaptions in body functions will be described as they relate to cardiovascular, respiratory, metabolic, glandular, renal, hepatic, hematologic, gastrointestinal, and reproductive physiology. Descriptions of development of the fetus, beginning as an embryo, and the formation of the placenta will follow. Antepartum nursing assessments directed at promotion and maintenance of health will be described as they relate to laboratory studies, physical assessment, and nutritional requirements.

ADAPTATIONS IN BODY FUNCTIONS
Cardiovascular adaptations

Body fluid is compartmentalized into cellular space, interstitial space, and blood space. Water and solutes exit from the capillaries into the interstitial space where they are continually exchanged with water and solutes in the cellular space.

Blood, which consists of a suspension of various specialized cells in plasma, exerts a pressure on vessel walls. The pressure exerted depends on blood volume and distensibility of the vessel walls. Blood flow is related to the pressure gradient and the resistance of the vessel walls. Flow is measured as cardiac output and the pressure gradient is measured as arterial blood pressure. During pregnancy specific adaptations occur in these functions. These adaptations are ultimately aimed at fetal sustenance.

Total body fluid increases during pregnancy, but blood volume, in particular, increases by approximately 45% over prepregnant levels. The increase occurs in the cells and in the plasma of the blood. Plasma volume expands roughly 2.5 L to a total of 3.7 L. This increase in plasma volume results in increased intracapillary pressure and decreased oncotic pressure. The red blood cell mass may not increase in as great a proportion as the plasma.

To respond to the enlargement of the vascular volume, greater demands are placed on the heart to promote increased blood flow. Cardiac output rises from 4.5 to 5.5 L/min to 6 to 7 L/min. Cardiac output is a combination of stroke volume and heart rate; this is increased by 10 to 15 beats per minute (bpm).

Theoretically it might be assumed that arterial pressure would increase, but it does not because of hormonal and neurogenic influences. Both estrogen and the autonomic nervous system (ANS) promote vasodilation. Therefore arterial pressure actually decreases, with the diastolic pressure decreasing more than the systolic pressure. Venous pressure, however, increases as a reflection of resistance to blood return from the lower limbs because of partial obstruction of femoral veins.

Provided that diseases or pregnancy complications do not affect cardiac function, blood volume changes, or peripheral vascular resistance, the utero-placental unit serves as a reservoir for the additional volume. Estimates of uterine blood flow are from 500 to 750 ml/min by term. Conditions such as cardiac disease, anemia, or hypertension can cause profound deficiencies in adaptive responses. Influences such as changes in the autonomic nervous system can also have profound effects on vasoconstrictive factors. Such changes may be seen with anesthesia. Simple changes in posture can reduce cardiac output. Obstruction of the inferior vena cava occurs when the pregnant woman is placed in a supine position.

In fact, at all times of crisis the uteroplacental unit is considered expendable to the mother. Any force competing against the cardiovascular adaptations will surely reduce blood flow to the uteroplacental unit and thus the fetus.

Respiratory changes

Respirations occur so that oxygen can be utilized in chemical processes for cellular proliferation and maintenance. This is accomplished through the processes of ventilation and gas transport and exchange between lungs, blood, and tissues.

Blood gases, primarily carbon dioxide and oxygen, remain in solution because of their individual or partial pressures. The partial pressures of each are changed in the alveoli of the lungs during inspiration and expiration. The gases move from the side of greater concentration to the side of lesser. This exchange occurs again between blood and tissues. Normal partial pressure of oxygen (pO_2) is 80 to 100 mm Hg and that of carbon dioxide (pCO_2) is 40 mm Hg. Oxygen, because of its low solubility, is carried by hemoglobin. Most carbon dioxide is carried in the plasma, becoming carbonic acid and increasing free hydrogen ions.

Since pregnancy increases cell numbers, requiring increased oxygen, changes are directed at facilitating oxygen availability. Hormonal influences and anatomic changes accomplish this.

Progesterone stimulates respiratory rate. The mother, however, increases her rate in excess of oxygen demand. In the process excess carbon dioxide is blown off. The resulting decrease in carbonic acid creates a pH difference in pregnancy. Normal pH is 7.38 to 7.42; in pregnancy the pH tends to rise to 7.40 to 7.42.

Anatomic changes also influence respiration. The upward displacement of the diaphragm by the gravid uterus causes a lateral expansion of the chest wall. Hormonal influences are thought to dilate the airways and to cause increased chest wall elasticity, which promotes these anatomic changes.

Changes in metabolism

Substrates for cellular metabolism are derived from ingested foods. They consist of carbohydrates, lipids, proteins, vitamins, and inorganic substances. These substrates are utilized to form new cells, to synthesize new substances, or to be burned as fuel for energy.

Carbohydrate is normally present in the blood primarily in the form of galactose and fructose. Galactose is converted to glucose, and fructose goes directly through the same pathways as glucose. Glucose can be utilized directly or can be converted and stored as glycogen. When glucose is not available, amino acids are the main source of glucose.

Glucose can be oxidized to carbon dioxide and water. Glucose can also be changed to glucose-6-phosphate, then channeled into glycogen formation or synthesized into other metabolites through degradation to pyruvate. Pyruvate enters the tricarboxylic Krebs cycle, in the presence of oxygen, and is converted to acetyl-CoA. Acetyl-CoA can also be formed by amino acids and fatty acids. Thus the Krebs cycle is a common junction in the metabolism of fats, proteins, and carbohydrates.

Lipids are hydrolyzed to form glycerol and fatty acids. Fatty acids are also synthesized from glucose and keto acids and can be stored as depot fat in the adipose tissue. When carbohydrates are not available, depot fat is mobilized so that fatty acids, easily oxidized, can be utilized as energy by cells. Fatty acids can also enter the Krebs cycle. In the liver, fatty acids may be used, in the absence of glucose, to spare amino acids. When this occurs, ketones are produced by fatty acid breakdown and are used as an alternative energy source.

Proteins are hydrolyzed to form amino acids. Amino acids are used for building new protein or for forming other nitrogen compounds. In order to supply energy, amino acids must be converted to carbohydrates or fats. Liver cells provide their own energy by converting amino acids into a carbohydrate form, keto acids, for entry into the Krebs cycle.

Insulin is necessary for utilization of glucose in oxidation and for the formation of glycogen and fats. It provides a carrier system for taking glucose into the cells and across the cellular membrane.

During pregnancy, there is an acceleration in the use of glucose because of rapid fetal cell and organ growth requiring a rapid source of energy. Complicating this is a diminished maternal sensitivity to insulin. As a result pregnancy has been said to produce a diabetogenic state.

Because the fetus is a continuous feeder from the mother, who is a periodic feeder, a starvation-like situation increases the potential for ketonemia. Placental hormones contribute to this by promoting insulin resistance and forcing the woman into utilizing fats for energy needs. The entire metabolic rate increases in pregnancy, as does the need for increased caloric intake to supply the fetus while maintaining maternal needs.

Glandular developments

The pituitary gland enlarges during pregnancy. This is presumably a result of its function as the master for all other glandular functions. It must aid in stimulating each of the following:

1. Thyroid function to meet the increased metabolic demands of pregnancy
2. Pancreatic function in the production of increased insulin
3. Ovarian function to aid in hormonal maintenance of the pregnancy
4. Adrenal function to increase cortisol

In addition, the pituitary produces oxytocin and antidiuretic hormone (ADH). Oxytocin improves uterine contractility in labor. ADH aids in increasing fluid volume in pregnancy.

The thyroid gland also enlarges during pregnancy and produces a physiologic goiter. This is a response to the need for increased metabolism. Initially there is increased thyroid binding globulin. Then T_4 uptake increases and T_3 uptake decreases.

The adrenals increase cortisol and catecholamine production. Cortisol contributes to the increase in catecholamines (epinephrine and norepinephrine), which contribute to the increase in maternal cardiac rate. Cortisol also mobilizes glucose and free fatty acids, thereby contributing to improved metabolism.

To counteract some of the effects of vasodilation, the adrenals produce increased amounts of renin and angiotensin. To aid in blood volume expansion aldosterone levels are also increased, contributing to sodium retention.

Renal adaptations

Increased blood volume circulates through the kidneys. This forces glomerular filtration of waste substances to increase. Renal blood flow constitutes about one fifth of the cardiac output. The entire plasma volume is filtered about 60 times per day. Substances to be retained by the body are first filtered and then reabsorbed in the tubules. Substances to be excreted are added to the fluid and flow to the distal portion of the tubule. In pregnancy, larger quantities are filtered in the glomerulus because of the greater capillary pressures associated with the increased blood flow.

In pregnancy, the glomerular filtration rate rises about 50%. Glucose and nitrogenous waste products of metabolism are therefore excreted in the urine in greater quantities. In turn, blood levels of nitrogenous waste products decrease. During pregnancy, normal laboratory values indicating renal function must be adjusted. A blood urea nitrogen (BUN) greater than 13 mg/100 ml is abnormal even though it is within the nonpregnant normal range. Serum creatinine levels greater than 0.8 mg/100 ml also require further investigation of renal function.

Renal function is affected too in pregnancy by anatomic changes. As the gravid uterus displaces other organs in the abdomen, it causes a physiologic hydroureter and hydronephrosis. This is usually more pronounced on the right side than on the left. The dilation of the ureters is further facilitated by estrogen.

During pregnancy the bladder has decreased tone because of hormonal influences. This factor and the distended ureters cause the pregnant woman to be more vulnerable to urinary tract infections. The increased glucose excretion into the urine also promotes bacterial growth.

Hepatic adjustments

In pregnancy there is no change in hepatic size or blood flow. However, the changes in metabolism during pregnancy lead to liver storage and conversion changes. Serum albumin is lower, cholesterol increases 40% to 50%, free fatty acids increase 60%, and phospholipids increase 35% to provide for the nutritional needs of the fetus.

Liver enzymes also reflect changes. While SGOT and SGPT do not change, alkaline phosphatase and leukocyte alkaline phosphatase (LAP) markedly increase.

Hematologic changes

White blood cells, or leukocytes, are primarily responsible for fighting infections. Leukocytes are described either as granulocytes or nongranulocytes. When infection occurs, granulocytes increase and nongranulocytes migrate to inflammatory areas through the circulatory system. During pregnancy the number of neutrophils that are granulocytes increases. This increase is stimulated by estrogen and plasma cortisol.

Normally there is a coexisting potential for coagulation and fibrinolysis. This might also be described as clotting and lysis of clots simultaneously. Coagulation occurs when a platelet comes in contact with a damaged vessel surface.

This contact triggers a cascade of events. First prothrombin activator causes prothrombin to be released in the liver and converted to thrombin. Then thrombin is converted to fibrinogen, which forms fibrin, causing the red blood cells and plasma to mesh. A clot is thus formed. The clot triggers release of activators for plasminogen formation. Plasminogen converts to plasmin and the clot is lysed.

In pregnancy the equilibrium for coagulation-fibrinolysis is skewed toward coagulation. Plasma fibrinogen rises throughout pregnancy. Platelet count can remain normal or can be reduced insignificantly. Circulating activators of plasminogen, however, are reduced, and therefore fibrinolytic activity is diminished. What cannot be explained, however, is the rise in fibrin breakdown products despite apparent diminished fibrinolytic activity in the normal pathways. Factors in pregnancy promoting the increased fibrin breakdown include entry of placental thrombin into maternal circulation, increased amounts of fetoplacental hormones, and perhaps the effect of immunologic complexes present for the fetus.

Gastrointestinal responses

Gastrointestinal changes primarily result from the anatomic shifting of abdominal contents. There is decreased gastric motility and prolonged stomach-emptying time. Constipation is frequently a problem in pregnancy.

The gallbladder is influenced by estrogen and becomes hypotonic. This causes an increased concentration of bile. An increased incidence of gallstones can result.

Adaptations of the reproductive system

Changes in the reproductive system during pregnancy are the result of increased vascularity and increased hormone production. The vulva and vagina become more vascular during pregnancy. Increased estrogen promotes elasticity. The increased vascularity and elasticity can result in vulvar varicosities. Increased estrogen also increases vaginal secretions and promotes a more alkaline pH, which can predispose to increased vaginal infections.

The cervix becomes softer and shorter and appears cyanotic (Goodell sign). Near term the cervix becomes even softer and shortens because of the influence of prostaglandins released from the stretching uterine musculature.

The muscle of the uterus increases in weight from approximately 60 to 800 g. It does this through hyperplasia, hypertrophy, and stretching. There is a marked increase in uterine vasculature. Vascular resistance is considerably reduced and uterine blood flow increases in the absence of disease. The increased uterine blood flow occurs because of the influences of progesterone, estrogen, and prostaglandins. It is also influenced by vasodilation from the autonomic nervous system and by the trophoblastic replacement of the muscular and elastic elements in the placental vessel walls.

The ovaries may be enlarged in early pregnancy. The corpus luteum becomes cystic and begins an increased production of progesterone and estrogen to maintain the nutritive lining in the myometrium of the uterus. As the placenta assumes the role of hormone production, by 14 to 16 weeks, the ovaries and corpus luteum return to normal size.

Breast tissue also responds to increased hormonal production of estrogen and progesterone. There is increased vascularity, and veins become more prominent. There is usually an increase in pigmentation and in the size of the areolae. The periareolar glands enlarge to provide greater lubrication during lactation.

DEVELOPMENT OF THE MATERNAL-FETAL UNIT

Knowledge of the growth and development of the maternal-fetal unit provides a basis for the care of the mother and fetus at risk for disease or pregnancy complications. This knowledge can provide a basis for early detection of maternal or fetal problems. Prevention of more serious complications can then ensue. (See also Chapters 9 and 10.)

Embryo

During the luteal phase of the menstrual cycle, cervical mucus becomes receptive to spermatozoa. Ejaculation of sperm into the vagina is aided by mucoid receptivity, which allows rapid migration of spermatozoa through the cervix, into the uterine cavity, and into the fallopian tube.

Active spermatozoa can reach the outer portion of the fallopian tube within 75 minutes. The sperm and ovum meet in the distal portion of the fallopian tube. Fertilization occurs when the sperm penetrates the vitelline membrane of the ovum. Cell division begins, forming a small cell mass called the *morula*.

The morula is passed through the fallopian tube by tubal peristalsis and ciliary propulsion. The outer cell layer of the morula secretes a fluid, which pools in a segmentation cavity. Now the cell mass is called a *blastocyst*.

The blastocyst takes approximately 6 to 7 days to form. Implantation takes place at the blastocyst stage, usually occurring high in the uterine fundus. At this time the outer cells on the blastocyst are called the *trophoblasts*.

The trophoblasts then invade the endometrium. It is thought that the reason that the trophoblast cells are not treated as foreign and rejected by the mother is an exchange of fetal and maternal cytoplasmic and nuclear material from the trophoblastic cells. This allows the maternal immunologic system to tolerate the fetus as a part of the body rather than as foreign to it.

Progesterone from the corpus luteum provides stored nutritive substances

in the endometrium, now called the *decidua*. The trophoblasts secrete proteolytic and cytolytic enzymes, permitting them to destroy vessels, glands, and
stroma in the endometrium.

Placenta

The trophoblasts proliferate rapidly after implantation and three layers of
cells appear. These send out fingerlike projections called *villi*. The outer layer
of cells, or the *syncytiotrophoblast;* the inner layer, or *cytotrophoblast;* and the
dividing layer of thin connective tissue, the *mesotrophoblast,* are formed within
these fingerlike projections. The mesotrophoblast forms the support for the
villi and fetal vascular tissue. The syncytial cells then synthesize proteins, glucose, and hormones for utilization by the embryo.

After 2 or 3 weeks, the chorion begins to develop within the villi. While the
chorion is developing, the amnion and its cavity are forming. Two cavities
form in the embryonic pole. The ventral cavity is the yolk sac. The dorsal
cavity becomes the amniotic cavity. As it enlarges, it forces the formation of
the body stalk, the allantois, the blood vessels, and the beginning of the umbilical cord.

The decidua basilis, the layer beneath the embryoblast tissue, comes into
contact with the villi, which then multiply rapidly. During villi multiplication,
the decidua basilis is called the *chorion frondosum.* By 14 weeks the chorion
frondosum organizes into the discrete organ called the *placenta.* The placenta
has segments, called *cotyledons,* which are connected by vascular channels to the
umbilical cord. The placental surface is exposed to the maternal blood in the
intervillous space and thins to a single layer of cells called the *placental membrane.* The exposure of fetal blood to maternal blood across this membrane
provides for fetal oxygenation, nutrition, and excretion of fetal wastes. The
two umbilical arteries carry carbon dioxide and other wastes from the fetus to
the mother. The vein carries nutrition and oxygen to the fetus.

Transfer of oxygen, carbon dioxide, nutrition, and wastes is dependent on
molecular size. Smaller molecules such as O_2, CO_2, electrolytes, and water
transfer by simple diffusion, moving passively from the side of greater molecular concentration to the side of lesser molecular concentration. Their transfer
is largely dependent on the adequacy of uterine blood flow into the intervillous
space.

Larger molecules such as glucose are selectively transferred by a more complex process called *facilitated diffusion.* This process occurs against a large concentration gradient and requires a carrier system. Energy expenditure can also
provide for selective transfer. Both are more dependent on placental surface
area and thickness for their diffusion.

In addition to simple and complex diffusion, the placenta also assumes an endocrine function. Early in the pregnancy it assumes responsibility for maintenance of the pregnancy. The principal hormones produced are estrogen, progesterone, human chorionic gonadotropin, and human placental lactogen.

Fetus

The first trimester is a period of tremendous growth and organogenesis from an embryo into a fetus. By the end of the second week, the three embryologic germ layers develop to form body organs and systems. The formation of these layers is called *gastrulation*.

The ectoderm gives rise to the skin, hair, and nails; the epithelium of the internal and external ear, nasal cavity, mouth, and anus; the nervous tissues; and the glands. The mesoderm forms connective tissue, blood vessels, lymphatic tissue, kidneys, pleura, peritoneum, pericardium, muscles, and skeleton. The endoderm forms the respiratory tract, bladder, liver, pancreas, and digestive tract.

By 6 weeks a single-chamber heart is functioning and lung buds appear, as do a rudimentary kidney and gut. By the end of the first trimester, the heart has compartmentalized into four chambers; the lungs have bronchi; the gut, liver, pancreas, and the spleen have developed; and the sex can be distinguished.

During the second trimester, facial features become defined. Fine body hair, lanugo, appears, and vernix is produced to protect fetal skin. Meconium begins to appear in the gut. Maturation of organs allows some immature functioning.

In the third trimester, the fetus rapidly gains weight and final maturation of the organs for extrauterine life occurs. Subcutaneous fat deposits appear and the body has a rounded appearance.

Assessments of fetal well-being have become more sophisticated. In addition to estimating fetal well-being by maternal well-being, fetal assessment can be made biochemically through laboratory studies and physically through observation of fetal heart activity on the fetal monitor. Visual examination of the fetus can be provided by ultrasound techniques.

ANTEPARTUM MATERNAL ASSESSMENTS
Laboratory studies

Initial laboratory studies give baseline data regarding previous maternal disease, existing maternal disease, or a predisposition to disease or complications in pregnancy. A typical prenatal profile includes a number of laboratory studies.

CBC. A complete blood count gives information regarding leukocyte and erythrocyte levels and plasma volume ratio. It also provides information regarding platelets and erythrocyte formation. If leukocytes are high, infection may be present and thus can be treated early. Shifts in the granular and non-granular leukocyte counts can aid in determining whether or not viral or bacterial infections are present. If the erythrocyte count is low or hemoglobin and hematocrit levels are low, anemia may be a problem; it should be treated vigorously with nutritive and iron supplements. If the woman is from the black or Mediterranean races, further screening for sickle cell disease or thalassemia may be needed. All women should have repeat hemoglobin and hematocrit determinations at 28 to 32 weeks.

Urinalysis. A urinalysis and culture and sensitivity of the urine can offer information about renal function and urinary tract infection. If renal function is in question, further evaluation for creatinine, protein, and uric acid may be done of the urine and serum. If infection is present, appropriate treatment can be instituted before the renal function is impaired or the pregnancy is threatened by premature labor.

Blood type and Rh. Blood type and Rh are important for prevention or treatment of erythroblastosis in the fetus. If the mother is Rh-negative and unsensitized, preventive Rh immune globulin should be given at 28 weeks.

Antibody screen. Screening should be done regardless of the Rh type because other hemolytic incompatibilities may be present.

Rubella screen. A rubella screen gives information about immunity against the disease rubella. A titer of less than 1:16 indicates that the mother has insufficient immunity against the disease. She cannot be vaccinated during pregnancy because the vaccine contains a live virus and could cause fetal anomalies. She should be instructed to avoid contact with groups who could potentially infect her.

VDRL. A serology test to screen for syphilis should be done on all mothers because this has implications for the treatment of the mother and for potential congenital syphilis in the fetus caused by maternal infection. The prenatal health examination may be the first opportunity for the woman to realize that she is infected. Treatment with antibiotics and follow-up serology must be undertaken.

Glucola-load blood sugar. Blood sugar must be evaluated if the family history is strongly positive for diabetes or if the woman is over 35 years of age, is extremely obese, has had a previous infant weighing over 9 pounds, has had a previous unexplained stillbirth, or has had numerous spontaneous abortions. The glucola-load test should also be done if the woman spills sugar into her urine on two consecutive office visits. If the 1-hour blood sugar is greater than 149 mg/100 ml, a 3-hour glucose tolerance test must be done to determine if insulin dependency is necessary during the pregnancy. Three-hour glucose tolerance fasting blood sugar levels are lower than normal (110 mg/100 ml or less) and at subsequent hours are usually higher during pregnancy. This must be taken into consideration when evaluating the test results in a pregnant woman.

Renal function laboratory studies are usually ordered if there are diseases such as collagen diseases, diabetes, or chronic hypertension. These include serum and urinary determinations of creatinine, uric acid, and total protein. Urinary determinations must be 24-hour collections but can be done on an outpatient basis.

Plasma progesterone. Plasma progesterone determinations can be done serially during the first 16 weeks when the woman has a history of frequent first trimester spontaneous abortions. The laboratory must adjust usual normal values to fit early pregnancy, and values vary from one laboratory to another. The tests are done weekly and must be compared to the normal range as well as to each other. If low or falling levels are found, natural progesterone in vaginal suppositories may be utilized to maintain the pregnancy until placental production is sufficient.

Papanicolaou smear. A Pap smear should be done on all pregnant women at the time of their first prenatal visit if one has not been done in the previous year. If third trimester bleeding develops, a Pap smear can be repeated in order to rule out bleeding caused by carcinoma. Pregnancy may increase cervical cancerous growth because of hormonal influences. In the presence of cervical cancer, pregnancy might need to be terminated for the treatment of the mother.

Other diseases such as *Monilia* infection may be detected on the Pap smear. These should be treated even if the woman is asymptomatic. Organism proliferation, if found on the Pap smear, may become great enough to cause pregnancy loss or premature rupture of membranes if left untreated.

Antepartum assessments and interventions

Physical assessments during a high-risk pregnancy are usually similar in nature to those during any other pregnancy. The first tool for assessment is a thorough history form that includes past pregnancy history for maternal, fetal, or neonatal complications and evaluates past and current medical or surgical complications. It should also assess current health status. Assessment for social habits such as smoking and alcohol or drug abuse should be included.

Ongoing physical assessments should be made more than once a month. In a high-risk pregnancy, the development of even a minor problem can be devastating to either the mother or the fetus. Therefore it is imperative that continued in-depth assessment be conducted.

1. Maternal weight gain of at least 1 to 2 pounds per week after the first trimester and no more than 6 pounds in 1 week is desired. Total weight gain for a normal woman should be 25 to 40 pounds. Adjustments

should be made for the underweight or overweight woman. Rapid, excessive weight gain may be a warning of pregnancy-induced hypertension.

2. Fundal height should be measured each visit after 22 to 24 weeks. Growth, in centimeters, roughly approximates from the symphysis pubis to the fundus the week of gestation. Thus at 28 weeks it should measure 28 cm. Another way of evaluating growth is 1 cm per week. When measurements are done by different evaluators, they can vary from week to week but should average out over a month.

3. Blood pressure measurements should be done each visit in the same arm and in the same position. It is expected that a slight decrease will occur during the second trimester, especially in the diastolic pressure, with a return to the patient's nonpregnant level near term. Blood pressure measurements also may warn of developing pregnancy-induced hypertension.

4. Assessment for edema should include inspection of the lower extremities and questions regarding facial edema or edema of the hands. Pathologic edema may be a warning of pregnancy-induced hypertension or other cardiovascular complications.

5. The fetal heart rate should be assessed with a Doppler device by 12 weeks and at each visit thereafter. It usually cannot be heard with a fetoscope until at least 18 weeks of gestation.

6. The urine specimen should be tested for glucose, protein, and nitrites. This allows screening for diabetes, renal function, and infection.

7. After 20 weeks, the woman should be questioned about fetal activity. By 26 to 28 weeks all high-risk pregnant women should be using a fetal activity chart to document this.

Special physical assessments such as blood sugar levels, chest sounds, maternal cardiac rate, or presence of premature labor signs may be included depending on the disease and the complications.

Educational needs of the woman must also be assessed early and throughout the pregnancy. Physical limitations may require adjustments for prepared childbirth classes. Certainly assessment for educational needs should include knowledge about the disease process and skills necessary for self-care in order to prevent hospitalization if at all possible.

Assessment of sleep, diet, and exercise can aid in determining unwarranted anxieties and anticipatory grief. Specific interventions directed at realistic understanding and reassurance can then be offered. Passive exercises should be taught to the woman treated with bed rest for prolonged periods. The box on page 15 describes appropriate passive exercises.

Changing life-styles have led to increased participation by pregnant women in exercise and sports. During exercise the normal physiologic effect of shunt-

PASSIVE EXERCISES FOR BED REST OBSTETRIC PATIENTS

1. KEGEL EXERCISE

Lying on your back or sitting up, tighten your pelvic floor muscles (as if stopping and starting your urine). Hold for 3 count, then relax.

2. ABDOMINAL BREATHING

Lying on your back with knees, bent, breathe in deeply letting your abdominal wall rise. Exhale slowly through your mouth as you tighten your stomach muscles.

3. BRIDGING

Lying on your back with knees bent, raise your hips up off the bed while keeping your shoulders down.

4. CURL-UPS

Lying on your back with knees bent, put your hands on your stomach. Lift head and shoulders up (tuck your chin); keep small of back against bed.

5. LEG SLIDING

Lying on your back with knees bent, slide your leg out, slowly straightening your knees. Keep small of back flat against the bed. Slowly pull both knees back up.

6. MODIFIED LEG RAISES

Lying on your back with one knee bent, bend opposite knee up toward your chest; then straighten leg by kicking up toward ceiling and lower leg to the bed. Repeat with first bent knee.

7. ABDUCTION

Lying on your back with knees bent, let your knees come apart, then squeeze them back together.

8. ANKLE CIRCLES

Pump ankles up and down. Circle in both directions while resting right ankle on left knee. Repeat with left ankle on right knee.

9. ARM LIFTS

Exhale deeply through your nose as you lift one arm up to the side over your head. The sides of your chest should expand. Exhale as you bring your arm down. Repeat with opposite arm.

Modified from instructions for passive exercises by physical therapists at Good Samaritan Medical Center, Phoenix, Arizona, 1982.

ing of blood flow from a nonpriority organ such as the uterus occurs. The fetus, therefore, can potentially suffer. If the exercise is not lengthy, in fact, a flush-back effect actually occurs when exercise ceases and maternal pulse rate returns to normal. This effect protects the fetus (Ketter and Shelton, 1984). Exercise testing and research are scanty and evidence is conflicting. However, testing for uteroplacental insufficiency (UPI) before an exercise program is attempted and periodically throughout the pregnancy might be a good guideline.

A woman who practices social habits such as smoking, alcohol consumption, or taking drugs should be instructed regarding the potential harm to herself and the fetus. Referrals to appropriate programs can then be made.

NUTRITIONAL ADAPTATION

Nutrition plays a significant role in fetal well-being and in prevention and treatment of high-risk pregnancy. The nurse caring for the high-risk patient must have a knowledge of nutritional needs, modifications, and risks of potential deficiencies if adequate counseling is to be given.

Adequate nutrients are critical in order for cell growth to take place during pregnancy. A 25% deficit in needed calories and protein can interfere with the synthesis of DNA. The cells that are undergoing rapid division at the time of insult will be most damaged (Worthington-Roberts, Vermeersch, and Williams, 1985). During the first 2 months of pregnancy, a deficit in adequate nutrients can have teratogenic effects or cause a spontaneous abortion. After the second month, a nutritional deficit can impede fetal growth causing a small-for-gestational-age infant or a small-brain-growth infant. These infants may be unable to attain their potential in stature, intellect, and future health. Cell division occurs by two processes:

1. Hyperplasia, an increase in cell number
2. Hypertrophy, an increase in the size of the cell

If the insult occurs during hyperplastic cell division, the number of cells will be permanently reduced. According to Bessman (1979), this can cause severe mental retardation, even in the United States, where nutritional concerns are frequently overlooked. Malnutrition during pregnancy can also increase the risk of pregnancy-induced hypertension, abruptio placentae, placenta previa, premature rupture of membranes, and preterm labor (Naeye, 1983).

Deficiency in various nutrients can have deleterious effects also. Protein, 75 to 100 gm daily, is very important in supporting the increased embryonic-fetal cellular growth, in promoting the increased maternal blood volume, and possibly in facilitating the prevention of pregnancy-induced hypertension. In order to prevent the development of anemia, an adequate intake of iron, folic acid, and vitamins B_6 and B_{12}, as well as protein, is needed. Supplemental iron usually is also necessary during pregnancy to provide the fetus with at least 300 mg of maternal stores of iron upon which to draw. This also will boost the mother's stores in case excessive bleeding occurs during delivery or in the early postpartum period.

During pregnancy, the diet should contain 30 to 50 mg of zinc each day. Zinc is commonly found in such foods as nuts, meats, whole grains, legumes, and dairy products. A deficiency of zinc during pregnancy increases the risk of premature rupture of membranes and preterm labor. This may be the result of a deficiency in the antibacterial properties of the amniotic fluid (Naeye and Ross, 1982). Jameson (1975) also found an increased risk for bleeding disorders and protracted labor related to incoordinate uterine activity when zinc deficiencies were present in the mother.

Restricted sodium intake, as well as excess intake, can cause problems during pregnancy. According to Nolten and Ehrlich (1980), a restricted sodium intake can interfere with adequate maternal blood volume increase and can activate the renin-angiotensin-aldosterone cycle, which can lead to vasoconstriction. Jaspers, de Jong, and Mulder (1983) demonstrated through their study that an excess sodium intake can increase the sensitivity of the blood vessel wall to angiotensin causing vasoconstriction. Thus an average sodium intake of 6 gm per day is considered therapeutic during pregnancy.

According to Whitney and Cataldo (1983), other nutrients should be increased considerably to facilitate fetal well-being and decrease maternal complications. These nutrients are calcium, phosphorus, magnesium, and folic acid.

Not only should the patient's pattern of weight gain be monitored, but daily diet should be evaluated as to caloric intake and recommended daily allowances. To meet the growing needs of the fetus and the changing needs of the mother while facilitating maternal storage of fat and protein, a 300 calorie increase is recommended per day. This should be started at approximately 3 months of gestation. The actual caloric increase will depend on the activity level of the woman to some degree. However, the formation of fatty and lean body tissues is important. These act as a reserve for energy that the fetus can draw upon during the last part of pregnancy and provide a source of energy for labor and delivery and during lactation.

To ensure that the body receives the needed additional nutrients, a pregnant woman should be encouraged to take the vitamin and mineral supplement prescribed by her health care provider and to select high-nutrient foods utilizing the basic four food groups. She should select four servings from each of the four food groups: protein, grains, milk and milk products, and fruits and vegetables. In the grain group, at least two servings should be of whole grains. In the fruit and vegetable group, at least one should be a vitamin C food, one a dark green leafy vegetable, and five times a week one should be a yellow vegetable. Calorie-laden foods, void of nutrients, and fried foods should be avoided. These foods increase the number of calories but do not supply the body with any nutrients. Thus they promote an abnormal weight gain. Additionally, social habits such as alcohol intake, smoking, and drug abuse, if continued during pregnancy, will interfere with adequate absorption and intake of various nutrients such as vitamin C.

When obvious deficiencies cannot be met using a balanced meal plan, dietary consultation with a registered dietician should be sought. Cultural or religious practices can also influence and complicate nutritional intake. Careful planning in such situations may positively allow for alternative selections of foods that provide adequate nutrition while still meeting cultural and religious practices. Financial aid agencies can be utilized if income is inadequate for purchase of healthful foods.

To determine if the pregnant woman is obtaining adequate nutrition and to prevent nutrition-related complications, the nurse must conduct an ongoing assessment. To assess the nutritional needs and status of the pregnant woman, her pattern of weight gain, her prepregnancy weight, her daily activities, and her dietary intake should be evaluated throughout the pregnancy.

An average weight gain during pregnancy should be between 25 and 40 pounds (Shearer, 1980). During the first 2 months, a 2 to 4 pound weight gain is considered average with a gain of ¾ of a pound to 1 pound per week during the remainder of the pregnancy. Individual differences in fat deposition and water retention, as well as in body frame, influence the amount and rate of gain. Tall, thin women tend to gain more fat. Overweight women tend to gain fluid. A woman whose prepregnancy weight is 20% or more below the standard weight for her height and age should gain more than the average in order to offset the increased risk she has of fetal mortality and maternal complications of pregnancy (Naeye, 1983). A woman whose prepregnancy weight is 20% or more above the standard weight for her height and age may need to gain less than average. However, she should never fast or be on a weight-reduction program during pregnancy. If either of these is practiced, the body's carbohydrate level is considerably reduced, which forces the body to use fat and protein for its energy sources. This would reduce the primary fetal energy source, carbohydrate, and reduce the protein needed for fetal tissue building. Ketones, a potential teratogen to the fetus, are increased also.

REFERENCES

Astedt, B., and others: Fibrinolytic activity of veins during pregnancy, Acta Obstet. Gynecol. Scand. **49**:171, 1970.

Beer, A.E., and Billingham, R.E.: Immunobiology of mammalian reproduction, Englewood Cliffs, N.J., 1976, Prentice-Hall, Inc.

Bessman, S.: The justification theory: the essential nature of the non-essential amino acids, Nutr. Rev. **37**:209, 1979.

Biezenski, J.J.: Maternal lipid metabolism, Obstet. Gynecol. Annu. **3**:203, 1974.

Bonica, J.J.: Maternal respiratory changes during pregnancy and parturition, Clin. Anesth. **10**:1, 1973.

Brewer, D.W., and Aubry R.H.: The physiology of pregnancy: clinical pathologic correlations, Part I, Postgrad. Med. **52**:110, 1972.

Brewer, D.W., and Aubry, R.H.: The physiology of pregnancy: clinical pathologic correlations, Part II, Postgrad. Med. **53**:221, 1973.

Brobeck, J.R. (ed.): Best and Taylor's physiological basis of medical practice, ed. 9, Baltimore, 1973, Williams & Wilkins.

Burt, R.L., and Davidson, I.W.F.: Insulin half-life and utilization in normal pregnancy, Obstet. Gynecol. **43**:161, 1974.

Burt, R.L., Leake, N.H., and Rhyne, A.L.: Glucose tolerance during pregnancy and the puerperium, Obstet. Gynecol. **33**:634, 1969.

Chesley, L.C.: Plasma and red cell volumes during pregnancy, Am. J. Obstet. Gynecol. **112**:440, 1972.

Committee on Maternal Nutrition, Food and Nutrition Board, National Research Council: Maternal nutrition and the course of pregnancy, Washington, D.C., 1970, National Academy of Sciences.

Eng, M., Butter, J., and Bonica, J.J.: Respiratory function in pregnant obese women, Am. J. Obstet. Gynecol. **123**:241, 1975.

Flowers, C.E.: Nutrition in pregnancy, J. Reprod. Med. **7**:201, 1971.

Fomon, S.I.: Infant nutrition, Philadelphia, 1967, W.B. Saunders, Inc.

Freinkel, N., and others: Facilitated anabolism in late pregnancy: some novel maternal compensations for accelerated starvation. In Malcusse, W.J., and Pirant, J., editors: Proceedings, VIII Congress of the International Diabetes Federation, Amsterdam, 1974, Excerpta Medica.

Goldstein, A. (ed.): Advances in perinatal medicine, New York, 1977, Stratton Intercontinental.

Greenhill, J.P., and Friedman, E.A.: Biological principles and modern practice of obstetrics, Philadelphia, 1974, W.B. Saunders, Inc.

Hansen, J.M., and Ueland, K.I.: Maternal cardiovascular dynamics during pregnancy and parturition, Clin. Anesth. **10**:21, 1973.

Holey, E.: Promoting adequate weight gain in pregnant women, MCN **2**(2):86, 1977.

Hytten, F.E., and Leitch, I.: The physiology of human pregnancy, Oxford, 1966, Blackwell Scientific Publications.

Jameson, S.: Zinc and copper in pregnancy: correlations to fetal and maternal complications, Acta Med. Scand. [Suppl.] **593**:21, 1976.

Jaspers, W., de Jong, P., and Mulder, A.: Decrease of angiotensin sensitivity after bedrest and strongly sodium-restricted diet in pregnancy, Am. J. Obstet. Gynecol. **145**(7):792, 1983.

Jepson, J.H.: Factors influencing oxygenation in mother and fetus, Obstet. Gynecol. **44**:906, 1974.

Ketter, D., and Shelton, B.: Pregnant and physically fit, too, MCN 9(2):120, 1984.

Knuttgen, H.G., and Emerson, K.: Physiological response to pregnancy at rest and during exercise, J. Appl. Physiol. 36:549, 1974.

Kobayashi, Y.: Illustrated manual of ultrasonography, Philadelphia, 1974, J.B. Lippincott.

Leader, A., Wong, K., and Deitel, M.: Maternal nutrition in pregnancy, Obstet. Gynecol. Surv. 37(4):229, 1982.

Lemasters, G.: Zinc insufficiency during pregnancy, JOGN 10(2):124, 1981.

Lim, V.S., Katz, A.I., and Lindheimer, M.D.: Acid-base regulation in pregnancy, Am. J. Physiol. 231:1764, 1976.

Lindheimer, M.D., and Kath, A.I.: Pregnancy and the kidney, J. Reprod. Med. 11:14, 1973.

Marshall, G.W., and Newman, R.L.: Roll-over test, Am. J. Obstet. Gynecol. 127:623, 1977.

Metzger, B.E., Unger, R.H., and Freinkel, N.: Carbohydrate metabolism in pregnancy. XIV. Relationship between circulating glucagon, insulin, glucose and amino acids in response to a mixed meal in late pregnancy, Metabolism 26:151, 1977.

Moghissi, K., and Hafez, E.S.E.: The placenta: biological and clinical aspects, Springfield, Ill., 1974, Charles C Thomas.

Naeye, R.: Effects of maternal nutrition on fetal and neonatal survival, Birth 10(2):109, 1983.

Naeye, R.L., Blanc, W., and Paul, C.: Effects of maternal nutrition on the human fetus, Pediatrics 52:494, 1973.

Naeye, R., and Ross, S.: Amniotic fluid infection syndrome, Clin. Obstet. Gynecol. 9:593, 1982.

Niswander, K.R.: Obstetrics: essentials of clinical practice, Boston, 1976, Little, Brown, & Co.

Nolten, W., and Ehrlich, E.: Sodium and mineralocorticoids in normal pregnancy, Kidney Int. 18(8):162, 1980.

Pernoll, M.L., and others: Oxygen consumption at rest and during exercise in pregnancy, Respir. Physiol. 25:285, 1975.

Pike, R.L., and Smicklas, H.A.: A reappraisal of sodium restriction during pregnancy, Int. J. Gynaecol. Obstet. 10:1, 1972.

Pritchard, J.A., and MacDonald, P.C.: Williams obstetrics, ed. 15, New York, 1976, Appleton-Century-Crofts.

Scott, D.B., and Kerr, M.G.: Inferior vena caval pressure in late pregnancy, J. Obstet. Gynaecol. Br. Commun. 70:1044, 1963.

Shearer, M.: Malnutrition in middle-class pregnant women, Birth Family J. 7(1):27, 1980.

Shearman, R.P. (ed.): Human reproductive physiology, London, 1972, Blackwell Scientific Publications.

Sorensen, B., and others: Changes in cardiac function during and after pregnancy expressed by systolic time internals, Acta Obstet. Gynecol. Scand. 55:447, 1976.

Suonio, S., and others: Effect on the left lateral recumbent position compared with supine and upright positions on placental blood flow in normal late pregnancy, Ann. Clin. Res. 8:22, 1976.

Ueland, K., Novy, M.J., and Metcalfe, J.: Cardiorespiratory responses to pregnancy and exercise in normal women and patients with heart disease, Am. J. Obstet. Gynecol. **115:**4, 1973.

Whitney, E., and Cataldo, C.: Understanding normal and clinical nutrition, New York, 1983, West Publishing Company.

Wohl, M.G., and Goodhard, R.S.: Modern nutrition in health and disease, Philadelphia, 1968, Lea & Febiger.

Worthington, B.: Nutrition in pregnancy: some current concepts and questions, Birth Family J. **6**(3):181, 1979.

Worthington-Roberts, B., Vermeersch, J., and Williams, S.: Nutrition in pregnancy and lactation, ed. 3, St. Louis, 1985, The C.V. Mosby Co.

CHAPTER 2

Identification of a high-risk pregnancy

Apregnancy becomes high risk when it is complicated by disease or health conditions that place the mother or the fetus at risk for illness or death. Diseases can be preexisting or can be provoked by the pregnancy, such as gestational diabetes. There may also be maladaptive physiologic conditions, such as pregnancy-induced hypertension or Rh isoimmunization. Psychosocial factors can complicate both disease and maladaptive processes.

The identification of a high-risk pregnancy is initially accomplished by obtaining a complete past and current history from the pregnant woman. Ideally, this should be at the time of preconception counseling or during the first prenatal visit within 2 weeks after the first missed menstrual period. Factors that arise during the pregnancy must also be evaluated for risk potential to the mother, fetus, or neonate. Even obtaining a careful history during labor can provide past and current history information that will alert health care providers to potential risk to mother, fetus, or neonate and facilitate preparations for appropriate interventions.

The nurse's role in obtaining the history varies with the setting. The physician is often primarily interested in the physical and disease-related aspects of the history and in some information regarding the psychosocial history. The nurse must understand and appreciate the physiologic risk factors but focus on psychosocial factors that either complicate the accomplishment of optimal care or can be utilized fully to ensure optimal care.

As can be expected, comprehensive histories are quite time-consuming to obtain. In busy outpatient settings, the history obtained may be inadvertently incomplete or the significance of important risk factors may be overlooked. To avoid this, medical model scoring systems have been devised to identify women at risk in general or to identify specific risk categories.

COMMON SCORING SYSTEMS
Maternal Child Health Care Index

Nesbitt and Aubry (1969) published an eight category scoring system called the *Maternal Child Health Care Index* (MCHC Index). The eight categories examined are maternal age, race and marital status, parity, past obstetric history, medical and obstetric disorders and nutrition, generative tract disorders, and an emotional, social, and economic survey. Each category has assigned points for factors within.

Maternal age. A score of 0, 5, 10, or 20 is assigned to maternal age ranges.

Under 15 years—20 points
15 to 19 years—10 points
20 to 29 years—0 points
30 to 34 years—5 points
35 to 39 years—10 points
Over 40 years—20 points

Race and marital status. A score of 0 or 5 is assigned to race and marital status.

White—0 points
Nonwhite—5 points
Single—5 points
Married—0 points

Past obstetric history. Past history of abortions, premature births, fetal death, neonatal deaths, or congenital anomalies is considered according to the number of occurrences. Points of 10, 20, and 30 are assigned to one, two, or three occurrences, respectively. The type of infant damage during the birth process is separately considered as physical (10 points) or neurologic (20 points) damage.

Medical/obstetric disorders and nutrition. Systemic illnesses, if present, are categorized by acute (mild or serious) or chronic (nondebilitating or debilitating). A score from 0 to 20 is assigned.

Specific infections such as acute and chronic urinary tract infections or untreated or at-term syphilis are assigned 5 to 35 points. Insulin-dependent and non-insulin-dependent diabetes, chronic hypertension with or without renal disease, heart disease by classes I through IV, and endocrine disorders such as adrenal, pituitary, or thyroid disorders or infertility are assigned points from 5 to 30 points.

Anemia is considered a risk based on degree. A hemoglobin of 10 to 11 gm is 5 points, 9 to 10 gm is 10 points, less than 9 gm is 20 points, Rh isoimmunization is 30 points, and ABO incompatibility is 20 points.

Nutrition is categorized by weight and adequacy of diet. Being malnourished or underweight is 20 points, whereas obesity is 30 points. Inadequate dietary intake in calories or nutrients scores 10 points.

Generative tract disorders are categorized by prior fetal malpresentation, prior cesarean delivery, and uterine or ovarian anomalies. Scores from 5 to 30 points are assigned.

The emotional survey scores fears, attitudes, biases, hostilities, motivations, behavioral patterns, prior pregnancies without adequate prenatal care, time of first prenatal visit, standard of child care and responsibilities, family unit and marital relationship, and history of psychiatric illness in the family. Scores from 0 to 20 points are assigned.

The social and emotional survey is based on the stability of employment, annual income or public assistance adequacy, education of the woman and her family, the location and quality of housing facilities, and the neighborhood environment.

The total score in all eight categories is added together and subtracted from 100 for the MCHC Index. If the index is below 70 points, the woman is considered a high-risk obstetric patient. Each category must then be analyzed for specific risk factors so that a medical management plan can be formulated.

Edwards's (1979) simplified index

Edwards (1979) simplified a scoring system, which considers some factors not included in the MCHC Index and scores individual items under demographics, miscellaneous, and medical categories. Scores from 2 to 7 points are assigned to diseases, infections, pregnancy complications, and psychologic factors. Women are scored at the first visit, at 16 weeks, and on admission to the labor and delivery unit. A score of 7 or more places the pregnancy in the high-risk category.

Hobel's (1973) scoring system

Hobel (1973) utilized another scoring method for his population of pregnant women. Categories were divided into prenatal factors and intrapartum factors.

Prenatal factors include cardiovascular and renal factors, metabolic factors, previous history factors, anatomic abnormalities, and miscellaneous factors. Scores of 1, 5, or 10 points are assigned.

Cardiovascular and renal factors. Hypertension, renal disease, and class II to IV cardiac disease are assigned 10 points each. A history of these in milder forms is assigned 5 points each. A history of bladder infections, a current bladder infection, and a history of pregnancy-induced hypertension are assigned 1 point each.

Metabolic factors. Insulin-dependent diabetes is assigned 10 points, thyroid disease and gestational diabetes are assigned 5 points each, and a family history of diabetes is given 1 point.

Previous histories. Rh isoimmunization and previous affected infants, previous stillborn or postterm infants, previous prematurity, or neonatal death are assigned 10 points each. Previous cesarean delivery, habitual abortion, an infant greater than 10 pounds, grand multiparity greater than 5, and epilepsy are all assigned 5 points each. Previous fetal anomalies receive 1 point.

Anatomic abnormalities. Uterine malformation, cervical incompetence, abnormal fetal position, and polyhydramnios are assigned 10 points each. A small pelvis scores 5 points.

Miscellaneous. Abnormal cervical cytology, multiple gestation, and sickle cell disease are assigned 10 points each. Maternal age greater than 35 years or less than 15 years; viral disease; Rh isoimmunization without a previously affected infant, positive serology; pulmonary disease; use of drugs, alcohol, or smoking; weight less than 100 pounds or greater than 200 pounds; influenza; and anemia of less than 9 gm hemoglobin are scored 5 points each.

• • •

A score from all five categories of 10 or more places the pregnancy in the high-risk category during the prenatal period. In the intrapartum period, factors are separated into maternal, placental, and fetal.

Maternal factors. Moderate to severe pregnancy-induced hypertension, increased or decreased amniotic fluid, amnionitis, or uterine rupture score 10 points each. Elective induction, prolonged latent phase, or uterine tetany score 1 point.

Placental factors. Placenta previa, abruptio placentae, postterm birth, or dark meconium fluid score 10 points each. Marginal separation scores 1 point.

Fetal factors. Abnormal presentation, multiple gestation, bradycardia or tachycardia longer than 30 minutes, prolapsed cord, or fetal weight less than 2500 gm score 10 points each. Spontaneous breech delivery, operative forceps, or general anesthesia score 5 points each. Outlet forceps or shoulder dystocia score 1 point each. A score of 10 points or more places either the mother or fetus at high risk.

Application of scoring systems

While all of these scoring systems claim high rates of ability to identify the high-risk pregnancy, each has faults. All three were used with clinic populations and so might be criticized for general use. All have in common a systematized manner of collecting comprehensive history about each woman and evaluating the relative importance of each factor.

The purpose of reviewing the three scoring systems is to familiarize the nurse with important areas that need to be considered in assessing each pregnant patient in order to recognize the high-risk patient. Professional nursing care in the high-risk obstetric setting demands skill in obtaining comprehensive histories and evaluating the significance of risk factors in a timely and efficient manner. Only with this skill can a plan of care be established that recognizes the importance of a holistic view of the high-risk pregnant woman, her fetus, and her family. The holistic view considers physiologic and psychosocial concepts and aids in establishing collaborative efforts with the woman, her family, and the health care team to effect optimal maternal and neonatal outcome.

NURSING MODELS

Nursing has attempted to respond to the need for a holistic view of patients in any setting and to establish its practice as a scientific discipline. The development of conceptual models in nursing provides the framework for nursing practice. A review of three nursing conceptual models is directed at outlining the elements of nursing practice as they relate to the role of nurses in obtaining patient histories. Each of these three models can be utilized in the identification of a high-risk pregnancy and provides a framework for the collaborative efforts of health care professionals with the woman and her family.

Models require that the nurse consider values, goals of nursing action, the recipient of care, and nursing intervention. Nursing models are logical, symbolic representations of persons in the health care system and force a holistic view based on scientific theory.

Roy adaptation model

The Roy adaptation model (Riehl and Roy, 1974) had its beginning in 1964 and has been operationalized and developed gradually over time. It is based on eight assumptions about man.

1. Man is a biopsychosocial being.
2. Man is in constant interaction with a changing environment.
3. To cope with a changing world, man uses innate and acquired mechanisms that are biologic, psychologic, and social in origin.
4. Health and illness are one inevitable dimension of man's life.
5. To respond positively to environmental changes, man must adapt.
6. Man's adaptation is a function of the stimulus he is exposed to and his adaptation level.
7. Man's adaptation level is comprised of a zone that indicates the range of stimulation that leads to a positive response.
8. Man is conceptualized as having four modes of adaptation: physiologic needs, self-concept, role function, and interdependence relations.

The goal of nursing is to facilitate adaptation utilizing the four modes of adaptation. To do this, the nurse must assess patient behaviors and factors that influence adaptation level and intervene by manipulating influencing factors (Riehl and Roy, 1974).

Application of the Roy adaptation model. The physiologic mode considers behaviors surrounding nutrition, elimination, circulation, fluids and electrolytes, exercise and rest, oxygen, and regulatory mechanisms. The self-concept mode considers behaviors acknowledging the physical self, the personal self, and the interpersonal self. The physical self includes behaviors such as contractions, pain, or bleeding. The personal self includes behaviors surrounding hygiene, appearance, and marital status. The interpersonal self is concerned with social relationships. The role function mode considers behaviors for attachment. The interdependence mode considers behaviors associated with independence/obstacle mastery, initiative taking, satisfaction, dependence/help seeking, attention seeking, and affection seeking.

Johnson behavioral system model

The Johnson behavioral system model (Riehl and Roy, 1974) considers behavior as a basic concept. The assumptions about man are:
1. Man is seen as a dynamic whole responding to an ever-changing environment both internal and external.
2. Through learned patterns of habitual responses, man can adjust to daily stresses and strains.
3. Man's ability to modify behavior patterns maintains the growth and development of new adaptive responses.
4. At times stressors impinging upon man are beyond his ability to cope with or without assistance.
5. If this instability arises when the stressor is related to health or illness, nursing's assistance may be beneficial in helping the patient achieve the previous level of stability.

The basic elements considered in the model are affiliation, achievement, aggression, dependency, elimination, ingestion, restoration, and sex. Each subsystem has goals:

Achievement—to achieve mastery and control

Aggression/protection—to achieve self-protection and self-assertion

Dependency—to gain trust and reliance

Elimination—to externalize the internal biologic environment

Ingestion—to internalize the external environment

Restoration—to redistribute energy

Sex—to procreate, to care for others, and to be cared about by them

These goals are observed by analyzing the action of the individual, the choice of alternative behaviors the individual views as possible, and the predisposition to act in a certain way. Behavior in each subsystem is related to categories of variables. These are biologic, developmental, cultural, environmental, familial, pathologic, psychologic, sociologic, and level of wellness.

Application of the Johnson behavioral system model. Disorders within any subsystem are manifested by insufficiency in functional capacity or discrepancy in behavior that meets the intended goal. Disorders within more than one subsystem are either incompatible with each other or place one subsystem in domination over another.

To apply this model to the pregnant woman, the nurse must observe behaviors in each of the eight subsystems, through speech, word usage, descriptions of feelings, habits, and covert and overt behaviors. The assessment is made over a period of time and not in one contact. Once all subsystems have been observed, a nursing diagnosis of disorders can be made, interventions can be planned and implemented, and outcome can be evaluated based on the objectives. Clinical data must be categorized into the subsystems and the nursing process utilized.

Orem model of self-care *(Kinlein, 1977)*

Orem's conceptual framework for nursing provides a basis for holistic assessment of the patient and identifies the nurse's function as assisting the patient toward optimal self-care. *Self-care* is defined as the activities a person initiates and performs in his/her own behalf in order to maintain life, health, and well-being (Kinlein, 1977). The patient's assets rather than deficits are assessed. Orem's model assumes that man, as a self-care agent, is capable of making decisions and taking purposeful action toward goals.

Nursing care is needed when disease or disability alters functions and interferes with the ability to care for oneself. Orem identifies three categories:
1. Wholly compensatory
2. Partially compensatory
3. Supportive/educative

Some terms commonly used in Orem's model are:
1. Universal self-care requirements. These requirements are defined as basic human needs such as air, food, water, excretion, activity, rest, safety, solitude, and social interaction (Orem, 1971).
2. Health alteration or deviation requirements. These include demands and actions that result from injury, disease, or exposure to disease-producing agents (Orem, 1971).
3. Therapeutic self-care demands. These include actions performed to support life processes and promote normal functioning; maintain normal growth, development, and maturation; prevent, control, and cure disease processes; and prevent or compensate for disability (Orem, 1971).
4. Self-care deficits. These include conditions in the patient or environment that limit accomplishment of self-care (Orem, 1971).

Application of Orem's model of self-care. Tables 2-1 and 2-2 describe the nursing process using Orem's self-care model with examples related to the high-risk pregnant woman.

TABLE 2-1. *Assessment of self-care for the high-risk pregnant woman*

Universal self-care requirements	Health alterations	Therapeutic self-care demands	Self-care assets	Self-care deficits
Increased caloric, protein, and iron intake	Diabetes	Recognizes need for control of blood sugars	Motivated, knowledgeable about disease	Inadequate knowledge about effects of pregnancy on disease
Control of blood sugars in normal range	Early pregnancy nausea and vomiting	Seeks education for self and family member; has been practicing home blood glucose monitoring	Supportive family member; pregnancy planned	Limited financial resources for supplies

Modified from Woolery (1983).

TABLE 2-2. *Interventions for self-care for the high-risk pregnant woman*

Goals for health care	Assistance	Evaluation
Establish improved nutrition meeting pregnancy demands	Education for effects of disease on pregnancy	Blood sugars at home between 80 and 120 mg % Dietary intake 2200 calories
Prevent nausea and vomiting	Education for nutritional needs of pregnancy	Husband participated in educational aspects
Educate family member and patient	Supportive measures to relieve nausea and vomiting	

Modified from Woolery (1983).

Orem's model encourages the woman to be responsible for her own care while creating a helping relationship rather than a maternalistic relationship.

Although medical models of assessment and nursing models differ in their focuses on disease versus health, the identification of a high-risk pregnancy and the interventions promoting optimal outcome depend on the efforts of both. The systematic collection of data regarding disease and complications as well as a nursing conceptual framework for assessment, intervention, and evaluation is essential for promotion, maintenance, and restoration of health in pregnancy.

REFERENCES

Edwards, L.: A simplified antepartum risk scoring system, Obstet. Gynecol. **54**:237, 1979.

Hobel, C.: Prenatal and intrapartum high risk screening, Am. J. Obstet. Gynecol. **117**:1, 1973.

Kinlein, M.: Independent nursing practice with clients, Philadelphia, 1977, J.B. Lippincott Co.

Nesbitt, R., and Aubry, R.: Maternal child health care index, Am. J. Obstet. Gynecol. **103**:972, 1969.

Orem, D.: Nursing concepts of practice, New York, 1971, McGraw-Hill Inc.

Riehl, J., and Roy, C.: Conceptual models for nursing practice, New York, 1974, Appleton-Century-Crofts.

Snyder, D.: The high risk mother viewed in relation to a holistic model of the childbearing experience, JOGN **8**(3):164, 1979.

Woolery, L.: Self care for the obstetrical patient: a nursing framework, JOGN **12**(1):33, 1983.

CHAPTER 3

Antepartum and intrapartum assessment of fetal well-being

Antepartum and intrapartum assessment of the fetus is relatively new, having only gained momentum in the last 10 to 15 years. In the past, nurses and physicians caring for pregnant women could only hope that if the mother was well the fetus was also; there are now many means of surveillance of the fetus. In modern obstetrics there are two patients requiring care. They are the mother and the fetus.

Sophisticated technology and laboratory analysis aid in the care of both patients. Nurses working in modern obstetric units must understand a myriad of technological and laboratory data in order to effectively care for the mother and fetus. Some of the technological and laboratory data available now are listed below.

1. Fetal heart rate (FHR) monitoring
2. Antepartum fetal surveillance
3. Obstetric ultrasound
4. Amniocentesis
5. α-Fetoprotein evaluation
6. Estriol determination
7. Chorionic villi sampling
8. Fetal activity charts

FETAL HEART RATE MONITORING

Fetal heart rate monitoring is actually a continuous observation of human oxygenation. Continuous monitoring with appropriate acid-base evaluation of the fetus is one of the most convenient and accurate means of assessing fetal well-being and thus reducing perinatal morbidity and mortality.

Recent statistics (U.S. Census Bureau, 1975) indicate that there are 25 perinatal deaths for every 1,000 births. Approximately two thirds of those occur in the antepartum period and the rest during labor. The morbidity figures may be even higher. Whereas certain hypoxic morbid outcomes are easy to recognize, others such as moderate decreases in IQ and learning disabilities are more difficult to recognize and attribute to specific causes (Freeman and Garite, 1981).

31

Hypoxic mortality and morbidity are related to the failure of the placenta to transport sufficient oxygen to the fetus. The solution to prevention of hypoxic morbidity and mortality lies in being able to predict the sufficiency of placental function. When inadequacy is recognized, appropriate intervention can be of great benefit to the fetus.

Historically, the technique for evaluation of fetal heart rate has been auscultation of the fetal heart rate. Benson and others (1968) concluded from a computerized evaluation of 24,863 deliveries that auscultation is not reliable in indicating fetal distress in terms of fetal heart rate except in extreme, sustained bradycardia, which is a late and often terminal sign of fetal distress. Under optimal conditions during labor, if one listens to the FHR every 15 minutes for 30 seconds, only 3% of the available information is gathered. In addition, the rate is averaged during that time interval and beat to beat variations, which are critical in the evaluation of hypoxia, cannot be detected at all.

It has been shown in numerous studies that only 50% of fetal morbidity and mortality occurs in an already identified high-risk population. This means that morbidity and mortality statistics are from the normal population and will often be missed.

Although one cannot ethically conduct studies comparing at-risk monitored patients with at-risk unmonitored patients, intuitively it becomes clear that at present continuous fetal heart monitoring for at-risk intrapartum patients is of benefit in decreasing morbidity and mortality. In addition, periodic antepartum continuous monitoring should aid the two thirds of the fetal population who suffer irreversible hypoxic damage before reaching the intrapartum period. Finally, because we now know that one tenth of all morbidity and mortality occurring in the intrapartum period cannot be predicted by present screening methods, we become obligated to monitor continuously the entire population during the intrapartum period.

With research findings supporting the overwhelming value of continuous electronic fetal monitoring over intermittent auscultation, it becomes readily apparent that all nurses caring for antepartum and intrapartum obstetric patients must become skilled in interpreting continuous electronic fetal monitoring. To do this, the perinatal nurse must be fully acquainted with:
1. The physiologic basis for fetal heart rate monitoring
   a. The maternal circulatory and cardiovascular adaptations to pregnancy
   b. The uteroplacental fetal exchange
   c. Fetal capabilities for withstanding stressors
2. Application of the monitor
3. Instrumentation, arrhythmia versus artifact
4. Recognition of fetal heart rate patterns and nursing intervention for fetal distress
5. Skills and techniques for antepartum evaluation of fetal well-being

Physiologic basis for fetal heart rate monitoring

Maternal circulatory and cardiovascular adaptations. The tremendous maternal blood volume increase is one of the more dramatic adaptations to pregnancy. Blood volume is known to increase gradually beginning the tenth week and to plateau at about 32 to 34 weeks of gestation. The plasma volume increases more than does the cellular volume and is reported to increase variably from 20% to 100%, with an average increase of 45%. Plasma increases in response to cell growth and proliferation of the uterus, placenta, and fetus.

To supply the growth and proliferation of cells, the vascular system in the pelvic region greatly enlarges. Under nonstress conditions the vasculature remains widely dilated. It is, however, very responsive to the autonomic nervous system and is capable of marked constriction in the presence of any stressor. Because the uterus and thus the fetus are considered physiologically expendable to maternal circulatory needs, great care must always be taken to eliminate and avoid stressors. Those stressors are any mechanical obstruction to adequate uterine blood flow and any activation of the autonomic nervous system that might cause vasoconstriction.

The usual state of uterine vasculature is one of low resistance to flow. This occurs in part because of new vascularization of the uterus but also because of the systemic influence of estrogens, which leads to an overall vasodilation. It is estimated that uterine blood flow is approximately 50 cc/min in the early weeks and increases to 700 cc/min by term.

Because of the vasodilation and the increased volume itself, the cardiac output (stroke volume × heart rate) is also increased. This further facilitates uterine blood flow during pregnancy. Heart rate increases from 10 to 15 beats and stroke volume increases 15% over the prepregnant state.

Uteroplacental-fetal exchange. The placenta performs several major organ functions for the fetus. It acts as:

1. A lung for exchange of CO_2 and O_2
2. A gastrointestinal tract for supply of nutrients and exchange of wastes and electrolytes
3. Skin for heat exchange
4. A kidney for excretion of wastes and maintenance of acid-base balance
5. An endocrine organ functioning for self-perpetuation
6. A barrier to blood and bacteria

After implantation, the placenta begins to form from the chorionic tissues. By the fourteenth week, the placenta is a discrete organ. It is at this point that segments of the placenta, called *cotyledons,* form and connect by vascular channels to the umbilical cord. The surface of the placenta then thins to a membranous single layer of cells. Fetal blood and maternal blood, though not mixing, are exposed to one another across this membrane and fetal respiration, nutrition, and excretion take place. The space in which these organs function is the intervillous space, which contains maternal blood. The fetus is therefore dependent on its mother for most homeostatic mechanisms.

Transfer and exchange of molecules occur in the maternal intervillous space, and molecules enter through the epithelial surface of the villi and move through the villous stroma and into the fetal capillary vessels within the villi. Molecules pass through tissue from the mother to the fetus and in reverse order from the fetus to the mother. The process is accomplished by means of diffusion, either simple or selective.

Simple diffusion is, as the phrase implies, a relatively uncomplicated process responsible for the rapid exchange of small molecules. From the side of greater concentration to lesser, small molecules such as O_2, CO_2, water, electrolytes, creatinine, and uric acid cross the placental membrane. Simple diffusion also allows drugs such as antibiotics, narcotics, barbiturates, and anesthetic agents to cross quickly to the fetus. Simple diffusion is totally dependent on uterine blood flow and its adequacy and on the concentration of the molecules.

Selective transfer is a more complex process and therefore occurs more slowly. It can occur against a large concentration gradient by an energy-dependent process. Glucose, for instance, is transported in this manner from stores within the placenta until it is needed by the fetus. Selective transfer can also be actively facilitated by specific enzyme systems. It is in this manner that amino acids as well as buffering substances are transferred. Both processes are more dependent on placental surface area and thickness than on uterine blood flow.

Because simple diffusion is faster, taking only minutes, one can now begin to understand that O_2 and CO_2 can quickly be exchanged to correct fetal oxygenation problems provided uterine blood flow and umbilical blood flow are unimpeded. On the other hand, the more complex processes of selective transfer, taking hours, cannot be utilized to correct acid-base imbalance from O_2 deficit.

Fetal capabilities for withstanding stressors. The fetus has certain remarkable capabilities that enable it to withstand stressors. These stressors can be caused by maternal adaptation failures, disease, or mechanical or physiologic obstruction of the blood flow through the uterus and into the intervillous space. The fetus is equipped with a higher concentration of hemoglobin in plasma (60% Hct) and each hemoglobin molecule can be supersaturated with O_2. However, the pO_2 of the blood reaching the fetus is approximately 40 mm Hg, whereas the adult has 90 to 96 mm Hg; therefore the fetus needs these capabilities.

The fetal heart must have significant hypoxia before myocardial depression occurs. This is partly due to the well-supplied, unimpeded blood flow through healthy coronary arteries. Impulses travel through the heart originating at the SA node, traveling across the AV junction, down the bundle branches, and out the Purkinje fibers in the ventricles. When myocardial depression occurs because of hypoxia, arrhythmias can occur.

Regulation of the fetal heart rate originates in the central nervous system (CNS). By the tenth week of fetal life both the central nervous and cardiac systems are developed enough to begin the beating of the fetal heart. Initially the sympathetic portion of the autonomic nervous system is active. It is responsible for the rate of each beat. Normally the fetal heart rate is from 120 to 160 beats per minute, tending toward the upper range in earlier fetal life and the middle to lower range toward term. The sympathetic system serves as a reserve throughout intrauterine life, speeding up the fetal heart rate in response to various stimuli as needed for fetal circulation. This is a healthy response.

As the fetus becomes more mature, the other portion of the autonomic nervous system, the parasympathetic, begins to affect the fetal heart rate. It functions as an opposing force against the steady beat provided by the sympathetic system and tugs at each beat to slow it. Its effects vary from one beat to the next and this is responsible for beat to beat variation.

Application of the fetal monitor

Electronic fetal heart rate monitoring gives us clear and precise information about the oxygenation and the health of the CNS. It does this by calculating and recording an average rate per minute, by indicating beat to beat variations,

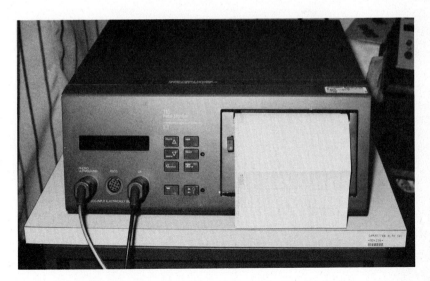

FIG. 3-1. Fetal monitor (Corometrics Model 115).

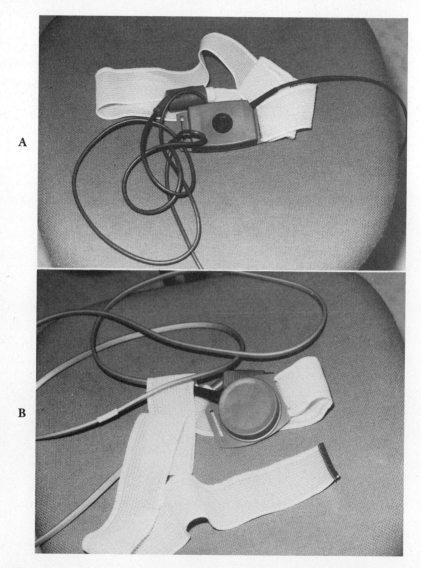

FIG. 3-2. A, Corometrics tocotransducer to be located near the umbilicus. **B,** Corometrics ultrasound transducer to be located in lower quadrant of abdomen.

and by giving periodic patterns in response to stimuli. To fully appreciate patterns it is necessary to have a continuous record for interpretation. Therefore correct application of the monitor and knowledge of how it operates are necessary. Fetal monitors generally have capabilities for indirect or external monitoring and for direct or internal monitoring (Fig. 3-1).

External monitoring. To place the external monitor in position, it is important to ascertain by abdominal palpation how the baby is positioned. The external monitor parts recommended for continuous monitoring are the tocotransducer (Fig. 3-2, *A*) and the ultrasound transducer (Fig. 3-2, *B*).

The tocotransducer should be placed over the fundus of the uterus slightly off center from the umbilicus and opposite the fetal small parts. The tocotransducer has a small pressure-sensitive button on its underside that detects the rise and fall of the uterus against the abdominal wall as it contracts and relaxes. It is secured in place with an elastic belt put around the mother's abdomen and comfortably stretched to a tightness that will allow it to trace at 5 to 15 mm Hg on the monitor paper with the uterus in resting tone. Resting tone should be indicated near 10 mm Hg on the monitoring paper. Table 3-1 describes advantages and disadvantages of external monitoring for contractions.

The ultrasound transducer has sending and receiving crystals enclosed in a disk-shaped casing. This should be placed over the fetal chest wall for best signal. Some detect the signal through a cone of focus. In this case the signal travels a specific distance and is transmitted and received over a specific width. Newer, more sophisticated models have a sweeping ability that enables them to detect the signal. The signal detected by an ultrasound transducer is the motion of the closure of the heart valves. To differentiate between that motion and other movements, the monitor has a logic system. If motion is detected that the machine does not recognize as logical it will fill in by averaging the last 3 to 6 beats and give that rate. The logic system therefore causes the appearance of greater beat to beat variability than may actually be present. Table 3-2 describes advantages and disadvantages of external monitoring of FHR.

TABLE 3-1. *Advantages and disadvantages of external contraction monitoring*

Advantages	Disadvantages
1. Noninvasive	1. Cannot measure strength accurately
2. Convenient	2. Loses some of the information at beginning and end of contractions
3. Continuous record of frequency and duration of contractions	3. Restricts patient movement in that it must be adjusted with change in position

Modified from Tucker (1978).

Internal monitoring. Direct or internal monitoring utilizes different components. These components are an intrauterine pressure catheter (Fig. 3-3, *A*) and a fetal spiral scalp electrode (Fig. 3-3, *B*).

The uterine pressure catheter is inserted in an aseptic manner. The perineal area, thighs, and under the buttocks are draped with sterile towels after a Betadine scrub. The catheter is filled with sterile saline and a syringe is left con-

---

TABLE 3-2. *Advantages and disadvantages of external FHR monitoring*

Advantages	Disadvantages
1. Noninvasive	1. Cannot accurately assess beat to beat variation
2. Does not require rupture of membrane or dilatation	2. Tracing quality is affected by change in maternal position
3. Convenient	
4. Continuous recording of FHR	

Modified from Tucker (1978).

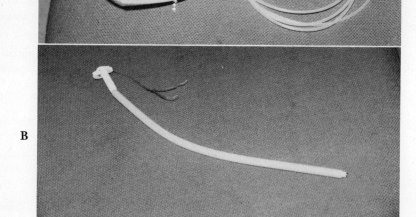

FIG. 3-3. A, Corometrics intrauterine pressure catheter. **B,** Corometrics fetal scalp electrode for attachment to leg plate.

nected at the distal end. The catheter is a flexible narrow-gauge tube with holes at the proximal end. It is partially enclosed in a firmer plastic catheter introducer. The examiner's hand carefully lifts the presenting part, and inserts the introducer with catheter just into the dilated cervix. Then the fluid-filled catheter is carefully advanced to a specific marker visualized on the outside of the perineum. The introducer is drawn back toward the distal end and the catheter is taped to the patient's thigh and abdomen. As the uterus contracts and relaxes the intracavity pressure is reflected against the fluid-filled catheter. The distal end of the catheter is connected to a strain-gauge pressure transducer with a pressure dome and a three-way stopcock. The cable of the transducer is then connected to the monitor where the changes in pressure are calculated in mm Hg and printed out on the monitor strip. The three-way stopcock has the catheter in one terminal and a saline-filled syringe in another. One terminal is opened to air for zeroing the line tracing on the monitor paper. This last terminal is capped and the stopcock opened to the patient. The syringe is left on the remaining terminal for flushing of the catheter as needed.

The fetal spiral electrode is attached to the presenting part of the fetus avoiding the fontanels and facial features or the genitals if breech. The spiral electrode has two color-coded wires attached to it. These are twisted together and all are encased in an introducer. The examiner identifies the area of the presenting part and inserts the introducer between the fingers and flush against the presenting part. The distal ends of the wires are rotated counterclockwise and the spiral attaches to the presenting part. The leg plate is then strapped to the patient's upper thigh after ECG paste is applied to the underside and the cord from the leg plate is plugged into the fetal ECG (FECG) receiver on the monitor. The monitor in this way can directly count every beat from the fetus and therefore does not need to respond to or disregard other sounds because none are received. What is printed on the monitor is the exact rate from beat to beat counted for 1 minute. Thus the direct fetal cardiac monitoring is the only completely accurate means of assessing beat to beat variability. Table 3-3 describes advantages and disadvantages of internal monitoring.

TABLE 3-3. *Advantages and disadvantages of internal monitoring*

Advantages	*Disadvantages*
1. Contractions are measured accurately for: 　Strength 　Duration 　Frequency 　Resting tone 2. Can assess beat to beat variation 3. More comfortable for the patient	1. Requires ruptured membranes and dilatation 2. Carries a small increased risk of infection 3. Could possibly cause injury to uterine wall 　or fetus if forcefully introduced

Modified from Tucker (1978).

Instrumentation

In order to understand the accuracy, dependability, and predictability of the printed data on the monitor strip, it is very important to understand how the monitor processes the information it receives.

All monitors have a logic system for FHR processing. With external monitoring the logic system is always engaged. The monitor processes the ultrasound response to valvular motion in the heart. Because there are two sets of valves moving at different times, the machine will not respond to other detected motion for a period of time preset in milliseconds. The monitor, through the use of a cardiotachometer, plots a new rate (in beats per minute) after each heart beat. If, for instance, each set of valves closes farther apart than the preset milliseconds range, the cardiotachometer will respond to both and give the appearance of a faster beat and more beat to beat variation than was really present. If, instead, the valves close within the preset time, the cardiotachometer will respond to only one set of closures. When the variation of beats appears decreased it must be remembered that the machine cannot take away information about variability, so what appears on the strip is real.

When participating in the purchase or selection of monitors, it is apparent that the more sophisticated a monitor is in its ability to differentiate the motion of the valves the more accurate the information received on external monitoring for FHR. This is true also for the tocotransducer. The more sensitive the pressure button, the more accurate the information about the relative strength, the onset, and the end of contractions. Monitors vary in all of these capabilities from manufacturer to manufacturer and from one model to another.

When internal monitoring is used, it is usually possible and always desirable to disengage the logic system. Monitors with capabilities for internal monitoring should have the means for disengaging the logic system with the push of a button, preferably on the front of the monitor, if internal modes are frequently used. By disengaging the logic system, all available data including arrhythmias can be printed about the FHR.

Arrhythmia versus artifact *(Freeman and Garite, 1981)*

Fetal arrhythmias occur fairly frequently, although significant fetal or neonatal morbidity is rare. Arrhythmias can never be recorded when the logic system is in operation and therefore cannot be detected when external modes are used. Although morbidity is rare, it is important to recognize an arrhythmia when present in order to initiate correction measures in utero or at the time of delivery for those cases associated with otherwise poor fetal or neonatal outcome. The common fetal arrhythmias are listed with their clinical significance in Table 3-4.

TABLE 3-4. *Arrhythmias and their significance*

Arrythmia	Significance
Premature atrial contractions	None except for possible increased cardiac anomalies
Premature ventricular contractions	Not a sign of hypoxia; no intervention
Paroxysmal atrial tachycardia	May lead to fetal heart failure, ascites, generalized edema; cannot treat in utero so must deliver and treat the neonate with prematurity considered
Congenital heart block	Associated with congenital cardiac anomalies requiring a pacemaker at time of birth

Modified from Freeman and Garite (1981).

TABLE 3-5. *Artifact versus arrhythmia*

Instrument	Artifact	Arrhythmia
Oscilloscope	Horizontal line between P, QRS, and T waves is wavy	Horizontal line between P, QRS, and T waves is smooth
Monitor paper	Vertical lines are disorganized	Vertical lines are organized as though purposefully drawn

Modified from Freeman and Garite (1981).

To recognize that an arrhythmia is present rather than attempting to diagnose which one it is becomes the nurse's responsibility. When a premature beat occurs there will be a momentary rise in rate. A compensatory pause following the rise in rate will be reflected as a sudden momentary drop in rate with characteristic vertical lines being drawn through the FHR tracing. Since electrical noise or maternal ECG artifact can lead to the same vertical line due to the interruption of the electrical signal received, it is important to examine the fetal ECG tracing on the oscilloscope.

Even on internal monitoring it must be remembered that the monitor paper reflects rate from beat to beat whereas the oscilloscope represents the actual fetal ECG. There are some differences in the monitor tracings between artifacts and arrhythmias (Table 3-5, Fig. 3-4).

Basic FHR pattern recognition and nursing interventions for fetal distress

The FHR reflects the CNS response. The CNS response is a reflection of fetal oxygenation. Therefore fetal heart rate monitoring is a continuous observation of fetal oxygenation.

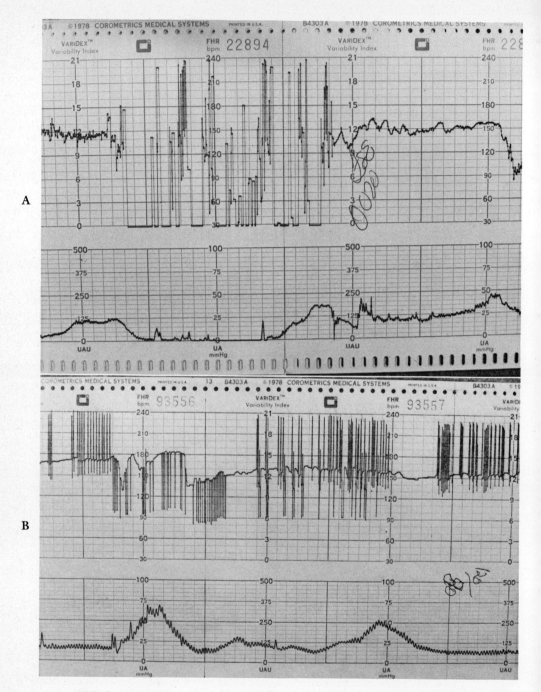

FIG. 3-4. A, Artifact. Note the disorganized scattering of impulses traced by fetal scalp electrode. **B,** Arrhythmia. Note the organized distribution of impulses traced by fetal scalp electrode.

Each examination of a fetal monitor strip should follow the same systematic steps:

1. Observe and describe the baseline FHR
2. Observe and describe the beat to beat variability
3. Observe and describe periodic changes in or patterns of response to documented stimuli
4. Initiate appropriate nursing interventions for observations of fetal distress

Baseline FHR (Freeman and Garite, 1981; Fig. 3-5). The baseline FHR can be defined as an average rate lasting at least 10 consecutive minutes. It should be observed between contractions. If contractions are occurring so close together as to make this difficult, the usual place to look is just prior to each contraction.

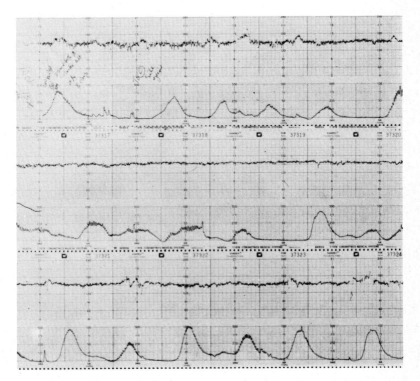

FIG. 3-5. Normal baseline FHR. Baseline FHR found between contractions, in the absence of periodic changes, and observed in 10 minute segments (panels 37317 through 37319 in center) is 150 to 155. This is a normal range. (Courtesy John P. Elliott, M.D., Phoenix, Arizona.)

TABLE 3-6. *Summary of baseline FHR abnormalities*

TACHYCARDIA (Fig. 3-6)

Description	Rate greater than 160 for at least 10 consecutive minutes
Etiology	Acute, short-term hypoxia
	Drugs given to the mother such as beta-sympathomimetics (Terbutaline, Ritodrine)
	Recovery from stress
	Arrhythmia
	Maternal fever
	Maternal hyperthyroid disease
Mechanism	Sympathetic response
Significance	Ominous when greater than 180 beats/min
Nursing intervention	Look for cause
	Turn patient to left side
	Hydrate to improve circulating volume
	O_2 at 8 to 10 L/min by tight face mask
	Reduce stressors (turn off Pitocin, treat maternal fever, etc.)

BRADYCARDIA (Fig. 3-7)

Description	Rate less than 100 beats/min for at least 10 consecutive minutes
Etiology	Chronic long-term hypoxia
	Drugs such as beta-blockers (Inderal)
	Arrhythmias
	Can be a terminal event after severe stress
	Prolapsed cord
Mechanism	Parasympathetic response
Significance	Ominous when lasting longer than 10 to 15 minutes
Nursing intervention	Turn side to side or to knee chest position
	O_2 at 8 to 10 L/min by tight face mask
	Correct maternal hypotension
	Look for cause such as prolapsed cord
	Prepare for delivery by most expeditious means

Modified from Freeman and Garite (1981).

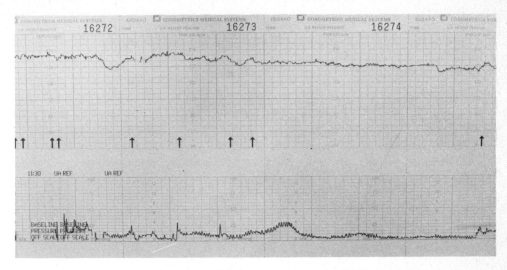

FIG. 3-6. Tachycardia. Baseline FHR between panels 16272 and 16274, in the absence of accelerations indicated by *arrows* in the center of the strip, is 180 to 190 beats/min.

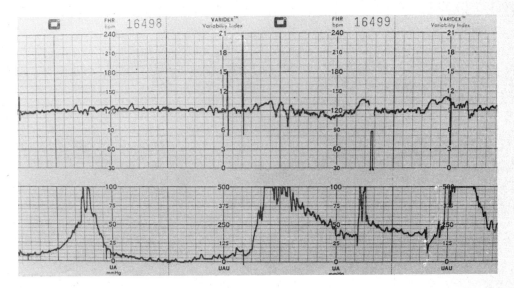

FIG. 3-7. Bradycardia. Baseline FHR between contractions is 110 to 115 beats/min.

TABLE 3-7. *Abnormalities of baseline variability*

INCREASED VARIABILITY (Fig. 3-8)

Description	Beat to beat variation of 15 or more beats/min for 10 minutes or more between periodic changes in the baseline FHR
Etiology	Acute short-term hypoxia
	Healthy response to fetal stimulation
Mechanism	Increased interplay of sympathetic and parasympathetic nervous systems
Significance	If episodic, benign
	If prolonged, consider it a warning
Nursing intervention	Look for cause of hypoxia and correct if prolonged

DECREASED OR ABSENT VARIABILITY (Fig. 3-8)

Description	Beat to beat variation of 3 or fewer beats/min for more than 10 to 15 minutes in the baseline FHR
Etiology	Chronic hypoxia
	Fetal sleep
	Drugs that depress the CNS (narcotics, sedatives, tranquilizers)
Mechanism	Lack of parasympathetic interplay with sympathetic nervous system
Significance	Could be ominous if longer than 20 to 40 minute fetal sleep cycle or duration of medication effect
Nursing intervention	Look for cause
	Stimulate the fetus by attempting to move
	Do not medicate mother with CNS depressants if not due to fetal sleep
	Place mother on left side
	Give O_2 8 to 10 L/min by tight face mask
	Improve circulating volume by hydrating mother
	Observe FHR pattern closely for other signs of fetal distress

Modified from Freeman and Garite (1981).

Baseline rate should be 120 to 160 beats per minute. Rates for 10 or more consecutive minutes above the baseline rate are termed *tachycardia* and those below are termed *bradycardia*.

Variability (Freeman and Garite, 1981). The variability described should be beat to beat variability. It is assessed in the baseline FHR. Average or good beat to beat variability is a variation of 5 to 10 beats, decreased or absent variability is 3 or fewer beats variation, and increased variability is 15 or more beats variation. When recording the rate observed on a monitor strip, a range of beats per minute will describe the beats of variation. Therefore recording of an exact rate of the moment from the monitor is misleading rather than accurate. A recorded range of 140 to 148 would thus reflect both a normal base-

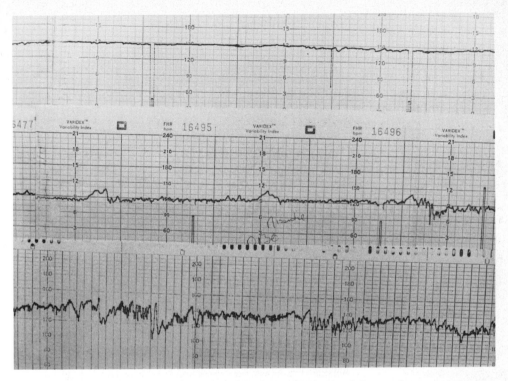

FIG. 3-8. Variability of beat to beat is depicted in each of the panels top to bottom. Top panel shows poor to absent beat to beat variability. Middle panel shows average beat to beat variability of 5 to 10 beats. Bottom panel shows increased variability of 15 to 20 beats. All are traced from fetal scalp electrodes.

line and average or good beat to beat variability. Variability expresses fetal reserve.

FHR patterns (Freeman and Garite, 1981). FHR patterns or periodic changes express the mechanisms of insult to the fetus. Knowing the mechanisms of insult enables nurses to know what action to take and to predict whether or not a change can be effected and how long it will take to accomplish. The periodic changes are in response to some documented stimuli. These are commonly fetal movement or maternal contractions. The FHR can either accelerate or decelerate in response to stimuli. Accelerations may be described as either *uniform* or *nonuniform*. Decelerations are described in terms of when they occur, that is, early or late or variable decelerations.

TABLE 3-8. *Summary of accelerations and decelerations*

UNIFORM ACCELERATIONS (Fig. 3-9, *A*)

Description	Uniform in shape
	Begins when the contraction begins and ends when the contraction ends
	Often mirrors the intensity of contractions
Mechanism of insult	Sympathetic response to stimuli
Significance	Healthy CNS response
	Often associated with breech presentations
Nursing intervention	Totally benign so none needed

NONUNIFORM ACCELERATIONS (Fig. 3-9, *B*)

Description	Nonuniform in shape
	Usually occur in response to fetal movement so vary in the contraction cycle
Mechanism of insult	Sympathetic response to stimuli
Significance	Healthy CNS response
Nursing intervention	None

EARLY DECELERATIONS (Fig. 3-10, *A*)

Description	Uniform in shape
	Frequently mirror contraction intensity
	Begin when contraction begins and end when contraction ends
	Occur only between 4 and 7 cm dilatation of cervix
Mechanism of insult	Head compression
	Parasympathetic (vagal) reflex due to pressure on the fontanels against the resisting cervix
Significance	Although not normal, since it does not occur in all fetuses, it is benign
Nursing intervention	Differentiate these from late decelerations
	No action necessary or helpful

LATE DECELERATIONS (Fig. 3-10, *B*)

Description	Uniform in shape
	Sometimes reflect the intensity of contractions
	Begin anywhere in the contraction cycle, although common near the peak
	End after the contraction has ended with a slow, sloping return to baseline
Mechanism of insult	Uteroplacental insufficiency leading to CNS hypoxia or myocardial depression
Significance	Always ominous regardless of depth of deceleration or degree of variability
	Acute episodes usually demonstrate good variability and are more likely to be correctable
	Chronic episodes usually are accompanied by decreased or absent variability and are less likely to be correctable
Nursing intervention	Turn patient to left side
	Administer O_2 at 8 to 10 L/min by tight face mask
	Infuse rapidly intravenous fluid
	Correct hypotension
	If Pitocin used, turn it off
	Expect expeditious delivery if not corrected within 30 minutes

---

Modified from Freeman and Garite (1981).   *Continued.*

TABLE 3-8. *Summary of accelerations and decelerations—cont'd*

VARIABLE DECELERATIONS (Fig. 3-10, *C*)

Description	Variable in shape, often V- or W-shaped
	Variable in placement with contractions; may occur between or with contractions
	Heart rate falls abruptly and rises abruptly
Mechanism of insult	Cord compression
Significance	Benign if:
	Infrequent occurrence
	Low point is within normal heart rate range
	Lasts less than 45 seconds
	Ominous if:
	Repetitive
	Falls below 90 beats/min
	Lasts longer than 50 seconds
	Followed by tachycardia
	Has a slow return to baseline
	Has loss of variability between decelerations
Nursing interventions	Turn side to side or to knee chest position
	Give O_2 at 8 to 10 L/min by tight face mask
	Improve circulating volume
	Expect expeditious delivery if ominous

*PROLONGED DECELERATION** (Fig. 3-10, *D*)

Description	Abrupt deceleration lasting 2 to 10 minutes
	Usually falls below 90 beats/min
Mechanism of insult	Prolonged cord compression
Significance	If lasts longer than 10 minutes, fetus becomes acidemic and myocardial depression occurs
Nursing interventions	Notify physician or midwife of first occurrence
	Check for cord prolapse
	Turn patient side to side or to knee chest position until change is effected
	Give O_2 at 8 to 10 L/min by tight face mask
	Correct maternal hypotension; increase intravenous fluids
	Continuous observation until delivery
	Be prepared for emergency delivery

Although a prolonged deceleration is not technically a pattern, if it occurs once it should be of concern. It must be suspected that if it occurs once it is likely to occur again and the return to baseline heart rate may or may not occur.

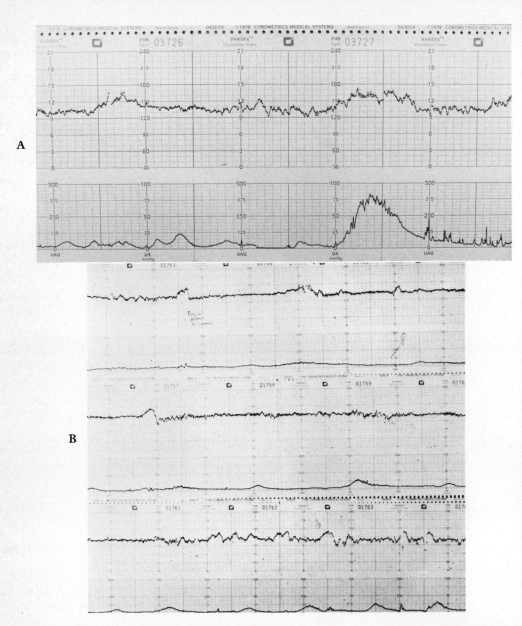

FIG. 3-9. A, Uniform acceleration is noted beginning in panel 03727 in response to the contraction beneath. **B,** Nonuniform accelerations can be seen between contractions. Baseline FHR 150 to 155 beats/min with accelerations to 170 beats/min. (**B,** courtesy John P. Elliott, M.D., Phoenix, Arizona.)

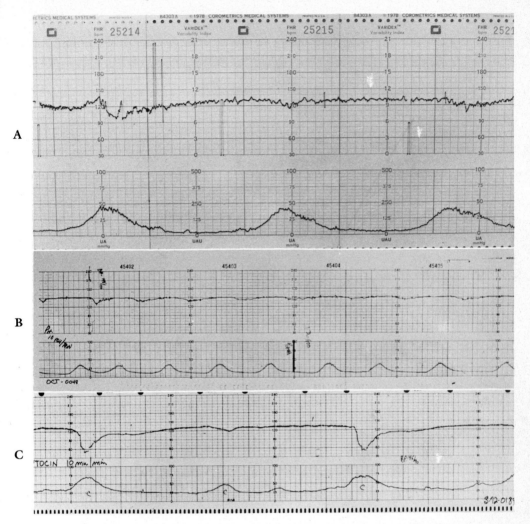

FIG. 3-10. A, Early decelerations. Baseline FHR 130 beats/min. Gradual decelerations to 120 beats/min are seen in panels 25215 and 2521. Both have returned to baseline FHR of 130 beats/min by the end of the contraction. **B,** Late decelerations. Baseline FHR 150 beats/min. Subtle decelerations are seen with each contraction beginning near or just after their peak and not returning to baseline until 30 to 40 seconds after the contraction has ended. Note the poor to absent variability that accompanies the baseline and is transmitted by external ultrasound. **C,** Severe variable decelerations. Note the abrupt fall in the heart rate from baseline of 130 beats/min. Note also the depth of the deceleration to 55 to 60 beats, the sloping return to baseline, and the absent variability. Those features make these severe and the prognosis for the fetus poor.

Continued.

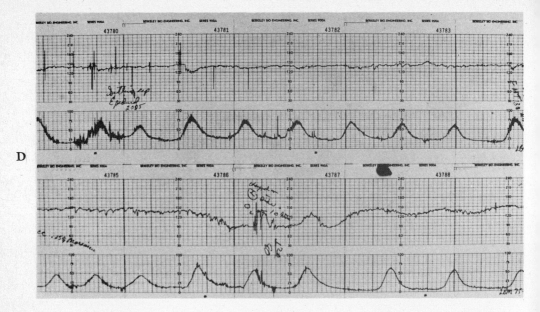

FIG. 3-10, cont'd. D, Prolonged deceleration in panels 43786 through 43787. This deceleration follows the initiation of epidural anesthesia and frequently can be avoided with IV fluid preload. Note the occurrence of late decelerations with good baseline variability following the recovery period. (**B to D,** courtesy John P. Elliott, M.D., Phoenix, Arizona.)

ANTEPARTUM FETAL SURVEILLANCE
Antepartum fetal heart rate monitoring *(Freeman and Garite, 1981)*

The latest census statistics estimate that two thirds of fetal deaths occur in the antepartum period. Certainly a means of surveillance that allows detection of that risk before damage occurs could greatly benefit those pregnancies. Antepartum fetal heart rate monitoring provides a means for doing just that. The objectives of antepartum FHR monitoring are:

1. To prevent fetal death
2. To prevent fetal damage
3. To avoid unnecessary premature intervention

Those patients who are candidates for antepartum FHR monitoring have a maternal or fetal condition that places the fetus at risk for respiratory or nutritive uteroplacental insufficiency (UPI). Generally a fetus undergoes nutritive compromise before respiratory compromise. The rapidity of progression varies with conditions. It may happen gradually as with chronic hypertension, abruptly as in abruption of the placenta, or bypass the nutritive stage entirely beginning with respiratory or hypoxic effects as in diabetes. The term *uteropla-cental insufficiency* relates specifically to inadequate exchange within the placenta. This can result from decreased uterine blood flow, decreased placental surface area, or increased membrane thickness. The term can also be applied to fetal uptake insufficiencies such as anemia, postmaturity, or discordant twins.

Some of the common maternal conditions associated with UPI are listed below.
1. Pregnancy-induced hypertension (PIH)
2. Chronic hypertension
3. Diabetes
4. Postterm pregnancy
5. Collagen vascular disease
6. Renal disease
7. Rh isoimmunization
8. Multiple gestation
9. Third-trimester bleeding

The decision as to when to test is usually made based on viability (not before 26 to 28 weeks), severity of the condition, and when the condition is recognized. With the availability of regionalized centers and transportation capabilities, as well as long-distance telemetry, early detection of UPI is possible, and desirable, for optimal treatment and outcome.

Nonstress test *(Freeman and Garite, 1981)*

The nonstress test (NST) is a test of fetal well-being. Well-being is demonstrated by the fetus as accelerations following stimuli; this is usually documented as fetal activity. The patients for whom this test is appropriate include those previously described. However, because loss of ability of the FHR to accelerate is usually demonstrated after profound hypoxic damage has resulted, the NST has some definite disadvantages. Thus it is often selected only for those patients whose maternal condition precludes contractions or whose condition is so labile as to warrant frequency of testing greater than twice a week. Patients who have had a previous classical cesarean section, who are currently being treated for premature labor, or who have had third-trimester bleeding should have an NST. Other reasons for choosing an NST might be a maternal condition such as diabetes or preeclampsia requiring stabilization and involving an immature fetus who might benefit from more time in utero. Then a daily NST would prove useful for assessing the effect of care on the mother and the well-being of the fetus. See the box on the following page for procedures, criteria for interpretation, and management of NST.

NONSTRESS TEST: PROCEDURE, CRITERIA FOR INTERPRETATION, AND MANAGEMENT

PROCEDURE
1. Document the date and time the test is started, make and model of monitor, the external modes used, patient name, reason for test, and maternal vital signs when in a semi-Fowler position.
2. Place patient in semi-Fowler position.
3. Apply both the ultrasound transducer and the tocotransducer to obtain all available data.
4. Record maternal blood pressure every 10 to 15 minutes.

CRITERIA FOR INTERPRETATION
1. Run the strip for 20 minutes. If there are at least two accelerations of at least 15 beats/min over the baseline heart rate lasting for at least 15 seconds, the test is called reactive.
2. Other reassuring features such as good variability and absence of ominous periodic changes with any spontaneous contractions or fetal movement should also be described and expected for a test to read as reactive (Fig. 3-11).
3. The recording must be of adequate quality for a reasonable determination of variability to be made. Because the logic system is in effect on the external mode, the model of monitor used should be the most sophisticated.
4. If at the end of the first 20 minutes the above criteria are not met, the fetus should be stimulated by moving it externally and waiting an additional 20 minutes for criteria to be met. If the NST remains nonreactive (Fig. 3-12) after the second 20 minutes or if any ominous periodic change is present, either a contraction stress test should be done or another more definitive evaluation of the fetus such as ultrasound for a biophysical profile should be carried out if inducing contractions is contraindicated.

MANAGEMENT
A reactive NST should be repeated every 3 or 4 days for continued prediction of fetal well-being. There are disadvantages of the test in that:
1. Studies vary in criteria used for the end point of 20-minute cycles and in criteria for the amplitude and duration of accelerations.
2. Studies vary in frequency of testing recommended. When testing is recommended every 3 or 4 days, it is usually more expensive than a contraction stress test.
3. When a test is truly nonreactive, a much later sign of hypoxia has been detected and fetal outcome is often poor. The NST therefore does not meet the objective of preventing fetal damage as well as some other fetal surveillance methods.
There are advantages of the test in that:
1. It is noninvasive, requiring no initiation of contractions.
2. There are no equivocal interpretations when criteria are followed.

Modified from Freeman and Garite (1981).

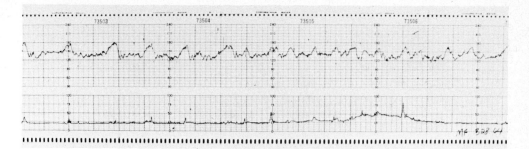

FIG. 3-11. Reactive nonstress test. Baseline FHR of 130 to 140 beats/min with numerous accelerations of greater than 15 beats lasting for more than 15 seconds. The small spikes in the tocotransducer tracing are fetal activity. (Courtesy John P. Elliott, M.D., Phoenix, Arizona.)

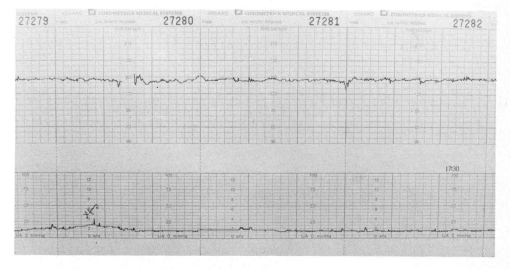

FIG. 3-12. Nonreactive nonstress test. Although there is apparent adequate beat to beat variability, no accelerations are seen that can be described as meeting the criteria of 15 beats over baseline for 15 seconds.

Contraction stress test *(Freeman and Garite, 1981)*

The contraction stress test (CST) can also be called a *stress test* or an *oxytocin challenge test* (OCT). All are synonymous in terms of the data documented on the monitor strip regarding FHR and uterine contractions. This section will refer to the test as a CST, meaning any one of the three.

The CST is a challenge to uteroplacental sufficiency and resultant fetal well-being. It does this when contractions are stimulated to a frequency of three in

10 minutes. The FHR tracing is observed for periodic changes. Candidates for testing are patients at risk for UPI either by history of previous pregnancy UPI or current maternal/fetal conditions such as hypertension, diabetes, intra-uterine growth retardation, or congenital fetal anomalies. See the box on page 57 for procedures, criteria for interpretation and management of CST.

ULTRASOUND

Ultrasound uses pulsed sound waves of very high range under directional control. It displays these on a cathode ray tube or screen. It can be viewed in real time or saved by taking a Polaroid picture.

Obstetric ultrasound has had some controversy surrounding its routine use and potential risk to the fetus. When indications are present, it can be a valuable means of making assessments. All high-risk or at-risk pregnancies can be considered for the benefits ultrasound examinations can provide.

Ultrasound is considered essentially noninvasive. It differs from X-ray in that ultrasound views a cross section of organs giving a two-dimensional aspect, whereas X-ray views the projected surface.

Ultrasound can be of benefit in obtaining the following information:
1. The Booking examination for confirmation of gestational age, diagnosis of multiple gestation, exclusion of major congenital anomalies
2. Diagnosis of problems of placental placement or abruption
3. Location of fetal and placental structures and amniotic fluid for amnio-centesis
4. Biophysical profile for fetal well-being
5. Assessment for abnormal fetal growth patterns

The Booking examination is widely used in the United Kingdom as a routine procedure to provide an accurate means of determining gestational age. It consists of assessment for the gestational sac, measurement of the crown-rump length, biparietal diameter, and femur length. It also assesses for the presence of multiple pregnancies and placental localization and rules out certain congenital anomalies (O'Brien, 1982). The value and accuracy of this examination begin as early as 5 weeks. Between 17 and 20 weeks the ability to do a physical examination of the fetus improves. The examination loses accuracy in estimating gestational age after 20 weeks.

Assessment of placental location or accidents can aid in the decisions for continued management and mode of delivery when a third-trimester bleed is suspected. Assessment for localization of the placenta, fetal structures, and a pocket of amniotic fluid is also invaluable during an amniocentesis.

The biophysical profile is a set of evaluations of the fetus to confirm or

CONTRACTION STRESS TEST: PROCEDURE, CRITERIA FOR INTERPRETATION, AND MANAGEMENT

PROCEDURE

1. Run a 20 minute NST for baseline information regarding FHR and uterine contractions.
2. Stimulate contractions either with intravenous oxytocin or by nipple stimulation of endogenous oxytocin.

Stimulation of contractions with oxytocin

1. Start mainline intravenous of normal saline.
2. Piggyback oxytocin diluted so that increments of 0.5 mU/min can be delivered.
3. Start at 0.5 mU/min double amount every 15 to 20 minutes until 4 mU, then increase by 2 mU, until three contractions occur in 10 minutes or maximum dose of 16 mU is reached.

Initiation of contractions with nipple stimulation

1. Place warmed moist cloths across breasts, replacing as needed, for 10 minutes.
2. On one side begin nipple rolling through the cloth. Continue until a contraction begins or for 10 minutes.
3. If no contraction in 10 minutes of rolling, change sides and continue for 10 minutes. If still not effective, roll both nipples simultaneously.
4. Replace warmed cloths throughout as needed.
5. Continue nipple rolling on effective side(s) until a contraction occurs. Stop until contraction is over and then begin again until three contractions occur in 10 minutes.
3. Keep patient in semi-Fowler position.
4. Record maternal blood pressure every 15 minutes.

CRITERIA FOR INTERPRETATION

1. *Negative:* (Fig. 3-13) No late decelerations noted on entire strip. Usually good apparent variability is also present and there is an absence of any other nonreassuring patterns.
2. *Equivocal:* A test may be equivocal for one of three reasons.
   a. *Suspicious:* Less than 50% of the contractions on the entire strip have late decelerations. Variability is usually good (Fig. 3-14, *A*).
   b. *Hyperstimulation:* A contraction frequency greater than four in 10 minutes, less than 60 seconds between contractions, or a contraction lasting longer than 90 seconds with a late deceleration occurring (Fig. 3-14, *B*).
   c. *Unsatisfactory:* The quality of the tracing is too poor to accurately interpret FHR with contractions or the frequency of three contractions in 10 minutes cannot be obtained for an endpoint of the test (Fig. 3-14, *C*).
3. *Positive:* (Fig. 3-15, *A* and *B*) Fifty percent or more of the contractions on the strip have late decelerations associated with them even if the endpoint of three contractions in 10 minutes is not obtained. If associated with decreased variability, the prognosis is poor.

MANAGEMENT

A negative CST predicts continued fetal well-being for 7 days and need only be repeated weekly provided maternal well-being is the same. An equivocal CST should be repeated in 24 hours. If a test remains equivocal for 3 days consecutively, NSTs are usually used from then on instead of CSTs. A positive CST necessitates more vigorous management. If the variability is good and the fetus is mature by the proper dates and in a vertex position a very carefully monitored induction can be attempted. If the fetus is immature, treating the maternal condition that might have precipitated the problem may be the treatment of choice to give the baby its best chance. When variability is poor, delivery by an emergency cesarean is the only chance for optimal outcome for the baby regardless of maturity.

Modified from Freeman and Garite (1981).

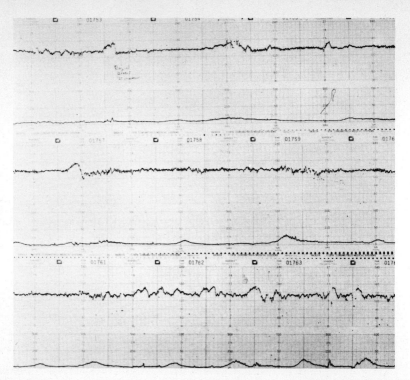

FIG. 3-13. Negative and reactive contraction stress test obtained with breast stimulation. There are no late decelerations noted in any panel. Good apparent beat to beat variability is present and the FHR accelerates periodically. Three contractions are present in 10 minutes (panels 01761 through 017630). (Courtesy John P. Elliott, M.D., Phoenix, Arizona.)

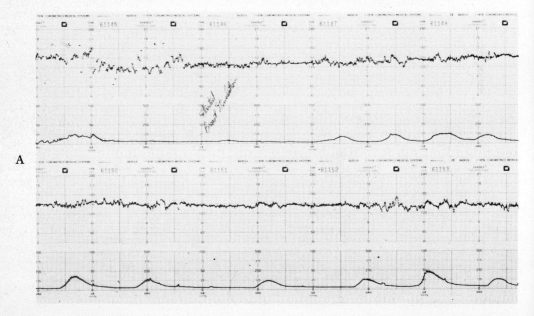

A

FIG. 3-14. A, Equivocal contraction stress test because of one late deceleration in panel 61145. Breast stimulation was started to further challenge the placental function and determine if late deceleration would persist. Because the remainder of the test was negative for late decelerations and reactive the test was repeated the following day.

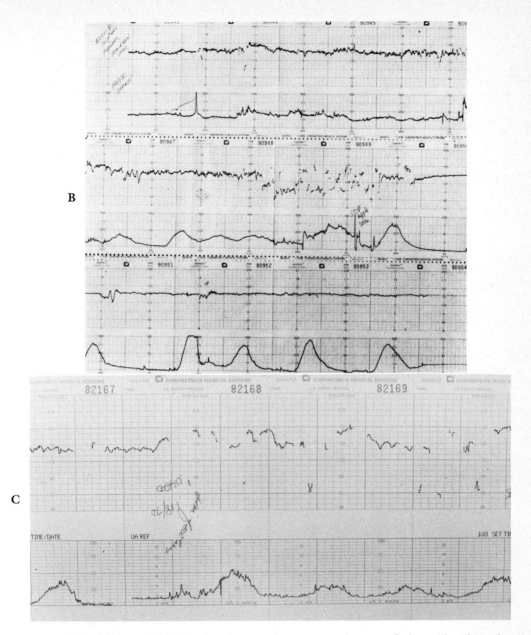

FIG. 3-14, cont'd. B, Equivocal contraction stress test because of a late and prolonged deceleration with excessive and hyperstimulated uterine activity in panels 90948 and 90949. The previous portion of the strip had good apparent variability and reactivity, although the remaining portion, during recovery, demonstrates poor variability. The tracing was continued until adequate recovery was evidenced. Then the test was repeated the following day. **C,** Equivocal contraction stress test because the tracing immediately following each contraction is unsatisfactory for accurate interpretation of the FHR response. (**B,** courtesy John P. Elliott, M.D., Phoenix, Arizona.)

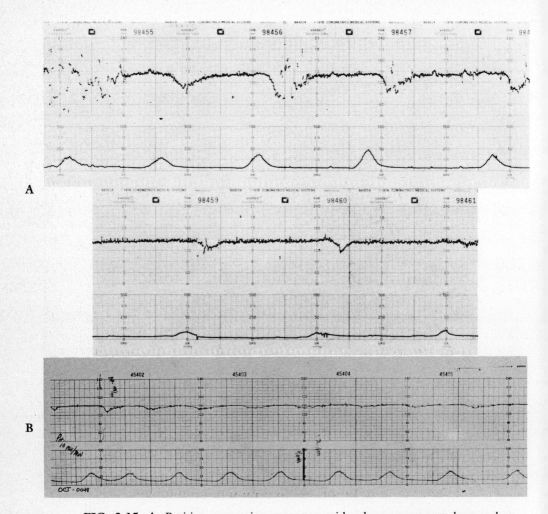

FIG. 3-15. A, Positive contraction stress test with adequate apparent beat to beat variability. Baseline FHR is 140 to 150 beats/min. The tracing was continued and reactivity was also noted while decisions were made for delivery in a postterm pregnancy. **B,** Positive, nonreactive contraction stress test with poor to absent variability. The baby was delivered by emergent cesarean birth with Apgar scores below 6. The mother was stable with PIH. (**B,** courtesy John P. Elliott, M.D., Phoenix, Arizona.)

diagnose stressors or distress in an immature fetus. It consists of a scoring of five facets of fetal well-being. Each gets a score from 0 to 2 for a possible total of 10 points. The parameters measured are as follows:

1. Biparietal diameter, femur length, chest and abdominal circumference to determine gestational age and appropriate size and assess for symmetry of growth
2. Amniotic fluid amount compared to normals for gestational age
3. Respiratory effort
4. Fetal heart rate and response to activity documented by an NST
5. Flexion and extension of all four extremities

A score from 7 to 10 indicates fetal well-being, 4 to 6 is questionable, and less than 4 means that the fetus is in jeopardy and usually must be delivered or will soon die in utero.

The nurse's role in caring for the patient having obstetric ultrasound focuses primarily on patient education. An understanding of why a particular patient might benefit from the information an ultrasound can give should enable the nurse to answer questions accurately.

Because of early ultrasound enabling mothers to recognize fetal viability and activity considerably before life is felt, a close relationship is often established earlier in the pregnancy. The father's participation in viewing the ultrasound can also aid in his early emotional attachment. In addition, detection and identification of fetal genitalia have enabled parents to feel personal sex-linked identity with the baby long before delivery. These attachment behaviors should be encouraged and supported by the nurse working with the couple.

AMNIOCENTESIS

Amniocentesis is a procedure for removing a small amount of amniotic fluid by insertion of a needle through the abdominal wall, the uterine wall, and the amniotic sac. It is done with ultrasonic visualization of uterine, placental, and fetal structures. An amniocentesis may be done for a number of evaluations, including the following.

1. Genetic evaluation
2. Evaluation of fetus in an Rh-sensitized mother
3. Evaluation of the fetus for lung maturity

Genetic evaluation is generally done between the weeks 14 and 18 when an adequate pocket of fluid can be tapped. It usually includes analysis for chromosomal disorders, biochemical disorders, and sex-linked disorders. Results often take as long as 3 to 4 weeks to obtain. During that time parents can experience varying degrees of anxiety.

Reasons why parents might elect to have a genetic amniocentesis are numerous. Commonly a genetic amniocentesis is indicated for a mother 40 years or older or when a family history indicates previous genetic disorders. Parents are not obligated to terminate a pregnancy with these disorders. They may view the genetic evaluation as a means of adequately preparing for a less than optimal outcome or they may use it to choose termination of the pregnancy.

Nursing responsibilities include psychologic support during the procedure and assistance in coping with anxiety during the wait for results. Some parents wish to know the sex of their baby and others do not. The parents' wishes should be established before results are discussed.

Evaluation of the fetus in an Rh isoimmunization mother is done for breakdown products from fetal hemoglobin hemolysis. These are bilirubin pigment measurements. It can be started as early as the week 22. Depending on the results, compared to gestational age, the amniocentesis is repeated every 1 to 3 weeks. If levels are extremely high, intrauterine blood transfusions may be necessary to gain additional time for the fetus to mature.

Nursing responsibilities include an assessment for any financial stress that repeated evaluation may cause. Social service referral may be necessary. Any anxieties revolving around the procedure and the potential results need to be discussed and realistic reassurances given.

Evaluation of the fetus for lung maturity is invaluable in the timing of delivery whether it be an elective repeat cesarean birth or whether it is an induction before term for medical indications. Lecithin is usually present in an unstable form until 35 to 36 weeks but can be measured in ratio to sphingomyelin (L/S ratio). Also measured for presence or absence is phosphatidyglycerol (PG), because its presence is a precursor to stable lecithin. When the L/S ratio is greater than 20% and PG is present, fetal lung maturity indicates that prematurity is no longer a consideration. Surfactant will be present in the alveoli so that expansion and contraction can occur.

When an amniocentesis is performed for the first time many women voice fear of the potential discomfort and possible trauma to the baby. The nurse can allay some of these fears by accurately describing the discomfort, procedure, and safeguards for the baby.

First an ultrasonic examination is done to locate the placenta, so that it can be avoided, and to locate a pocket of amniotic fluid large enough to prevent trauma to the baby. Next the abdominal area for puncture is cleansed with Betadine and draped with sterile towels. The physician is gloved and the tray of contents opened and made accessible for him or her. A needle the size of a spinal needle is inserted through the abdominal wall and the uterus and into the amniotic sac. The discomfort is described as similar to an injection, with some pressure and minor cramping. A syringe is attached and about 10 cc of fluid is withdrawn, placed in a container surrounded by ice, and sent to a center skilled in perinatal testing. The entire procedure is over in 5 to 10 minutes as a general rule. A small piece of tape is placed over the site.

The nurse's role in the procedure is to have the patient sign a permit for the procedure after being sure that last-minute questions have been answered. Baseline FHR should be documented before the procedure. Following the procedure, the mother should be sent for FHR monitoring for 20 to 30 minutes if the fetus is 26 weeks or more old.

The risks of spontaneous abortion, fetal trauma, and infection are areas of concern to the woman. These are best described by the physician.

Chorionic villi sampling

Prenatal diagnosis of genetic abnormalities has, until very recently, only been available in the second trimester. The decision for termination of the pregnancy, when diagnosis is positive, leads to a more physically traumatizing abortion procedure. It is also a more profoundly distressing dilemma because fetal movements are usually being perceived by the mother and abdominal girth increase has been noted by others.

Chorionic villi sampling can resolve much of this difficulty. The chorion is the most accessible fetal tissue in the first trimester and can be sampled through a special procedure. A specially designed 1.9 mm catheter is guided, under ultrasound direction, through the cervix and into an area outside the embryonic sac that represents the developing placenta. The cells obtained are of embryonic origin and reflect the genetic makeup of the embryo.

The fetal tissue can be immediately recognized under the microscope and completely analyzed in 4 hours for the immediate preparation and in 2 weeks for cultures. Amniotic fluid takes 3 to 4 weeks. The chorionic villi sampling therefore gives earlier and quicker results. Pooled data of worldwide investigators revealed a 12% pregnancy loss. Other data demonstrate a 0% to 6% loss, which rivals statistics for genetic amniocentesis and falls within the usual statistics for spontaneous abortion in the general population (Division of Medical Genetics, 1984).

α-Fetoprotein

Measurement of α-fetoprotein can be done either in the amniotic fluid or in the maternal serum. It is a substance found in increased amounts when an open neural tube defect is present in the fetus. If present in the serum in increased amounts between 15 and 19 weeks of gestation, an amniocentesis and further ultrasound evaluation must be done to be more certain whether a defect is present or not. Normal serum levels between 15 and 19 weeks are 0.4 to 2.5 moles/molecule (MoMs) (Southwest Genetic Center of Phoenix, 1983).

Estriol determinations

Estriol is produced by the placenta as a result of the metabolic activity of the placenta and the fetus. It can be measured in maternal serum or 24 hour urinary collections. However, other maternal factors can influence the results, such as metabolic rate, infection, or time of day; therefore the results must be compared serially to be of benefit in evaluating continued fetal well-being. Using an averaging formula, a 35% drop in quantity is considered significant and further testing with a CST is warranted.

Fetal activity chart

Perceptions and reports of fetal movement are the oldest and least expensive technique to monitor fetal well-being. Studies with ultrasonic monitoring report that mothers perceive 82% to 87% of documented fetal movement. Recommended lengths of time to count an acceptable number of fetal movements vary. Mothers are instructed each day to be on their left side for 1 hour and count fetal movements, recording them on a chart. If the number of fetal movements is less than four or five averaged over an hour, the mother is instructed to go into a health care facility for fetal heart rate monitoring. Mothers respond favorably to this self-monitoring when the significance of fetal activity and the chart is explained to them.

Fetal movement charts can effectively serve as a signal of impending fetal jeopardy. Some studies have suggested that as many as 81% of inactive fetuses require resuscitation at birth. Fetal activity patterns and response to various stimuli or lack thereof have not been well studied. It should not therefore be the only means of monitoring but simply a useful daily subjective observation of continued fetal well-being (Rayburn, 1982).

REFERENCES

Arbitol, M.M.: Aortic compression and uterine blood flow during pregnancy, Obstet. Gynecol. **50**:562, 1977.

Amato, J.C.: Fetal monitoring in a community hospital, Obstet. Gynecol. **50**:269, 1977.

Banta, H.D. and Thacker, S.B.: Assessing the costs and benefits of electronic fetal monitoring, Obstet. Gynecol. Surv. **34**:627, 1979.

Benson, R., and others: Fetal heart rate as predictor of fetal distress: a report from the collaborative project, Obstet. Gynecol. **32**:529, 1968.

Berne, R.M., and Levy, M.N.: Cardiovascular physiology, ed. 4, St. Louis, 1981, The C.V. Mosby Co.

Bernstine, R.L.: Safety studies with ultrasonic Doppler technique, Obstet. Gynecol. **34**:707, 1969.

Cetrulo, C.L., and Schifrin, B.S.: Fetal heart rate patterns preceding death in utero, Obstet. Gynecol. **48**:521, 1976.

Chez, R.A., and others: Symposium—once a section, always a section?, Contemp. Obstet. Gynecol. **15**(1):128, 1980.

Christie, G.B., and Cudmore, D.W.: The oxytocin challenge test, Am. J. Obstet. Gynecol. **118**:327, 1974.

Cordero, L. Jr., and Hon, E.H.: Scalp abscess: a rare complication of fetal monitoring, J. Pediatr. **78**:533, 1971.

Dgani, R., and others: Prenatally diagnosed blocked atrial premature beats, Obstet. Gynecol. **51**:507, 1978.

Division of Medical Genetics: CVS latest news, Philadelphia, 1984.

Eberhard, M., Caritis, S., and Edelstone, D.: Sinusoidal fetal heart rate pattern following intrauterine fetal transfusion, Obstet. Gynecol. **52**:43s, 1978.

Ewing, D.E., Farina, J.R., and Otterson, W.N.: Clinical application of the oxytocin challenge test, Obstet. Gynecol. **43**:563, 1974.

Freeman, R., and Garite, T.: Fetal heart rate monitoring, Baltimore, 1981, Williams & Wilkins Co.

Freeman, R.K.: The use of the oxytocin challenge test for antepartum clinical evaluation of uteroplacental respiratory function, Am. J. Obstet. Gynecol. **122**:481-489, 1975.

Freeman, R.K., and others: Fetal cardiac response to paracervical block anesthesia, Part 1, Am. J. Obstet. Gynecol. **113**:583, 1972.

Gabbe, S.G., and Hon, E.H.: New trends in fetal heart rate monitoring, the importance of variability. In Rooth, G., and Brattlby, L.E., editors: Perinatal medicine (5th European Congress of Perinatal Medicine, Uppsala, Sweden, June 9–12, 1976), Uppsala, 1976, Alniquist Wiksell.

Gaziano, E.P., and Freeman, D.W.: Analysis of heart rate patterns preceding fetal death, Obstet. Gynecol. **50**:578, 1977.

Gibbs, M.D., and others: Internal fetal monitoring and maternal infection following cesarean section, Obstet. Gynecol. **52**:193, 1978.

Gray, J.H., and others: Sinusoidal fetal heart rate pattern associated with alphaprodine administration, Obstet. Gynecol. **52**:678, 1978.

Haine, M., and Boehm, F.: A statewide program to teach nurses the use of fetal monitors, JOGN 7(3):29, 1978.

Harrigan, J.T., and others: Fetal cardiac arrhythmia during labor, Am. J. Obstet. Gynecol. **128**:693, 1977.

Havercamp, A.D.: A controlled trial of the differential effects of intrapartum fetal monitoring, Am. J. Obstet. Gynecol. **134**:399, 1979.

Haverkamp, A.D., and others: Evaluation of continuous fetal heart rate monitoring in high risk pregnancy, Am. J. Obstet. Gynecol. **125**:310, 1976.

Hobbins, J.C.: The fetal monitoring debate, Obstet. Gynecol. **54**:103, 1979.

Hobel, C.J. and others: Prenatal and intrapartum high risk screening: prediction of the high risk neonate, Am. J. Obstet. Gynecol. **117**:1, 1973.

Hon, E.H.: Placental dysfunction in obstetrics, ed. 13, New York, 1965, J.P. Greenhill.

Hon, E.H.: The human fetal circulation in normal labor. In Cassels, D.E., editor: The heart and circulation in the newborn and infant, New York, 1966, Grune and Stratton, Inc.

Hon, E.H., and Paul, R.H.: Quantitation of uterine activity, Obstet. Gynecol. **42**:368, 1973.

Hon, E.H.: An introduction to fetal heart rate monitoring, ed. 2, Wallingford, Conn., 1975, Corometrics Medical Systems, Inc.

Hon, E.H., Bradfield, A.H., and Hess, O.W.: The electronic evaluation of fetal heart rate v. the vagal factor in fetal bradycardia, Am. J. Obstet. Gynecol. **82**:291, 1961.

Hon, E.H., Zannini, D., and Quilligan, E.J.: The neonatal value of fetal monitoring, Am. J. Obstet. Gynecol. **122**:508, 1975.

Huey, J.R., Jr., Miller, F.: The evaluation of uterine activity: a comparative analysis, Am. J. Obstet. Gynecol. **136**:478, 1980.

Jung, A., and Stenchever, M.D.: Aplasia cutis congenita and the fetal scalp electrode, Am. J. Obstet. Gynecol. **129**:351, 1977.

Katz, M., and others: Neonatal heart rate reactivity following variable decelerations during labor, Am. J. Obstet. Gynecol. **136**:389, 1980.

Keegan, K., and others: Antepartum fetal heart rate testing v. the non-stress test—an outpatient approach, Am. J. Obstet. Gynecol. **136**:81, 1980.

Keegan, K., and Paul, R.H.: Antepartum fetal heart rate testing v. the non-stress test as a primary approach, Am. J. Obstet. Gynecol. **136**:75, 1980.

Kelso, I.: An assessment of continuous fetal heart rate monitoring in labor, Am. J. Obstet. Gynecol. **131**:526, 1978.

Klapholz, H.M., and others: Role of maternal artifact in fetal heart rate pattern interpretation, Obstet. Gynecol. **44**:373, 1974.

Lackritz, R., and others: Decelerations on fetal electrocardiography with fetal demise, Obstet. Gynecol. **51**:367, 1978.

Lee, W.K., and Baggish, M.S.: The effect of unselected intrapartum fetal monitoring, Obstet. Gynecol. **47**:516, 1976.

Manning, F., and others: Antepartum fetal evaluation: development of a fetal biophysical profile, Am. J. Obstet. Gynecol. **136**:787, 1980.

Mannor, S.M.: The safety of untrasound in fetal monitoring, Am. J. Obstet. Gynecol. **113**:653, 1972.

McCue, C.M., and others: Congenital heart block in newborns of mothers with connective tissue disease, Circulation **56**:82, 1977.

Mendenhall, H.,W. and others: The non-stress test: the value of a single acceleration in evaluation the fetus at risk, Am. J. Obstet. Gynecol. **136**:87, 1980.

Mendez-Bauer, C., and others: Relationship between blood pH and heart rate in the human fetus during labor, Am. J. Obstet. Gynecol. **97**:530, 1967.

Miller, F.: Monitoring uterine activity, Contemp. Ob/Gyn **13**(6):35, 1979.

Miller, F., and others: Significance of meconium during labor, Am. J. Obstet. Gynecol. **122**:573, 1975.

Mondanlou, H., and others: Complications of fetal blood sampling during labor. The pediatrician should always be informed when scalp samples have been taken, Clin. Pediatr. **12**:603, 1973.

Mondanlou, H., and others: Sinusoidal fetal heart rate pattern and severe fetal anemia, Obstet. Gynecol. **49**:537, 1977.

Nelson, K.S., and Broman, T.H.: Perinatal risk factors in children with serious motor and mental handicaps, Neurology **2**:371, 1977.

Neutra, R.R., and others: Effect of fetal monitoring on cesarean section rate, Obstet. Gynecol. **55**:175, 1980.

Niels, H., and others: Microfilm storage of fetal monitoring records: a practical solution, Obstet. Gynecol. **51**:632, 1978.

Nochimson, D., and others: The non-stress test, Obstet. Gynecol. **51**:419, 1978.

O'Brien, G.: The Booking exam for early fetal assessment, Contemp. OB/Gyn **20**(8):55, 1982.

Organ, L., and others: Indexes of heart rate variability, Am. J. Obstet. Gynecol. **130**:20, 1978.

Painter, M.J., and others: Fetal heart rate patterns and development in the first year of life, Am. J. Obstet. Gynecol. **132**:271, 1978.

Parer, J., and others: Fetal oxygen consumption and mechanisms of heart rate response during artifically produced late decelerations of fetal heart rate in sheep, Am. J. Obstet. Gynecol. **136**:478, 1980.

Parer, J.T.: Physiological regulation of fetal heart rate, JOGN **5** [Suppl.]: 26s, 1976.

Paul, R.H., and Petrie, R.H.: Fetal intensive care—current concepts, Los Angeles, 1973, University of Southern California.

Paul, R.H.: A practical system for storing and retrieving fetal monitoring data, Contemp. OB/Gyn 7(6):149, 1976.

Queenan, J.T.: Who's evaluating the efficiency of your monitor? Contemp. OB/Gyn 13(1):9, 1979.

Quilligan, E.J., and Paul, R.H.: Fetal monitoring: is it worth it?, Obstet. Gynecol. 45:96, 1975.

Rayburn, W.: Clinical implications from monitoring fetal activity, Am. J. Obstet. Gynecol. 144:967, 1982.

Renou, P., and others: Controlled trial of fetal intensive care, Am. J. Obstet. Gynecol. 126:470, 1976.

Rochard, F., and others: Non-stressed fetal heart rate monitoring in the antepartum period, Am. J. Obstet. Gynecol. 126:699, 1976.

Rodeck, C., and others: First trimester chorion biopsy, Br. Med. Bull. 39:338, 1983.

Scheider, H., and others: Fetal trigeminal rhythm, Obstet. Gynecol. 50 [Supplement]:58s, 1977.

Scheidt, P., and others: One year follow up of infants exposed to ultrasound in uterus, Am. J. Obstet. Gynecol. 131:743, 1978.

Schifrin, B.S.: Fetal heart rate monitoring during labor, JAMA 222:196, 1972.

Schifrin, B.S.: Fetal heart rate patterns following epidural anesthesia and oxytocin infusion during labor, J. Obstet. Gynaecol. Br. Commun. 79:332, 1972.

Schifrin, B.S.: Antepartum fetal heart rate monitoring. In Gluck, L., editor: Intrauterine asphyxia and the developing fetal brain, Chicago, 1977, Year Book Medical Publishers, Inc.

Schifrin, B.S., and Lapidus, M.: Contraction stress test for antepartum fetal evaluation, Obstet. Gynecol. 45:433, 1975.

Schifrin, B., and others: Routine fetal heart rate monitoring in the antepartum period, Obstet. Gynecol. 54:21, 1979.

Schneiderman, C.I., and others: Maternal-fetal electrocardiogram conduction with intrapartum fetal death, Am. J. Obstet. Gynecol. 113:1130, 1972.

Shenker, L., and others: Routine electronic monitoring of fetal heart rate and uterine activity during labor, Obstet. Gynecol. 46:185, 1975.

Sibai, B.M., and others: Sinusoidal fetal heart rate pattern, Obstet. Gynecol. 55:637, 1980.

Starkman, M.N.: Fetal monitoring psychologic consequences and management recommendations, Obstet. Gynecol. 50:500, 1977.

Sugarman, R.G., and others: Fetal arrhythmia, Obstet. Gynecol. 52:301, 1978.

Tucker, S.: Fetal monitoring and fetal assessment in high-risk pregnancy, St. Louis, 1978, The C.V. Mosby Co.

Tutera, G., and Newman, R.L.: Fetal monitoring: its effect on the perinatal mortality and cesarean section rates and its complications, Am. J. Obstet. Gynecol. 122:750, 1975.

Webster R.D., Cudmore, D.W., and Gray, J.: Fetal bradycardia without fetal distress, Obstet. Gynecol. 50:50s–53s, 1977.

Winkel, C.A., and others: Scalp abscess: a complication of the spiral electrode, San Francisco, 1975, Department of Obstetrics and Gynecology of Letterman Army Medical Center.

Zalar, R.W., Jr., and Quilligan, E.J.: The influence of scalp sampling on the cesarean section rate for fetal distress, Am. J. Obstet. Gynecol. 12:239, 1979.

UNIT II

PSYCHOLOGIC IMPLICATIONS OF A HIGH-RISK PREGNANCY

Recent research in nursing and the behavioral sciences (Colman and Colman, 1971) points to the need to consider the high-risk mother as a unique person who must cope with a complex group of problems, psychologic as well as physiologic. In addition to undergoing the normal maturational process of childbearing, the high-risk mother must cope with a great emotional burden and psychologic adjustment to a childbearing experience that may not culminate in a happy, healthy mother-infant dyad.

CHAPTER 4

Psychologic adaptations to high-risk pregnancy

T o understand the emotional work and psychologic adjustments a high-risk mother might go through, certain concepts should be examined. Understanding concepts of attachment, the tasks of pregnancy, and the concepts of adaptation in relation to crisis, loss, grief, anxiety, and frustration can be helpful in the nursing process when dealing with a high-risk mother.

ATTACHMENT AND DEVELOPMENTAL TASKS

Attachment is a process influenced by many complex factors and is a permanent interactional, emotional bond that exists for life. The process of mother-infant attachment begins when the idea of pregnancy is contemplated and continues throughout the lives of both. For the mother it is dependent on a myriad of factors. These factors include the following.
1. Emotional maturity
2. Experience in being nurtured
3. Interpersonal relationships with significant others
4. The ability to cope with physiologic and psychologic stresses
5. Desire for pregnancy and self-concept of motherhood
6. Fears and fantasies during the pregnancy

There is more support for the theory that there occurs a sensitive period when attachment develops (Klaus and Kennell, 1976). This is usually thought to be the period immediately postpartum. The interactions of mother and infant at that time are categorized into sensory levels that can be observed.

Tactile

Most mothers when given the opportunity will make immediate tactile contact with their infant. The touching follows a pattern graphically described by Rubin (1969). The initial contact is exploratory and is made with the fingertips. Progression of tactile contact follows an orderly pattern but can vary in its length of time. After the fingertips, the palms of the hand are used to stroke and massage the baby. Then the baby is drawn into close contact with the mother and encompassed.

Verbal

Some mothers make early verbal contact by carrying on a continual stream of soft, high-pitched verbalization. The context usually involves relating the infant to the mother and to the outside world.

Visual

Early eye to eye contact is sought even when the infant is not being held. The mother usually tries to position herself so that she and the infant are en face. If the infant does not open his or her eyes, the mother will implore him or her to do so.

Entrainment

The pattern of speech of the mother has a powerful influence on the infant's activity. The infant very soon forms activity patterns in a reciprocal relationship that resembles a dance. The infant's response in this manner seems to lock the mother and infant into repeating this over and over.

Synchrony

The first act of synchrony occurs in the feeding process. The mother responds to the infant's sucking bursts and pauses for breath. Mothers learn to respond in the cycles of sucking and pausing at the appropriate points to stimulate or discourage sucking.

·   ·   ·

A series of developmental tasks must be accomplished in pregnancy for the mothering, attachment behaviors to come about. Clark and Alfonso (1979) describe these tasks.
1. Pregnancy validation
2. Fetal embodiment
3. Fetal distinction
4. Role transition

In a high-risk pregnancy, there can be a great deal of interference with the accomplishment of these tasks. The woman's own illness and fears for her well-being can cause heightened ambivalence about the pregnancy. Previous pregnancy losses may be recalled and complicate acceptance of the reality of a current pregnancy. If there are signs of bleeding or other ominous physical signs, it might be difficult to validate the pregnancy. Feelings of self-worth can be poor when the maternal accomplishment of pregnancy is thwarted.

When there is maternal illness, hospitalization may cause prolonged separation from family. Dependency needs may not be fulfilled. Socialization with other pregnant women can be limited, and difficulty with fetal embodiment occurs. Ultrasound examinations, which are often done in a high-risk pregnancy, can facilitate fetal embodiment.

If hospitalization occurs during the time of fetal distinction, preparations for the baby may be halted. Prenatal education for self and partner also might not be an option offered to an ill or hospitalized mother. Unmet expectations for the pregnancy may be a source of frustration at a time when activities would otherwise be directed at preparation for motherhood.

Preparation for the birth process might be totally out of the mother's control if her well-being is in question. Fears about procedures and care may take precedence over usual plans. The growth rate of her body may be a great concern. Choices for infant feeding, the birth process, or the coach's support might be different from what she desires.

When all or any of the developmental tasks are thwarted or interfered with, attachment can be slow in the neonatal period. If either the neonate or mother is ill immediately after delivery, early contact may not occur. When the neonate is premature or is connected to machinery, the parents might fear to touch the infant. The appearance and behavior of the neonate can be so new to the parents that their visual inspection finds nothing to identify with. Finally, if the pregnancy was thought to be in jeopardy, efforts might have been devoted to "letting go" rather than "attaching to." If this is so, the parents must resolve those feelings before they can begin to attach. The depth of emotion surrounding the possible death of the baby can be so strong as to permanently interfere with attachment if feelings are not explored.

The nurse caring for the high-risk pregnant woman must assess for the accomplishment of the tasks of pregnancy. When the woman is hospitalized, it is important to provide flexible visiting hours and rooming-in privileges for the father when possible. Discussions with other pregnant women in the hospital can facilitate exploration of common concerns and meet needs for socialization. Special classes to meet the physical limitations and fulfill the quest for information about labor, delivery, and motherhood skills should be developed for this unique group. Focusing on the effort being put forth to obtain an optimal pregnancy aids in improving ideas of self-worth.

Early contact and information seeking should be encouraged and supported if the neonate is in intensive care. If breast feeding is the chosen method of feeding, it should be encouraged and supported with information and help in establishment of lactation. Lactation can help the mother feel positive about her mothering when other skills are not possible yet.

ANXIETY, FRUSTRATION, AND CONFLICT

Anxiety is an internally experienced form of discomfort. It arises from interpersonal transmission of anxious feelings and unmet expectations related to acquired needs. Interpersonal transmission of anxious feelings occurs when one has empathy for someone else.

Anxiety can arise when acquired expectations such as needs for status, esteem, or confirmation of self-views are not met. The strength of the unmet needs and degree of awareness about them determine the extent of anxiety.

Behaviors that result from anxiety may be expressed as helplessness, apathy, restlessness, irritability, or anger. These behaviors become automatic and are used repetitively to relieve anxiety. Thus each person has his or her own automatic manner of response to anxiety (Peplau, 1957).

When relief behaviors fail, anxiety can rapidly progress to panic. The nurse caring for the high-risk pregnant woman must assess for behaviors aimed at the relief of anxiety and aid the woman in the use of the energy anxiety evokes. Talking about the event can help in identifying, analyzing, and understanding the events causing the anxiety. Beginning such discussion with a mother can be facilitated with statements such as "Many women in your situation feel . . . ." Providing group sessions in which pregnant women can discuss these events may also help. Fathers must be encouraged in the relief of anxiety in positive ways. Couples who do not receive help together might otherwise increase each other's anxiety.

Frustration and conflict are closely related. Frustration occurs when obstacles prevent the achievement of a goal. The behavioral effects of frustration include anger, aggression, withdrawal, fixation, or finally even learning.

Frustration occurs in a high-risk pregnancy when such goals as a healthy pregnancy, having a perfect baby, or having the perfect birth experience have the obstacles of illness, separation, and rigid rules imposed on them (Yates, 1962).

Conflict results when there are simultaneous, opposing goals of equal strength. If the desired pregnancy causes physical restrictions requiring financial strains or imposes difficulty in mothering tasks with other children, conflict can result. The choices offered to the mother might all be unappealing. If her goal is to have a vaginal delivery and a cesarean delivery is the only safe way for her, conflict will occur (Yates, 1962).

The nurse caring for the high-risk pregnant woman must understand the behaviors exhibited and the situations that provoke them. Intervening through recognizing the behaviors and the feelings that led to them can help the woman in directing her energies in positive directions.

CRISIS, COPING, AND ADAPTATION

A crisis occurs when an individual faces a problem that he or she cannot solve immediately. This results in an inner tension with signs of anxiety and inability to function. The inability to function, or a state of disequilibrium, results in a need to restore equilibrium (Caplan, 1957).

The ability to restore equilibrium is dependent on three balancing factors (Aguilera and Messick, 1970). First, an individual must have a realistic perception of the event. Second, there must be adequate support from significant others. Third, an individual must have developed adequate coping mechanisms in the past.

According to crisis theory (Caplan, 1973), there are two categories of crisis. A maturational crisis is one in which developmental tasks must be accomplished. First-time parenthood is such a crisis. A situational crisis is an event such as illness or pregnancy. Caplan (1973) further describes pregnancy as a period of increased susceptibility to crisis. During pregnancy physiologic factors interact with psychologic factors precipitating stress in all areas.

A high-risk pregnancy, when the woman or her fetus is at potential risk for illness or death, can be a serious time of crisis. When the situational crises of illness and pregnancy are superimposed on each other or the maturational crisis of parenthood, the woman and her partner are called upon for coping mechanisms that might never have been developed.

Adaptation, in a general sense, is a dynamic, evolving, unending complex of processes bringing about and maintaining an organism-environment relationship that is useful. It is the means of restoring equilibrium when the relationship is in disequilibrium (Coelho et al., 1974).

In order to cope and effectively adapt to changing situations, three conditions must be met. First, information must be obtained. Second, satisfactory maintenance of physiologic and psychologic functions must be present to foster the processing of information. Third, there must be freedom to make decisions, and options must be present to choose among.

To deal with the multiple crises a high-risk pregnancy imposes, the mother must call on past coping mechanisms and must learn new ones. The nurse should discuss with parents ways they have responded in the past and encourage the use of tactics that have worked before. Previous pregnancy loss should be discussed early in a current pregnancy to assess for coping strategies.

Information must be provided repeatedly about the disease or the condition the woman is facing. Information should include maternal effects and fetal effects. Self-care modalities should be explained thoroughly to provide autonomy and choices where possible. Information will facilitate a realistic appraisal of the events and prepare the couple for potential future events.

The mother should be accompanied by significant people, especially her partner, when information is given. Hospitalization should include flexible rules for the father's presence whenever he can be there. Separations should be minimized whenever possible.

When both the woman and her partner can be given choices in care, personal strategies for coping will be less limited and thus more effective. Skill in encouraging these coping mechanisms is necessary in a high-risk obstetric setting because of the psychologic impact on the entire family. To maintain the unity of the family when the pregnancy is over, it is important to facilitate the sharing of events. Interventions in a crisis should be aimed at restructuring the present. They should suppress negative uses of energy and support efforts in a positive direction.

LOSS AND GRIEF

Throughout life, individuals experience losses. These can be loss of a significant relationship, loss of possessions, or loss of some aspect of self. During a high-risk pregnancy, the woman faces actual loss and potential loss.

There is the actual loss of a significant relationship if the fetus does not survive. There is also that potential loss involved in a precarious physical condition. During hospitalization, there is often the partial loss of the significant relationship with the father and other people close to the mother.

Financial loss can be experienced if the pregnancy results in an unexpected loss of the mother's income. Financial loss can also be experienced if the cost of care for the mother and or neonate exceeds the couple's resources.

Certainly a high-risk pregnancy can result in the loss of some aspect of the self. In our society, parenthood is usually highly valued. A woman might value her ability to conceive as proof of her femininity. The manner in which she conducts herself in pregnancy and labor may also be valued in terms of her role as a woman. If those values must be compromised, some aspect of the self may be lost.

The emotional state that results from loss or the threat of loss is grief. Grief work is the process of coping with the loss. Anticipatory grief is the emotional state demanding energy to work through a difficult loss before it occurs. It prepares the individual for the eventual real loss and strengthens the coping mechanisms needed to deal with the crisis that loss precipitates (Reed, 1974).

Grief work is similar regardless of actual or potential loss. From her work with grieving patients and their families, Kubler-Ross (1969) described five stages in the grief process. These include:

1. Denial and isolation leading to reactions of numbness, shock, denial, or inappropriate cheerfulness. Initially, this might be seen as failure to keep office appointments or to comply with recommended care.
2. Anger and fear, which can be displaced in all directions. This can be manifested as envy or resentment of other pregnant women not at risk or resentment of the fetus causing all the problems. Ambivalence of wanting the pregnancy over with and needing a good outcome becomes intertwined with guilt over the "death wish."
3. Bargaining. This is manifested as a sense of helplessness and a wish to be helped. Guilt again becomes intertwined as a cause is sought and blame can be placed on the self or significant others for minor incidents totally unrelated.

4. Depression. This can be manifested by despair and a feeling of emptiness for the loss and a sadness at preparing for life while sensing an impending loss.
5. Acceptance. This can lead to a reorganization of behavior and detachment from the loved one.

Although the concept of grief work is similar, there are some important differences between conventional grief as described by Kubler-Ross (1969) and anticipatory grief. One difference is the end point of the two types of grief. Conventional grief can be prolonged indefinitely depending as much on the mourner's psychology as on the nature of the loss. Anticipatory grief, however, has a finite end point dependent on the physical occurrence of the actual loss. Grief might continue after that, but it is no longer anticipatory grief (Aldrich, 1963).

Another important difference in anticipatory grief work is in acceleration. Under usual circumstances, conventional grief diminishes in degree as time passes. Anticipatory grief work, however, theoretically accelerates as the anticipated loss becomes more imminent. The direction and rate of acceleration are affected by the individual's mobilization of defense mechanisms such as denial and acceptance (Aldrich, 1963).

Conventional grief can be prolonged when, for any of several reasons, ambivalent feelings about the lost object are so unacceptable to the mourner that they are repressed or in other ways disguised, thus becoming inaccessible to conscious resolution. Ambivalent feelings may be unacceptable for a variety of reasons. First, there might be an unusually high component of hostility in the ambivalence. Second, there may have been early training forbidding the acknowledgment of hostility because of the persistent equation of a hostile wish with a hostile act. Finally, there may be a combination of these factors. Some mourners who cannot accept their ambivalence will persist in their grief as though to stop grieving would be equivalent to acknowledgment that they are glad for the loss.

Ambivalence has a special impact on anticipatory grief. The difference in the impact of ambivalence on anticipatory grief is that the target of the ambivalence is not only still alive but also vulnerable because he or she is balanced between life and death. This vulnerability makes the death wish appear potent and dangerous. Anticipatory grief, therefore, can be more readily denied (Aldrich, 1963).

Because life is still evident, hope accompanies anticipatory grief. Thus the mourner's actions might conceivably delay the loss or prevent it from happening. However, the anticipatory mourner with unacceptable ambivalence can increase guilt over the death wish by committing or having committed errors of omission or commission in the care of the loved one (Aldrich, 1963).

A period of anticipation can provide the mourner with an opportunity to carry out grief work in advance. At the same time, it complicates the process by giving the hostile component of ambivalence a more realistically destructive potential (Aldrich, 1963).

Johnson (1979) discussed anticipatory grief in high-risk pregnancy. Anticipatory grief work can both assist and hinder parents. It assists in resolving loss if the baby dies or is born less than the perfect child of their expectations. However, if the baby is born alive and perfect, they must then make the transition from grief work to the initiation of attachment. If the baby is born and

S U G G E S T E D   P L A N

Psychologic implications of a high-risk pregnancy

Potential patient problem	Outcome criteria

A. Potential lack of pregnancy validation first trimester related to:
    Previous pregnancy losses
    Signs of pregnancy loss
    Lack of uterine growth
	Verbalizes knowledge of pregnancy
	Discusses concerns for continuation of pregnancy

B. Potential difficulty with fetal embodiment related to:
    Previous pregnancy losses
    Signs of pregnancy loss
    Lack of fetal activity
	Discusses reality of fetus
	Notes first fetal activity
	Shares ultrasound examination, genetic amniocentesis, fetal activity, etc., with significant other

C. Potential negative attachment behaviors related to:
    Predominance of fear for fetal or own well-being
    Anticipatory grief
    Unmet expectations for birth experience or maternal role performance
	Speaks positively of own mothering
	Seeks early contact with neonate
	Speaks in high-pitched soft voice to fetus or neonate
	Seeks eye contact with neonate
	Strokes abdomen or strokes neonate

has difficulties of even a temporary nature, the parents must then continue unresolved anticipatory grief work for the loss of the perfect child while simultaneously initiating attachment to the actual child. There can be multiple attachment difficulties if detachment has begun prior to the birth; one cannot detach and attach simultaneously. Grief needs to be connected with something tangible to eventually be resolved. If the perfect child remains only in the dreams of parents and the actual child does not have the potential to meet these dreams, the loss is unreal and can remain unresolved for a prolonged time.

O F   N U R S I N G   C A R E

Assessment and intervention

Dx.	Assess for physical signs of pregnancy, such as:
	    fundal growth
	    first FHR
	    lack of bleeding
	    first fetal movement noted

Th.	Stress positive signs of pregnancy
Ed.	Instruct in early nutritional needs, means of relieving discomfort of pregnancy, embryologic and fetal growth, choices to be considered
Ref.	Prenatal educator for early bird classes
Dx.	Assess for fetal activity and fundal growth
Th.	Encourage discussion of potential or known fetal sex if genetic amniocentesis is done Discuss the visual and tactile experiences of fetal movement, ultrasound, and changes in own physical appearance Provide for sharing of these experiences with significant other
Dx.	Assess for positive feelings about own mothering Observe for tactile, visual, and verbal contact with fetus or neonate
Th.	Discuss verbal, tactile, and visual experiences parents have with fetus or neonate Discuss feelings surrounding sensory perceptions of fetus or neonate Stress normalcy of concerns, fears, anxiety, and commonality with other parents in similar situations
Ed.	Educate regarding common feelings
Ref.	To parent support groups, cesarean birth groups, and special prenatal education classes

Dx., diagnostic; Th., therapeutic; Ed., education; Ref., referral.

Continued.

Psychologic implications of a high-risk pregnancy—cont'd

Potential patient problem	Outcome criteria
D. Potential anxiety, frustration, conflict related to: Unmet maternal needs for socialization with other pregnant women Potential pregnancy loss Loss of control over birth experience Hospitalization and separation from family and friends Financial concerns	Participates in socialization with other pregnant women such as: rap sessions support groups special prenatal classes Seeks activities for preparation for childbirth and mothering skills Resolves financial concerns and arrangements for care of family if hospitalized
E. Potential failure to cope and adapt to altered situation related to: Separation from family and friends Previous inexperience with adequate coping Failure to gain information for reality confrontation	Verbalizes feelings Discusses new information Obtains frequent and prolonged contacts with family and special friends
F. Potential loss and anticipatory grief related to: Own illness Separation from family Negative birth experience Financial loss Neonatal anomaly or illness Potential or actual fetal or neonatal death	Progression through stages of grief work Reorganization of behavior Performs positive attachment behaviors with live or dead neonate Verbalizes feelings Seeks and accepts support of family, friends, and support groups

Assessment and intervention

Dx. Assess for social behaviors such as:
    absence or withdrawal
    anger
    aggression
    depression

Th. Encourage participation in those social activities that do not conflict with
    physical restrictions
    Establish special activities to meet needs for socialization and education of
    women with physical restrictions
    Give choices where possible

Ed. Instruct regarding the specific disease and its complications and effects
    Instruct in choices that can be made for the birth experience
    Keep explanations simple and realistic in times of crisis

Ref. Social service
    Special support groups and education classes

Dx. Assess for negative behaviors such as:
    withdrawal
    depression
    anger
    aggression

Th. Provide flexible visitation rules and rooming-in rights for fathers
    Provide control and choices where possible

Ed. Provide information about disease, maternal and fetal or neonatal effects
    Provide information about shared childbirth experiences

Ref. Prenatal educator for childbirth preparation
    Neonatal nursery personnel
    Clergy

Dx. Identify stages of grief work and assess for adaptive behaviors such as:
    acceptance of support
    seeking information
    sharing of feelings
    Assess for restoration of nutritional, rest, and exercise patterns

Th. Provide presence of supportive person
    Avoid clichés and statements such as "I know how you feel"
    Listen rather than talk
    Encourage contact with neonate whether ill or dead

Ed. Give simple, direct explanations
    Elaborate initially only when requested by parents

Ref. Parent support groups
    Grief support groups
    Clergy

In working with parents who are doing anticipatory grief work, the nurse must remember the three balancing factors that aid an individual in resolving a crisis and loss initiated by illness, death, or pregnancy.

1. The individual's realistic perception of the event
2. Adequate support from others, especially significant others
3. History of previous success with adequate coping mechanisms

When all three are present, the crisis can be resolved and equilibrium restored. It must be remembered that anticipatory grief is a period of intense involvement requiring suspension of normal roles in the family, work, and community systems. The nurse must provide the opportunity for an environment that allows for this suspension of roles, as well as for optimal facilitation of the three balancing factors. This can be done in the following ways.

1. Explore individual and family perceptions of the high-risk pregnancy.
2. Educate the individual and family to further understanding and perception of the event and to give them the capability to control and change some of the realistic aspects.
3. Define the role of significant others.
4. Provide a flexible environment allowing for support from significant others if the woman must be hospitalized.
5. Explore individual and family response to crisis.
6. Identify strengths and weaknesses in coping mechanisms used previously.
7. Provide an environment conducive to "pregnancy work" where possible. Rubin (1975) defines this as:
   a. Safe passage for the fetus
   b. Acceptance of the child by significant others
   c. Binding in
   d. Giving of oneself

In the hospital setting, these can best be accomplished when visiting hours are open for significant others, even to the point of encouraging overnight stays when possible. Regionalization of care, though providing for improved physiologic care, can produce failure in the area of psychologic care because of separation of families and the imposition of unnecessary institutional rules.

In the outpatient setting, the nurse can provide for the three balancing factors by providing prenatal education classes specifically designed for meeting the unique need for information and providing for any physical limitations the women might have. Special "rap sessions" might prove helpful in evaluating and validating feelings. Extensive use of referrals to professionals and community resources should be planned. Social service agencies, clergy, and grief support groups can provide help.

Anticipatory grief work is a natural process strengthened by family ties and good, compassionate interpersonal relationships. The universality of the experience can be productive and has the potential to bind individuals together.

REFERENCES

Aguilera, D., and Messick, J.: Crisis intervention: theory and methodology, ed. 4, St. Louis, 1982, The C.V. Mosby Co.

Aldrich, C.K.: The dying patient's grief, JAMA **184:**329, 1963.

Caplan, G.: Psychological aspects of maternity care, Am. J. Publ. Health **47:**25, 1957.

Caplan, G.: Psychological aspects of pregnancy. In Leif, N., editor: The psychologic basis of medical practice, New York, 1973, Harper & Row.

Clark, A., and Alfonso, D.: Childbearing: a nursing perspective, Philadelphia, 1979, F.A. Davis Co.

Coelho, G., Hamburg, D., and Adams, J.: Coping and adaptation, New York, 1974, Basic Books, Inc.

Colman, A., and Colman, L.: Pregnancy: the psychological experience, New York, 1971, Herder & Herder.

Johnson, S.: High-risk parenting: nursing assessment and strategies for the family at risk, Philadelphia, 1979, J.B. Lippincott Co.

Klaus, M., and Kennell, J.: Maternal-infant bonding, St. Louis, 1976, The C.V. Mosby Co.

Kubler-Ross, E.: On death and dying, New York, 1969, MacMillan Inc.

Neale, R.E.: Initiatory grief. In Schoenberg, B., and others, editors: Anticipatory grief, New York, 1974, Columbia University Press.

Penticuff, J.: Psychologic implications in high risk pregnancy, Clin. North Am. **17:**69, 1982.

Peplau, H.: Therapeutic concepts in aspects of psychiatric nursing, League Exchange **26B,** 1957.

Reed, A.W.: Anticipatory grief work. In Schoenberg, B., and others, editors: Anticipatory grief, New York, 1974, Columbia University Press.

Rubin, R.: Maternal tasks in pregnancy, Maternal-Child Nursing J. **4**(3):43, 1975.

Rubin, R.: Some cognitive aspects of childbearing. In Bergersen, B., and others, editors: Current concepts in clinical nursing, vol. 2, St. Louis, 1969, The C.V. Mosby Co.

Snyder, D.: The high risk mother viewed in relation to a holistic model of the childbearing experience, JOGN **8**(3):164, 1979.

Yates, R.: Frustration and conflict, New York, 1962, John Wiley & Sons, Inc.

U N I T I I I

HEALTH DISORDERS
COMPLICATING PREGNANCY

Various health disorders can complicate pregnancy. In the past, major medical disorders precluded pregnancy achievement either because maternal well-being could not be guaranteed or because the fetal effects were devastating. Now, with more sophisticated medical management of maternal conditions and with high technology for fetal surveillance, outcomes for both the mother and neonate have improved. Common health disorders complicating pregnancy that will be discussed in this unit are diabetes, cardiac disease, and renal disease.

CHAPTER 5

Diabetes and pregnancy

Diabetes is a disease characterized by the inability to produce or use sufficient endogenous insulin to metabolize glucose properly. The inability to metabolize glucose in quantities sufficient to supply the body leads to faulty metabolism of fats and proteins for energy.

Pregnancy is a diabetogenic state in and of itself. Metabolism of glucose, fats, and proteins is altered and antiinsulin forces are present.

In pregnancy, diabetes is classified according to the age at which it was diagnosed, the length of time the disease has been present, and what vascular changes have occurred. The classifications provide prognostic indicators for neonatal outcome (Table 5-1).

INCIDENCE

Diabetes with pregnancy has long been recognized as a serious problem for both the mother and fetus. Prior to the availability of insulin in the 1920s, diabetics rarely became pregnant. Those who did become pregnant rarely carried a fetus to viability. Diabetes occurs now in 1% to 2% of the pregnant population. Maternal survival is 99.5%. Fetal survival is approximately that of the general population, 95% to 97%, and is largely tied to adequate control before and during the pregnancy.

ETIOLOGY

The etiology of diabetes is inherent in pancreatic inability to produce sufficient insulin to transport glucose into the cells. The tendency to develop diabetes appears to be familial. In the absence of a positive family history for diabetes, childhood viral infections are implicated. As a result of damage to the beta cells in the islets of Langerhans, where insulin is produced in the pancreas, there is insufficient insulin production to meet cellular requirements for glucose transport.

PHYSIOLOGY
Normal

Pregnancy is a diabetogenic state in that it tends to increase the need for glucose. This occurs for a number of physiologic reasons. First, the rapid cell

TABLE 5-1. *Guide to classification of obstetric diabetes (White, 1978)*

Category	Description
NON-INSULIN-DEPENDENT	
Class A	Also known as *gestational diabetes,* characterized by an abnormal glucose tolerance test (GTT) without other symptoms (The treatment is diet control. The fetus is more prone to have congenital anomalies and an increased incidence of macrosomia is seen. If the mother is over age 25, 50% will have overt diabetes within 15 years.)
INSULIN-DEPENDENT	
Class B	Onset at age 20 years or older or of less than 10 years' duration; insulin dependency might occur only with pregnancy
Class C	Onset between ages 10 and 19 years or duration of 10 to 19 years
Class D	Onset at less than 10 years of age or duration of more than 20 years or evidence of vascular disease
Class F	Renal disease
Class R	Retinitis proliferans or vitreous hemorrhage
Class H	Arteriosclerotic heart disease
Class T	After renal transplant

Modified from Niswander, K.: Manual of obstetrics, Boston, 1980, Little, Brown & Co.

growth of the embryo increases maternal energy demands, which stimulates physiologic stress. The stress situation requires physiologic changes aimed at maintaining homeostasis. The changes stem from the increased secretion of adrenocorticotropic, growth, and thyroid hormones. These hormones are glucogenic, ketogenic, and antagonistic to insulin.

More specifically, these hormones cause an increased metabolism of fats and proteins to aid in the demand for higher levels of glucose by the growth and proliferation of cells in the embryo or fetus. The increased breakdown of fats and proteins for energy sources requires additional oxygen consumption for transport through the Krebs' cycle. In addition, increased fatty acid breakdown leads to increased ketone bodies. These in turn lead to ketoacidosis if quantities exceed the body's ability to utilize them. Increased metabolism of proteins leads to increased amino acids. Both fatty acids and amino acids contribute to acidemia.

At the same time, the hormones produce a factor that is antagonistic to insulin and that further reduces the utilization of glucose. Insulin acts as a transport system to carry glucose across the cellular membrane into the cell for energy needs. If there is not enough insulin to do this effectively, glucose builds up in the blood stream. The body, not realizing that glucose cannot get into the cell, still attempts to meet cell energy needs by increasing the break-

TABLE 5-2. *Manifestations and consequences of insulin lack*

	Adaptation to cellular starvation	*Urinary and blood alterations*	*Metabolic acidosis, water and electrolyte imbalance*	*Vascular effects*
Insulin lack	Decreased glucose utilization and storage	Hyperglycemia, glycosuria	Cellular dehydration, osmotic diuresis	Peripheral circulatory failure leading to decreased blood pressure, coma, and death
	Increased metabolism of fatty acids Increased breakdown of amino acids	Increased ketogenesis leading to increased ketonemia, increased ketonuria, and increased glyconeogenesis, in turn leading to aminoacidemia, nitrogen in the urine	Ketoacidosis, metabolic acidosis Catabolism leading to sodium and potassium loss	
	Signs and symptoms of insulin lack (hyperglycemia)			
Manifestations of hyperglycemia	Period of increased appetite, unusual thirst, loss of weight and strength and stamina, leg cramps or muscle fatigue, nausea and vomiting	Glycosuria, polyuria, ketonuria, ketonemia, aminoacidemia, hyperglycemia, pruritus	Kussmaul's respiration, increased nausea and vomiting, listlessness, dehydration, altered blood chemistries, increased hemoglobin	

Modified from Tepperman, J.: Metabolic and endocrine physiology, Chicago, 1973, Yearbook Medical Publishers, Inc., and Clark A., and Alfonzo, D.: Childbearing: a nursing perspective, Philadelphia, 1979, F.A. Davis Co.

down of fats and proteins to supply additional glucose. This complicates the process further.

Typically, the normally functioning pancreatic beta cells in the islets of Langerhans respond to this process by producing additional amounts of insulin to meet the cellular demands for glucose. Therefore the glucose levels in the blood stream are maintained between 80 and 120 mg/100 ml.

As the pregnancy advances, the placenta forms and begins to produce increasing amounts of estrogen and progesterone, human placental lactogen (HPL), and cortisol. These hormones enhance the forces already antagonistic to insulin. The healthy pancreas in the nondiabetic produces increasing amounts of insulin to counteract the antagonistic forces, and normal blood sugars are maintained. In the diabetic, exogenous insulin must be adjusted frequently, based on blood sugar levels, to accomplish the same homeostasis.

Pathophysiology

Theoretically the cause of faulty metabolism in the diabetic is one or more of the following.
1. Production of defective insulin
2. Overproduction of insulin antagonist
3. Increased tissue refractiveness (resistance) to insulin
4. Inadequate amount of insulin production

When insulin is not available or effective in transporting glucose into the cell, glucose remains in the blood stream in abnormal quantities. Because of cellular starvation the body begins breakdown of fats (ketogenesis) and proteins (glyconeogenesis) for energy. Table 5-2 describes the manifestations and consequences of insulin lack.

When lack of insulin becomes a chronic or recurrent event, there are long-standing vascular effects (Table 5-3).

When glucose is low in relation to the amount of insulin, a diabetic person experiences some different physiologic responses. This is manifested by hypoglycemia. Table 5-4 describes manifestations and consequences of an abundance of insulin in relation to glucose.

Hypoglycemia is characterized by its rapid onset and can result from several causes.
1. Too much insulin might have been prescribed or taken inadvertently, or the dose might be more than needed because of altered activity at the time.
2. Delays in mealtimes can cause the onset of insulin action to occur in the absence of adequate glucose.
3. Hypoglycemia can be caused by skipping meals or failure to eat all that is prescribed. (Numbers 2 and 3 are the most common causes.)

TABLE 5-3. *Long-standing vascular effects*

Consequences	Manifestations

Nephrosclerosis, retinopathies, cataracts, atherosclerosis, peripheral neuropathies	Untreated vascular effects lead to
	  Abdominal pain related to tissue hypoxia
	  Headaches and drowsiness related to cerebral hypotension
	  Hypotension related to hypovolemia
	  Oliguria and anuria related to decreased renal blood flow
	  Coma and death related to cardiac failure

Modified from Tepperman, J.: Metabolic and endocrine physiology, Chicago, 1973, Yearbook Medical Publishers, Inc., and Clark, A., and Alfonso, D.: Childbearing: a nursing perspective, Philadelphia, 1979, F.A. Davis Co.

TABLE 5-4. *Manifestations and consequences of relative abundance of insulin*

	Adaptation to decreased glucose	Urinary and blood alterations	Metabolic acidosis, water and electrolyte imbalance	Vascular effects
Insulin abundance	Increased release and depletion of glycogen stores from the liver	Hypoglycemia	Cellular death	Peripheral vascular circulatory collapse and decreased glucose to brain and other organ cells, coma, and death
	Increased metabolism of fatty acids	Increased ketogenesis leading to increased ketonemia, increased ketonuria	Ketoacidosis Metabolic acidosis	
	Increased breakdown of amino acids	Increased glyconeogenesis leading to aminoacidemia, nitrogen in urine	Catabolism leading to sodium and potassium loss	
	Signs and symptoms of insulin abundance			
Behavioral and physiologic manifestations of hypoglycemia	Increased appetite, sweating, lethargy, confusion, loss of consciousness, convulsions	Ketonuria, ketonemia, aminoacidemia, hypoglycemia	Rapid onset of coma, altered blood chemistries, brain death	

Modified from Tepperman, J.: Metabolic and endocrine physiology, Chicago, 1973, Yearbook Medical Publishers, Inc., and Clark, A., and Alfonso, D.: Childbearing: a nursing perspective, Philadelphia, 1979, F.A. Davis Co.

4. Placental failure leading to decreased levels of the insulin antagonists can increase the effectiveness of available insulin, leading to hypoglycemia. This is a warning sign in the third trimester and precedes intrauterine death.

5. Hypoglycemia can also be exaggerated in early control of hyperglycemia. This is called the *Somogyi effect*. A high blood sugar being brought down to normal ranges rapidly can cause overshoots in blood sugar response, and wide variations from low to high blood sugars can result. Somogyi effects can also be seen when inadequate treatment of a hypoglycemic episode has taken place. It is extremely important that hypoglycemia be treated with a measured amount of glucose and followed by a meat exchange or protein source borrowed from the next meal. This avoids causing the body to rapidly utilize the glucose and then drop blood sugars even lower than the previous levels, because no other source of glucose is being gradually formed and released from fats and proteins.

Signs and symptoms

Signs of preexisting diabetes in a previous pregnancy are listed below.
1. Prior delivery of a greater than 9 pound infant
2. Previous stillbirth or an infant with congenital defects
3. History of polyhydramnios
4. History of recurrent monilial vaginitis

Signs of diabetes in a current pregnancy include the following.
1. Glycosuria on two successive office visits
2. Recurrent monilial vaginitis

Signs suggestive of diabetes as the pregnancy advances are the following ultrasound findings.
1. Macrosomia of the fetus
2. Polyhydramnios
3. Congenital anomalies

In known diabetic pregnant women, diabetic symptoms vary by the trimester. Table 5-5 outlines the trimester manifestations and consequences.

Maternal effects

In general, the diabetic state in the mother does not deteriorate because of the pregnancy itself. In fact, most women, regardless of their classification during pregnancy, are in better control than when not pregnant. Despite the antagonistic forces of hormones, control is often better because of the close observation of blood sugar levels by the patient and health care team. If vascular deterioration does occur during pregnancy, the prognosis for fetal outcome is poor. Vascular deterioration can be seen in retinopathy and renal complica-

TABLE 5-5. *Trimester manifestations and consequences of diabetes*

	Insulin requirements	Blood glucose alterations	Complicating factors
First trimester	Decrease related to inhibition of anterior pituitary hormones Developing embryo is a glucose drain Decreased maternal caloric intake	Frequent low blood glucose levels leading to increased numbers of hypoglycemia episodes, increased incidence of starvation, ketosis, and ketonemia	Loss of appetite, nausea, or vomiting common in any early pregnancy Recovery from acidemic state more difficult because of insulin antagonists
Second trimester	Increase related to placental hormones and their antiinsulin properties	Hyperglycemia leading to ketonemia, amino acidemia	Decreased renal threshold from increased blood flow makes urine sugars meaningless Body produces lactose or milk sugar, which further increases urinary sugar
Third trimester	Markedly increased related to increased placental hormones	Hyperglycemia leads to ketonemia, acidemia	Same
Labor	Decreased related to workload of labor and increased metabolism	Hypoglycemia, acidemia from starvation ketosis	Usually kept NPO pending cesarean delivery
Postpartum	Decreased markedly related to loss of placental hormones	Hypoglycemia	Lactation can initially complicate as supply is established and scheduled

Modified from Clark, A., and Alfonso, D.: Childbearing: a nursing perspective, Philadelphia, 1979, F.A. Davis Co.

tions. Though it is not believed, in most well-managed diabetics, to be due to the pregnancy, diabetes can be in a more malignant state at that time.

A diabetic pregnancy is more vulnerable to certain complications. The diabetic women who develops hyperemesis gravidarum is at risk for severe metabolic disturbances. In addition to the obvious risk of dehydration and electrolyte imbalance always encountered with hyperemesis, starvation ketosis becomes a very real threat to the mother and the developing fetus. Hospitalization with appropriate intravenous therapy for fluids and calories is a must.

Pregnancy and diabetes lead to an increased vulnerability to and incidence of preeclampsia/eclampsia. This is particularly true when there is already evidence of renal and vascular compromise. Hypertension and the resultant vasospasm can be the final blow to an already marginally effective placenta.

Polyhydramnios is also more frequently encountered in the pregnant diabetic. Approximately 10% of all diabetics during pregnancy have more amniotic fluid than nondiabetics. Though the mechanism for this is not fully understood, fetal hyperglycemia is thought to result in increased fetal diuresis. The significance of polyhydramnios varies with sources. There may be a threat of premature rupture of the membranes because of the increased osmotic pressure, and polyhydramnios is known to be associated with an increased incidence of fetal anomalies. In severe polyhydramnios, repeated amniocentesis can be performed to relieve the pressure. This procedure, when repeated, places the mother at increased risk of rupture of the membranes and infection associated with the procedure.

The pregnant diabetic is also more susceptible to certain infections. Vaginitis, especially monilial, occurs more frequently. This is primarily related to the altered pH of the vaginal canal common to all pregnancies and glycosuria, which makes a prime medium for bacterial growth. Because of the increased incidence of vaginitis, the pregnant diabetic has an increased risk of urinary tract infections, which can be dangerous to her health and increase the likelihood of preterm labor.

The pregnant diabetic is more likely to deliver by a cesarean section because of concurrent complications, fetal distress, fetal macrosomia, and induction failures prior to term.

The frequently changing insulin needs and necessary modifications in daily living habits keep the patient and significant others continually preoccupied with the disease and the pregnancy, often to the exclusion of outside interests. When the incentive to maintain adequate control is high, it must be considered as taking a great emotional toll. Even the most minor deviations are fraught with expressions of guilt and fear for fetal well-being.

In addition to the great emotional concern, there is financial strain from the frequent testing and the expense of equipment. Often these have not been anticipated and frequently are not covered or are only partially covered by existing insurance.

The couple also faces anticipatory grief for the loss of the ideal pregnancy, for the potential loss of a perfect child, and for the potential of a less than perfect birth process. These added concerns must all be taken into consideration when caring for the pregnant diabetic.

Psychologic effects of the diabetes itself interplay with the effects of concern for the well-being of the pregnant woman and eventual neonatal outcome. Just as most women want to produce a perfect child, so do pregnant diabetic women. As a result, most pregnant diabetic women are highly motivated to gain and maintain good diabetic control during the pregnancy.

Those women who are childhood diabetics, however, can enter pregnancy with some psychologic impairment manifested by behaviors that are not conducive to good control. Some of these behavioral manifestations are:

1. Immaturity in taking responsibility for own care. This can be the result of overprotective parents who could not allow the person, as a child, to take responsibility for self-care.
2. Inability to take on "mothering tasks." This can be the result of an overprotective mother who continues the mother-child relationship into adulthood in matters affecting diabetic control.
3. Use of diabetes to control life situations. This can be manifested in bizarre food habits or in bulemic or anorexic behaviors to control blood sugars.

When any of these behavioral complications is present and a woman becomes pregnant, her psychologic impairment can be intensified with her changing body image and impending parenthood. Then, despite high motivation, the pregnant woman is sometimes unable to perform tasks and report signs and symptoms so that control of blood sugar is maintained.

Fetal and neonatal effects

The effects of diabetes on the fetus are dependent on previous vascular complications in the mother and on hypoglycemic and hyperglycemic episodes. If the mother has class D or more advanced disease, vascular deficits can affect the sufficiency of the placenta. Placental insufficiency can cause varying degrees of nutritional or hypoxic damage to the fetus.

Hypoglycemia has little effect on the fetus, provided the mother is treated before maternal brain damage occurs. The embryo draws its glucose from stores in the lining of the uterus and the fetus draws from stores in the placenta. Glucose is transferred across the placental membrane by selective transfer. The immediate effects of maternal hypoglycemia on the fetus therefore are minimized over time.

Hyperglycemia, however, can have numerous deleterious and sometimes fatal effects. Chronic hyperglycemia in the mother contributes to decreased synthesis of DNA and RNA and is thought to be a reason for an increased incidence of congenital anomalies. Faulty carbohydrate, protein, and fat metabolism also occurs in the embryo and adversely affects organ development. Common fetal anomalies seen in infants of diabetic mothers include the following.

1. Neural tube defects such as hydrocephalus, meningocele, and spina bifida
2. Congenital cardiac anomalies
3. Gastrointestinal malformations
4. Congenital renal anomalies or malformations

Congenital anomalies are directly related to diabetic control in the 3-month period prior to conception. Other fetal effects of maternal hyperglycemia are listed below*:

Increased fetal insulin production

Decreased production of fetal cortisol

Fetal ketoacidosis

Increased fetal adipose deposition and fluid retention

Deficient stable lecithin

Delayed lung maturity

Macrosomic infant

Fetal brain cell damage and decreased brain growth

Increased incidence of respiratory distress syndrome (RDS) even after 37 weeks

Increased incidence of learning disabilities, lower IQ, and intrauterine fetal demise

Neonatal morbidity is sometimes due to the effects of hyperglycemia. The fetus is programmed to produce high quantities of insulin and the neonate does not turn this off immediately. At birth the supply of increased glucose is suddenly cut off, but increased production of insulin continues resulting in hypoglycemic episodes. In addition, greater amounts of hemoglobin are present in the hyperglycemic infant, and increased neonatal breakdown frequently overworks the young hepatic system resulting in hyperbilirubinemia.

MEDICAL DIAGNOSIS

Women who have already been diagnosed as diabetic, either during a previous pregnancy or in the absence of pregnancy, usually will be classified as previously described (White, 1978). If insulin-dependent, the woman should be screened for renal, retinal, and cardiac involvement. Some commonly ordered tests are listed below.

1. Serum creatinine and 24-hr urine collection for creatinine clearance and total protein
2. Electrocardiogram
3. Ophthalmology examination for retinitis

Screening for a diagnosis of diabetes in pregnancy should be done in any pregnant woman who is at risk for diabetes. Risk factors for a diagnosis of diabetes include the following.

1. Positive family history in parents or siblings
2. Previous unexplained stillbirth
3. Prior traumatic delivery

---

*Modified from Clark, A., and Alfonso, D.: Childbearing: a nursing perspective, Philadelphia, 1979, F.A. Davis Co.

4. Prior infant with a birth weight of 9 pounds or greater
5. Prior fetal anomalies
6. Poor reproductive history, especially repeated spontaneous abortions
7. Obesity
8. Hypertensive disorder
9. Recurrent monilial vaginitis
10. Age over 35 years
11. Polyhydramnios without demonstrated fetal anomalies
12. Glycosuria on two consecutive office visits

Screening can be done by giving a 50 gm glucola load and 1 hour later testing the blood sugar. A blood sugar level of greater than 140 mg/100 ml should be investigated further to determine insulin dependency. Values on a glucose tolerance test must be interpreted differently in pregnancy than in a nonpregnant state. Value differences are related to the fact the fetus is a glucose and amino acid drain on maternal metabolism and to the increased glomerular filtration rate during pregnancy. Listed below are normal serum values in a 3-hour glucose tolerance test in pregnancy.

Fasting: 110 mg%
One hour: 220 mg%
Two hours: 150 mg%
Three hours: 130 mg%

Some physicians and diabetic women want some assurance of adequate control prior to conception. When control has been questionable prior to conception, anomalies are far more likely to occur. Hemoglobin A_1C is hemoglobin that has been "sugar coated" and therefore remains in the body for longer than normal (2 to 3 months) and can predict previous adequacy of control. Levels above 8 are associated with an increased incidence of congenital anomalies. Some endocrinologists will continue every 2 to 3 months to screen for adequacy of control, especially in those women who have demonstrated an inability to accept responsibility for self-care.

USUAL MEDICAL MANAGEMENT
Antepartum management

Usual medical management focuses on outpatient control of diabetes. This requires great effort on the part of the woman and her family but is less financially costly and certainly more emotionally rewarding than long hospitalization and separation from family. Management is usually provided through a team approach with an obstetrician and endocrinologist knowledgeable in effects of pregnancy and care of the mother and fetus.

Home monitoring and control consists of five areas in the insulin-dependent diabetic.

1. Blood glucose monitoring should be done two or more times per day. Ideally, this should begin before conception. If this is not possible, it should begin as soon as pregnancy is suspected or determined.
2. Urine testing for ketones must be done two to four times per week.
3. Multiple dose insulin or the use of the insulin pump should provide blood glucose control between 80 and 120 mg/100 ml.
4. Dietary control must be adhered to and rigid scheduling instituted. The diet should include 300 additional calories or be 1,800 to 2,400 calories, depending on size and activity of the woman, according to the American Diabetic Association (ADA).
5. Exercise and patterns of daily living must be modified to attain good control.

Each component of management will be described in the following sections.

Blood glucose monitoring. The aim of maintenance is euglycemia throughout each 24 hours. Blood glucose monitoring at home is the only way to determine a plan for best control. This can be done by one of two usual means.

1. A dry method with color-stable strips may be used. Accuracy depends on the individual's skill at color interpretation between given color changes on the chart provided and in accuracy of timing. Strips can be labeled and saved for office visit confirmation.
2. A glucostix and a glucose reflectance meter are a second option. Although this method requires a certain amount of skill and consistency of techniques, it yields results most closely resembling serum sugar levels. The complexity of technique varies with different manufacturers of machines as does the accuracy of results.

Urine testing. Because lactosuria (milk sugar) is present by week 20, only a glucose-specific testing material can be used. These are Testape, Clinistix, or Ketodiastix. Because ketones can be tested simultaneously with sugar, Ketodiastix are more commonly used. Urine testing has limited use for glucose monitoring but is necessary for ketones.

Urine testing should be done with double voided specimens. This means that the patient should empty her bladder 1 hour before meals and bedtime, then void ½ hour later and test this specimen. No more than two glasses of fluid should be taken in the interval between emptying and voiding again. Blood sugar should be checked if glycosuria is 1% or greater or if ketonuria is present. Ketonuria in two consecutive specimens should be reported to the physician. Ketonuria can occur when dietary intake is insufficient as well as when ketoacidosis is present.

Insulin management. Because intermediate insulins last a maximum of 18 hours, split doses of insulin are usually necessary to maintain a state of euglycemia throughout the 24 hours. The total dose is divided so that 66% to 75%

of the total amount is given in the morning and the remainder is given before the evening meal. When blood sugar levels are in the hyperglycemic range, it might be necessary to give additional doses of regular insulin to maintain adequate control. These additional regular insulin doses may be given routinely with the intermediate insulin for the effect on lunchtime and bedtime snack blood sugar levels. They may also be given alone in response to high blood sugars occurring episodically. Usual insulin changes recommended on an outpatient basis are described in Table 5-6.

Insulin pump. In the past, the only means of administering insulin at home was through multiple subcutaneous injections. Recently a devise for continuous infusion has been marketed. There are basically two types of systems that mimic the pancreas. There is a closed-loop system, which uses an implantable glucose sensor that feeds data to a computer. Via a double-lumen catheter, small amounts of venous bloods are withdrawn. The computer than calculates the amount of insulin or glucose that must be administered by measuring glucose concentration and its rate and direction of change over the last 4 minutes.

TABLE 5-6. *Changes with split dose insulin*

Time	Blood sugar level	Action
Fasting blood sugar	Less than 60	Call physician for adjustment
	60 to 120	No change in 4 PM dose
	120 to 150	Increase evening NPH insulin by 2U and check fasting blood sugar next day
	150 to 210	Increase evening NPH insulin by 4U and check fasting blood sugar next day
	Above 210	Call physician for adjustment
Lunch blood sugar	Less than 60	Call physician for adjustment
	60 to 120	No change in AM regular insulin
	120 to 150	Increase morning regular insulin by 2U
	200 to 240	Increase morning regular insulin by 6U
	Above 240	Call physician
PM dinner blood sugar	Less than 60	Call physician for adjustment
	60 to 120	No change in morning dose
	120 to 150	Increase morning NPH insulin by 2U and check 4 PM blood sugar next day
	200 to 240	Increase morning NPH insulin by 6U and check 4 PM blood sugar next day
	Above 240	Call physician for adjustment
Bedtime snack blood sugar	Less than 60	Call physician
	60 to 120	No change in PM regular insulin
	120 to 150	Increase PM regular insulin by 2U
	200 to 240	Increase PM regular insulin by 6U
	Above 240	Call physician

Private practice protocols of Drs. D. O'Keeffe and J. Elliott, perinatologists, Phoenix, Arizona, 1983.

This unit is about the size of a microwave oven and must be moved by cart, so it is only used in the hospital setting.

The other device is an open-loop system. It infuses insulin at a basal rate and, prior to meals, delivers a bolus. The basal rate is generally a 12.5 to 15 mU/kg/hr. Some open-loop systems require resetting after each bolus dose; others do this automatically. The open-loop systems are small and portable, usually worn around the waist with a belt.

Diet management. Adherence to dietary recommendations is also important in adequate control. Caloric intake should be increased by approximately 300 calories daily and modified to provide at least a 25-pound weight gain and additional nutrients for mother and fetus. Caloric intake should be 1,800 to 2,400 calories per day. These are usually distributed across three meals and two or three snacks (Table 5-7). In addition to increased caloric intake, protein should be increased by 30 gm to total 100 to 110 gm, calcium should be 1,200 mg, folic acid should be 0.4 to 0.8 mg, and ascorbic acid should be 60 mg. Iron supplementation is needed to meet additional requirements for that mineral.

Exercise recommendations. Regular exercise should continue during pregnancy unless contraindicated. The pattern should not, however, vary widely from day to day. If early signs of uteroplacental insufficiency (UPI) are present, it might be advisable to maintain bed rest to reduce the metabolic needs of the mother competing with the needs of the fetus.

Antepartum monitoring. Antepartum monitoring is essential to the physician to aid in the decision for the timing of the delivery. The development of ultrasonography and adequate antepartum monitoring has greatly altered the anticipated outcome in the pregnant diabetic. These tests allow for early and periodic evaluation of fetal condition and timing of delivery to coincide with optimal outcome. The purposes and usefulness of these tests vary and will be discussed separately.

Ultrasound. Ultrasound examinations are usually done at intervals throughout the pregnancy. As the pregnancy enters the second trimester, it is sometimes done to assist in accurately predicting gestational age and for reassurance about fetal organ development. At various intervals thereafter, it gives information about fetal growth rate, quality of activity, and volume of amniotic fluid.

Amniocentesis. The usual use of amniocentesis is to ascertain the lecithin/sphingomyelin (L/S) ratio and the presence of phosphatidylglycerol (PG), which is a precursor to L/S. An L/S ratio of 2.0 or greater when PG is present is sufficient to expect that surfactant levels are high enough in the fetus to prevent the development of respiratory distress syndrome (RDS). The amniocentesis is generally done after week 36 of gestation.

TABLE 5-7. *Sample meal pattern*

2200 calories
275 gm carbohydrates
110 gm protein
73 gm fat

BREAKFAST

1 fruit exchange	½ cup (4 oz) orange juice
1 bread exchange	1 slice toast with 1 teaspoon margarine
1 meat exchange	1 poached egg
2 fat exchanges	1 cup 2% milk
1 cup skim milk	
(2% milk uses 1 fat)	

LUNCH

2 meat exchanges	2 oz Swiss cheese
3 bread exchanges	2 slices rye bread
2 vegetable exchanges	tomato slices
2 fruit exchanges	½ cantaloupe
3 fat exchanges	1 teaspoon margarine
1 cup skim milk	1 cup whole milk
(whole milk uses 2 fats)	

AFTERNOON SNACK

1 fruit exchange	1 fresh apple
1 bread exchange	6 saltines
1 meat exchange	1 oz cheese
1 fat exchange	½ cup 2% milk
½ cup skim milk	

DINNER

3 meat exchanges	3 oz baked chicken with lemon
3 bread exchanges	½ cup rice w/soy sauce
1 vegetable exchange	1 dinner roll with 1 teaspoon margarine
1 fruit exchange	½ cup broccoli
3 fat exchanges	tossed salad with 2 teaspoons Italian dressing
1 cup skim milk	1 slice unsweetened pineapple
	1 cup skim milk

BEDTIME SNACK

2 bread exchanges	whole sandwich with 1 oz tuna packed in water
1 meat exchange	1 teaspoon mayonnaise
1 fat exchange	1 small apple
½ cup skim milk	½ cup skim milk
1 fruit	

Modified from Hartshorn, S., 1980, Outline of professional procedures.

Contraction stress test (CST). The CST gives two important pieces of information. First, it assures everyone of an energetic fetus doing well in its present environment. Second, it reassures everyone that the placenta continues to function adequately and that the dreaded complication of uteroplacental insufficiency (UPI) has not occurred. For classes B, C, and D diabetes the CST is started at or near week 34 and is done weekly until delivery. For more advanced disease it is started by week 28. For class A diabetes, it should be started by week 38. If CST results are not reassuring, delivery is necessary regardless of fetal lung maturity.

Nonstress test (NST). This test is done instead of the CST in settings less sophisticated in monitoring or when a CST is contraindicated. It does not assess for early UPI and is therefore not the test of choice. Because it can be done twice weekly, it can also be more costly to the patient. It is occasionally done between CSTs as term approaches or when the patient is hospitalized for control.

Estriol determination. The majority of placental estrogen is estriol and is excreted into the urine after being released into the bloodstream. A placenta that is failing to support the fetus might also fail to produce enough estrogen. Depending on the availability and reliability of special laboratory facilities, either 24-hour collections of urine are done or serum estriol levels are drawn. Both tests are done serially, usually daily by the time CSTs are started. In this way it is possible to keep a day by day watch for reassurance that all remains well with the fetus and its environment. If there is a 35% fall in levels, a CST is repeated within 24 hours for more specific information and to help make a reliable decision regarding delivery. Estriol determinations are quite expensive.

Fetal activity chart (FAC). FACs should be used for daily surveillance of fetal well-being from 24 weeks of gestation.

Intrapartum management

Intrapartum management requires tight control because of changing metabolic demands. The patient is usually admitted 1 or 2 days prior to a planned delivery. Unless contraindicated for other reasons, vaginal delivery is anticipated and accomplished with oxytocic induction of labor. There are several methods for intrapartum management depending on the patient's condition. If the patient is to have an elective cesarean birth, in the absence of marked hyperglycemia, no insulin is given until she is in the recovery room.

A continuous insulin infusion may be used for laboring patients by adding 5 U of regular insulin to each 500 ml of D5W. The initial infusion rate is 1 U of insulin and 5 gm of glucose per hour. This is started the day of the induction. Continuous insulin infusions must always be delivered through an infusion pump.

The ratio of glucose and insulin is titrated as hourly blood sugar levels indicate in order to keep the blood sugar within the normal range. The frequency of blood glucose checks may lessen when the patient stabilizes her blood glucose levels. The patient is given nothing by mouth. Fetal monitoring is continuous throughout.

All laboring patients should have blood glucose levels checked at least every hour because of the increased metabolic needs of labor. They should be on continuous fetal monitoring with close observation for decreased variability and other signs of fetal distress.

Postpartum management

The role of the placental hormones in determining the relative increase in insulin needs throughout the second and third trimesters should be acknowledged. This aids in the explanation for the apparent remission or decreased severity of symptoms in the postpartum period. There is removal of the antagonistic placental hormones and suppression of the anterior pituitary growth hormone. The insulin dose in the postpartum period then can be one half the prepregnancy dose or less. This effect can last from 3 days to 6 weeks. When good control is maintained during pregnancy and when the continuous infusion of insulin is used during labor there is generally less postpartum hypoglycemia. Lactation further decreases the need for insulin, and caloric needs can increase by approximately 300 to 500 calories/day.

NURSING PROCESS
Prevention

Diabetic women during the childbearing years need to be counseled that a planned pregnancy after adequate control will contribute to a healthier pregnancy and a better neonatal outcome. Nurses working in outpatient settings with such women should include this information in education classes.

Assessment

On the first prenatal visit, the nursing history should include assessment for presence of risk factors for diabetes. All diabetic women should be assessed for the classification of their disease. In addition, the history should include an assessment of what means are being used for diabetic control and what the woman understands about diabetes and its effects on pregnancy. Assessments for an accurate due date are essential to determine growth rate and ultimately to time delivery for optimal neonatal outcome. Assessment of emotional status regarding responsibility for self-care can facilitate the plan for patient education. The last major area of assessment in the history should include financial resources; the fetal surveillance measures, potential short-term hospitalizations for control, and increased cost of cesarean delivery should be preplanned.

Throughout the pregnancy and into the postpartum period, physical assessment should include determination of blood glucose levels, checking for urinary ketones, and assessment of the adequacy of dietary intake. The frequency of assessment of blood glucose levels and urinary ketones varies with the insulin management plan. A common plan is given below.

1. Assess blood glucose levels before each meal and at bedtime during the antepartum period.
2. Assess blood glucose levels each hour during labor and postpartum recovery.
3. Assess blood glucose levels each hour if the woman comes to the hospital in ketoacidosis.
4. Urinary ketones should be assessed twice weekly throughout the pregnancy.

If the woman has ketoacidosis from decreased dietary intake in the first trimester, she should be observed for signs of electrolyte imbalances, especially potassium, and for blood glucose control. An intravenous insulin infusion will be necessary, as will potassium replacement. After 25 weeks of gestation, if she has ketoacidosis from hyperglycemia, in addition to assessing for electrolyte balance and blood glucose control, fetal well-being should be continuously monitored until maternal glucose levels stabilize.

Other areas of assessment include fundal height measurements to aid in judgments of fetal growth rate and absence of polyhydramnios. Blood pressure, urinary protein, weight gain, and presence of edema are assessed in order to determine maternal well-being and detect the development of preeclampsia. Urine should also be inspected at each visit for signs of infection (protein and/or positive nitrites) and signs of vaginal yeast shedding, which indicates a monilial infection.

Throughout the pregnancy, the woman should be observed for her ability to prepare for parenthood as evidenced by preparations for the baby, talking about the baby as a separate being, and seeking early contact with the neonate. The couple should be assessed for their understanding of test results and diabetic control issues and expectations for neonatal outcome to allay unrealistic fears and anxieties.

Antepartum intervention

The goal in caring for the pregnant diabetic woman is to encourage and enable her to monitor her diabetes as an outpatient. Education of the woman aimed at accomplishing this and understanding the effects of pregnancy on diabetes is therefore the major antepartum nursing intervention. The nurse should teach the woman based on the assessment of measures already being used. The following should be taught and/or discussed.

1. How to determine blood glucose levels before each meal and at bedtime using a reflectance meter or color stable sticks
2. How to determine urinary ketones twice weekly
3. Changing diet to 2,000 or more calories because of increased nutrients necessary for pregnancy
4. Mixing intermediate and regular insulin and giving in divided doses as ordered
5. The effects of pregnancy and diabetes
6. Potential fetal surveillance studies to be done such as ultrasounds, amniocentesis, and fetal monitoring
7. Potential changes in daily activities such as short-term hospitalization for control and limited activities if early signs of uteroplacental insufficiency develop
8. Insulin adjustments to be made by the pregnant woman (Table 5-6)

Referrals should be made where appropriate and available to the following specialists.

1. Dietician for diet instruction
2. Social worker for aid in evaluating financial resources
3. Antepartum testing nurse for fetal surveillance
4. Perinatal nurse specialist for instruction in effects of pregnancy and diabetes and continued follow-up
5. Childbirth educator for preparation for labor, vaginal delivery, or cesarean delivery
6. Diabetic nurse specialist for instructions and follow-up if the insulin pump is to be used

Intervention—drug therapy

If the nurse caring for the pregnant diabetic woman is to accurately educate her and assist her in decisions for care, there must be an understanding of the use of insulin.

Insulin is a hormone synthesized and secreted by beta cells of the islets of Langerhans in the pancreas. Its purpose is to promote cellular uptake of glucose, fatty acids, and amino acids for their conversion to energy and to promote storage of glycogen. When blood glucose increases, insulin is released to transport the energy source into cells for immediate use or for future storage. In diabetes mellitus, there is a lack or relative lack of the body's own insulin, and therefore, it must be supplied exogenously.

Insulin for exogenous use is derived from the pancreas of a variety of animals. The usual insulin is a combination of beef and pork insulin. It can, however, come from beef alone, pork alone, fish, sheep or be biosynthetic human insulin (made by genetically programming *Escherichia coli* bacteria to produce insulin).

Adverse reactions to insulin include hypersensitivity and/or allergic skin reactions, lipodystrophy, and tissue resistance. When these occur, the exogenous derivative is usually changed from beef and pork combination to beef alone, pork alone, sheep, fish, or biosynthetic human insulin (the most expensive and difficult to obtain).

Although insulin remains active for long periods of shelf life, patients should be instructed to date the bottle after opening. To ensure continued sterility, bottles should be discarded after 3 months of use. All insulin in current use should be stored at room temperature to facilitate adequate absorption and utilization. To extend its shelf life, it should be protected from strong light and extreme temperatures.

The usual insulins utilized during pregnancy are rapid- and intermediate-acting insulins. Rapid-acting insulin commonly used is regular insulin that is a clear solution that can be given subcutaneously or intravenously. Regular insulin is the *only* insulin that may be given intravenously both because of its rapidity of action and because it is clear (not a suspension).

The intermediate insulins are NPH (neutral protamine Hagedorn) and lente (insulin zinc suspension). See Table 5-8 for onset, peak, and duration of all insulins.

The onset, peak, and duration of insulin allow one to plan and adjust insulin, diet, and exercise to coincide with metabolic needs. Knowing this for each

TABLE 5-8. *Insulin comparison chart*

Type	Preparation	Appearance	Onset (hr)	Peak (hr)	Duration (hr)
Rapid-acting	Regular insulin (crystalline zinc)	Clear solution	0.5 to 1	2 to 4	5 to 7
	Semi-lente (Prompt insulin zinc suspension)	Cloudy suspension	0.5 to 1	5 to 7	12 to 16
Intermediate-acting	NPH (neutral-protamine Hagedorn)	Cloudy suspension	1 to 1.5	6 to 10	18 to 22
	Lente (insulin zinc suspension)	Cloudy suspension	1 to 1.5	8 to 10	18 to 24

Modified from American Hospital formulary, American Society of Hospital Pharmacists, 1976.

type of insulin facilitates the timing and amount of insulin in relationship to the time and amount of meals and the amount of exercise.

Sulfonylureas and other oral antidiabetic agents are never used in pregnancy. This is because of their slow clearance and obvious difficulty with full 24-hour euglycemia and because of their suspected teratogenic properties.

Intrapartum intervention

During labor, the nurse must titrate intravenous insulin to the woman's blood glucose levels. This usually requires hourly changes. The fetus should be continuously monitored and interventions directed at improving uterine blood flow and fetal oxygenation (see Chapter 3). Preparation for potential cesarean delivery should be made early in labor. Referral should be made to the nursery personnel and pediatrician who will be in attendance at the time of delivery.

The nurse should provide birth choices for the couple, such as father in attendance and early breastfeeding if maternal and neonatal conditions permit. It is very important to provide a birthing atmosphere in spite of added medical care.

Postpartum intervention

Intravenous titration of insulin usually continues for the first 24 hours postpartum. Blood glucose monitoring can usually be spaced to every 3 to 4 hours as normal glucose levels are maintained.

If cesarean delivery was used, the postpartum care must include routine surgical care. Care should be directed at prevention of infection at the surgical site and through the Foley catheter into the urinary tract. As food is introduced by the first or second postoperative day, insulin can be reinstituted subcutaneously or by pump as the woman desires. If lactation is desired, diet should continue with the same calories and added nutrients as during the pregnancy.

Evaluation

The primary goal of nursing care throughout a diabetic pregnancy is to provide the woman with skills and knowledge that will enable her to manage her diabetes on an outpatient basis. This can best be accomplished through home blood glucose monitoring, adequate dietary intake, and a team approach with the woman and all necessary health care providers. During the intrapartum period, frequent blood glucose monitoring and insulin titration is necessary for optimal neonatal outcome. In the postpartum period, interventions must be aimed at reestablishment of insulin needs and glucose control while encouraging parenting tasks.

S U G G E S T E D   P L A N

Diabetes and pregnancy

Potential patient problem	Outcome criteria
Antepartum care	

A. Potential hypoglycemia or hyperglycemia related to:
    Drain of maternal glucose for fetal growth
    Maternal anorexia
    Increased levels of insulin antagonist hormones such as HPL, estrogen, and progesterone
	Plasma glucose values between 80 and 120 mg/100 ml
	No signs and symptoms of hypo- or hyperglycemia

OF NURSING CARE

Assessment and intervention

Dx. Assess patient's knowledge of disease, diet, urine and blood testing, and insulin administration
Evaluate normal daily activity
Assess for signs and symptoms of hypoglycemia such as
sweating
tiredness
nervousness
headaches
blurred vision
dizziness
shaking
hunger
irritability
Assess for signs and symptoms of hyperglycemia such as
weakness
dizziness
drowsiness
nausea/vomiting
excessive thirst
frequent urination
sugar and possibly acetone in urine

Th. No oral hypoglycemic agents should be used
Test second voided urine specimen for glucose and ketones two to four times per day with Testape, Ketodiastix, or Clinistix.
Monitor blood glucose two or more times each day with Dextrostix, Dextrometer, or B-G Chemstrip
Administer insulin via multiple dose or insulin pump as ordered (normally need less during first 3 months of pregnancy, and then needs gradually increase as pregnancy progresses)
Provide consistent meals and snack times
Maintain balance between diet, activity, and insulin

Ed. Explain that strict control of blood glucose is most important for a healthy newborn
Explain how pregnancy affects diabetes and diabetes affects pregnancy
Explain reason for increase in number of prenatal visits
Teach to treat mild signs and symptoms of hypoglycemia with a protein snack instead of carbohydrate snack to prevent Somogyi effect
Teach home glucose monitoring
Teach diet changes and significance of strict dietary control

Ref. Dietician

Dx., diagnostic; Th., therapeutic; Ed., education; Ref., referral.   *Continued.*

Diabetes and pregnancy—cont'd

Potential patient problem	*Outcome criteria*
B. Potential vaginal and urinary tract infections related to: 　　Increased amount of glucose in 　　　the urine 　　Altered vaginal pH	No signs and symptoms of an infection Prompt treatment if infection does develop
C. Potential preeclampsia related to: 　　Diabetic cardiovascular degenera- 　　　tion, which results from high 　　　glucose and lipid blood levels	No rise in baseline BP No proteinuria No pathologic edema
D. Potential growth retardation, con- 　genital malformation, mental or 　motor retardation, macrosomia re- 　lated to: 　　Premature aging of placenta 　　Prolonged hypo- or hypergly- 　　　cemia 　　Ketoacidosis	Reactive NST Negative CST Average fetal growth
E. Anxiety related to: 　　Fear of fetal outcome	Verbalizes fears and concerns Participates in decisions affecting care

Assessment and intervention

Dx.   Assess for abdominal and bilateral groin pain
      Assess for signs of vaginitis
Th.   Be prepared to administer an antibiotic if an infection occurs
Ed.   Teach ways to prevent an infection such as:
          drinking 6 to 8 glasses of water per day
          emptying bladder whenever feel urge
          wiping perineum from front to back
          wearing cotton underwear
          avoiding persons with colds, infections, or other sicknesses
          washing hands frequently
          importance of good oral hygiene, which includes flossing
          notifying physician of the first sign of an infection
      UTI can cause preterm labor

Dx.   Check vital signs as ordered
      Check weight daily
      Check urine for protein every day
      Assess level of edema
      Assess for signs and symptoms such as headache, changes in vision, epigastric
          pain
Th.   Encourage patient to rest on left side to promote circulation to kidneys and
          placenta
Ed.   Instruct regarding importance of 8 to 10 hr of sleep per night and rest pe-
          riod during the day on left side

Dx.   Assess number of fetal movements in 1 hr while patient is at rest
      Evaluate insulin needs (should gradually increase after 3 months of gestation)
      Assess FHR
Th.   Carry out as ordered:
          NST
          CST
          urine/serum estriols
          serial ultrasound
      Assist with amniocentesis when ordered to determine fetal lung maturity
Ed.   Instruct patient to count number of fetal movements felt in 1 hr (if less than
          four notify physician)
      Explain any ordered test

Dx.   Assess family's coping and mother's resources
      Identify diversional activity of interest
Th.   Encourage verbalization
      Provide diversional activity
Ref. Diversional therapist
      Clergy
      Social worker

Continued.

Diabetes and pregnancy—cont'd

Potential patient problem	Outcome criteria

Intrapartum care
A. Potential hypoglycemia related to:
    Vigorous work of labor
    Slowed digestion
	Plasma glucose values between 80 and 120 mg/100 ml

B. Potential fetopelvic disproportion related to: Fetal macrosomia	Labor progresses according to normal labor curve Fetal heart rate baseline between 120 and 160 bpm with no periodic deceleration patterns
Postpartum care A. Potential hemorrhage related to: Uterine atony caused by excessive amniotic fluid	Vital signs stable for patient Contracted uterus
B. Potential preeclampsia related to: Diabetic cardiovascular degeneration	No rise in baseline BP No proteinuria No pathologic edema

Assessment and intervention

Dx. Monitor blood glucose every 1 hr with Dextrostix, Dextrometer, or B-G
Chemstrip
Check urine for glucose and acetone every 4 hr
Th. Administer IV with glucose as ordered
Piggyback regular insulin via continuous infusion pump at ordered rate
Support patient
Ed. Keep patient informed of any treatments

Dx. Monitor contractions, labor progress, FHR via fetal monitor
Assess amount and character of amniotic fluid
Check vital signs every 15 min
Check for bladder distension every 2 hr
Th. Keep patient informed of progress
Allow for expression of fear due to increased anxiety
Coach as patient needs
Encourage patient to void every 2 hr
Ed. Prepare for possible cesarean delivery
Ref. Notify doctor of any FHR change from its normal pattern
Notify pediatrician and nursery

Dx. Record BP, pulse rate, and respirations twice every 30 min, twice every 1 hr,
twice every 4 hr, then qid
Check firmness of uterus and vaginal flow with each vital sign
Pad count
Th. Keep bladder empty
Manually massage relaxed, boggy fundus very gently until firm
Maintain oxytocics and IV fluids as ordered
Ed. Instruct mother on need to keep uterus contracted
Ref. Notify doctor if excessive vaginal bleeding occurs, drop in vital signs from
patient's baseline

Dx. Record BP as stated under hemorrhage
Check weight daily before breakfast
Check urine for protein every 4 hours
Assess level of edema
Assess for signs and symptoms such as headache, changes in vision, or epi-
gastric pain
Th. Encourage patient to continue to rest on left side for 4 days following deliv-
ery
Ref. Notify doctor of first sign of preeclampsia such as BP increased from base-
line, proteinuria, or increased edema

Continued.

Diabetes and pregnancy—cont'd

Potential patient problem	Outcome criteria
C. Potential infection related to: Diabetes	Temperature less than 38°C (100.4° F) No foul-smelling lochia No burning or pain on urination
D. Potential hypo- or hyperglycemia related to: Work of labor Removal of placental hormones Infection Trauma Surgery Oral contraceptives	Plasma glucose values between 80 and 120 mg/100 ml No signs and symptoms hypo- or hyperglycemia

REFERENCES

American Hospital Formulary, American Society of Hospital Pharmacists, 1976.

Beland, I.: Clinical nursing: pathophysiologic and psychosocial approaches, New York, 1974, MacMillan Inc.

Clark, A., and Alfonso, D.: Childbearing: a nursing perspective, Philadelphia, 1979, F.A. Davis Co.

Evans, H., and Glass, L.: Perinatal medicine, New York, 1976, Harper & Row, Inc.

Gabbe, S.: Optimal diabetes control = new techniques and physician interest + patient interest. Contemp. Ob/Gyn 18:105, 1981.

Javonovic, L.: Pump therapy offers conveniences for insulin dependent pregnant women, Infusion 1(3):2, 1982.

Johnson, S.: High-risk parenting, Philadelphia, 1979, J.B. Lippincott Co.

Assessment and intervention

Dx. Check temperature qid for 48 hr postdelivery, if greater than 100.4° F check
  every 2 hr
  Check vaginal discharge and lochia for odor every shift
  Ask patient regarding pain, burning on urination
Th. Use aseptic technique in care of patient
Ed. Explain pericare, good hand washing, and signs and symptoms of an infec-
  tion
Ref. Notify physician if temperature reaches 100.4° F (38° C) or any other signs
  of infection develop

Dx. Signs and symptoms of hypo- or hyperglycemia
  Check urine every 2 hr for glucose and ketone
  Monitor blood glucose immediately postdelivery, then as ordered
Th. Administer insulin as ordered
  Continue to monitor IV fluids
  Provide consistent meals and snacks
Ed. Teach diet and insulin changes postdelivery
  Teach that oral contraceptives alter carbohydrate metabolism; plan to use any
  other contraceptive device
Ref. Dietician

Diabetes, Elkhart, Ind., 1980, Eli Lilly Co.
Moore, M.: Newborn, family and nurse, Philadelphia, 1981, W.B. Saunders Co.
Niswander, K.: Manual of obstetrics, Boston, 1980, Little, Brown & Co.
Perez, R.: Protocols for perinatal nursing practice, St. Louis, 1981, The C.V. Mosby Co.
Pritchard, J., and MacDonald, P.: Williams' obstetrics, New York, 1980, Appleton-
  Century-Crofts.
Skillman, T., and Lzagournis, M.: The acute diabetic complications, diabetes mellitus,
  Kalamazoo, Mich., 1975, Upjohn Co.
Warshaw, J.: Insulin influences on fetal growth: the diabetic pregnancy and its out-
  come. Unpublished paper presented at the Mead-Johnson Symposium on Perinatal
  & Developmental Medicine, Vail, Colo., June 4-8, 1978.
White, P.: Classification of diabetes, 1978. In Niswander, K., editor: Manual of ob-
  stetrics, Boston, 1980, Little, Brown & Co.

CHAPTER 6

Cardiac disease and pregnancy

Pregnancy complicated with cardiac disease can be potentially dangerous to maternal well-being. The understanding of normal and abnormal cardiovascular physiology in pregnancy can aid enormously in anticipation of problems and prevention of complications.

INCIDENCE

The incidence of cardiac disease in the pregnant population ranges between 0.5% and 2%. Rheumatic fever, once responsible for 88% of cardiac disease in pregnancy, is now on the decline, responsible for only about 50% of cardiac disease in pregnancy. Congenital disease now plays a more prominent role. Mitral valve disease is still the most frequently seen valve defect in pregnant women. However, because of better childhood management of congenital heart disease, pregnancy outcomes are generally positive. Other cardiac diseases are rarely seen in pregnancy (Brinkman and Meldrum, 1980).

ETIOLOGY

Cardiac disease in pregnancy can take a variety of forms and can vary in functional severity. Some of the specific forms are listed below.
1. Rheumatic fever
2. Valve deformities
3. Congenital heart disease
4. Developmental abnormalities
5. Congestive cardiomyopathies
6. Cardiac arrhythmias

PHYSIOLOGY
Normal

In the antepartum period, cardiac output (the amount of blood pumped by the left ventricle into the aorta) rises significantly as early as the first trimester of pregnancy. It continues to rise and reaches a plateau between 28 and 34 weeks. It rises in response to the plasma volume increase, hormonal influences, and autonomic nervous system influences.

Blood volume increases by plasma volume expansion and red blood cell multiplication. The mean plasma volume increase is 45% over the prepregnant volume and red cell multiplication is in porportion to volume expansion if nutritional requirements are met. In early pregnancy it is the increased volume with each heart stroke that increases cardiac output. As pregnancy advances, the heart rate increases to offset continued increased stroke volume. The increased volume maintains a dilated systemic vasculature.

Hormonal influences affect resistance to blood flow and contractility of the myocardium. Estrogen increase leads to a systemic vasodilation. This facilitates increased cardiac output because of lowered peripheral resistance. Prolactin increases myocardial contractility.

During pregnancy autonomic nervous system (ANS) influences on blood flow become more prominent. In the nonpregnant state, when the ANS is blocked, there is little effect on blood pressure. However, in pregnancy, when the ANS is activated or blocked, dramatic changes in the maternal blood pressure can result. Thus the cardiovascular system is hyperfilled from increased blood volume and hyperdynamic because of the predominance of the ANS (see Chapter 1).

The cardiovascular system can respond to the physiologic adaptations in a number of ways. Increased venous pressure occurs especially in the lower extremities. This can lead to a normal finding of an accentuated jugular pulse. A slightly enlarged heart sometimes occurs because of the upward and leftward displacement of the heart anatomically. Benign arrhythmias can occur presumably because of the hormonal influences on myocardial contractility. Maternal position can have a profound effect on the cardiovascular system. When the weight of the gravid uterus lies against the inferior vena cava, partial or total occlusion reduces return volume to the heart and subsequent output.

The hemodynamic responses to labor are also important; this can be a critical period in the care of a pregnant woman with cardiac disease. Uterine contractions normally increase cardiac output and stroke volume because of increased intravascular volume. Some of this increase in workload of the heart can be relieved by positioning in the lateral position and by pain relief, especially with caudal or epidural anesthesia.

All cardiovascular adaptations, both anatomic and physiologic, can cause patients to report signs and symptoms that mimic, to some degree, those of cardiac disease. These include the following.

1. Dyspnea
2. Orthopnea
3. Dyspnea with exertion
4. Edema
5. Fatigability
6. Infrequent palpitations

In addition, the physician may note the following on examination.

1. Extrasystolic heart sounds
2. Chest x-ray findings of increased cardiac size
3. Benign murmurs

These all may be quite normal during pregnancy.

Pathophysiology

To understand the pathophysiology of cardiac disease in pregnancy, one must understand what functional lesion is present. It is also necessary to understand various terms describing cardiac function.

Stroke volume. Stroke volume is the amount of blood ejected with each contraction of the left ventricle. It is affected by four factors.

1. Diastolic filling pressure (preload)
2. Distensibility of the ventricle
3. Myocardial contractility
4. Aortic pressure, which is the amount of pressure the ventricle must overcome to push blood into the aorta (afterload)

Contractility. There is a direct relationship between diastolic volume and the amount of blood pumped during systole. The greater the diastolic filling pressure, the more the fibers of the left ventricle stretch during diastole and the harder they contract during systole, increasing stroke volume and cardiac output. However, if the muscle fibers are stretched beyond a certain point, there is a loss of distensibility. This loss decreases the force of contractions and therefore decreases cardiac output.

Preload. Preload is the force responsible for stretching the ventricular muscles. It can also be called *diastolic filling pressure*. If the preload is low, the ventricular muscle will not stretch enough for effective contractility. This leads to decreased stroke volume. If preload is too high, the muscle fibers will be overstretched. This also results in decreased contractility, leading in turn to decreased stroke volume.

Afterload. Afterload is the amount of pressure resistance in the aorta to the emptying of the left ventricle. It can also be called *systemic vascular resistance*. Systemic vascular resistance (or afterload) is measured by taking blood pressure readings. The higher the afterload, the greater the force required by the left ventricle to overcome aortic pressure with systolic pressure to force the aortic valve to open. A high afterload decreases stroke volume and cardiac output if the pressure cannot be effectively overcome.

Signs and symptoms

With cardiac disease in pregnancy, the actual lesion is responsible for the specific symptoms, but basically it causes problems with preload or afterload.

Listed below are the usual signs that the cardiac condition is deteriorating in a patient with preexisting cardiac disease.

1. Dyspnea severe enough to limit usual activity
2. Progressive orthopnea
3. Paroxysmal nocturnal dyspnea
4. Syncope during or immediately following exertion
5. Chest pain associated with activity

In addition, a pregnancy with preexisting cardiac disease can increase predisposition to thromboembolic changes, palpitations, and fluid retention. These complications sometimes require prophylactic treatment or increases in dosage of current drug therapy. Other conditions of the cardiovascular system such as chronic hypertension can also rapidly deteriorate. Patients with chronic hypertension may develop cardiac functional compromise during pregnancy because of the increased volume expansion.

Symptoms of cardiac disease in general are classified by the functional incapacity. The classification does not change in pregnancy although symptoms may worsen. The classifications of cardiac disease are outlined by Burrow and Ferris (1980).

Class I: asymptomatic at all degrees of activity
Class II: symptomatic with increased activity
Class III: symptomatic with ordinary activity
Class IV: symptomatic at rest

These are prognostic indicators of maternal and fetal complications.

Maternal effects

Sudden severe pulmonary edema can occur if afterload is high. If pulmonary hypertension is present in cardiac lesions such as mitral stenosis or tetralogy of Fallot, right-sided cardiac failure can occur with a resultant increase in preload and decreased stroke volume.

Quite independent of hemodynamic changes, systemic emboli can occur. Patients with atrial fibrillation or mitral valve problems causing atrial fibrillation are particularly susceptible to embolic episodes if not treated adequately with anticoagulants.

Cyanotic heart disease generally does not decrease the pregnant woman's ability to oxygenate herself unless there is pulmonary hypertension. In atrial or ventricular septal defects, pulmonary hypertension may progress and reverse existing shunts. If this occurs, maternal mortality is 50%.

A dissecting aneurysm, either with coarctation of the aorta or in Marfan's syndrome, is associated with a 50% maternal mortality. A dissecting aneurysm can develop suddenly as the pregnancy advances and fluid volume increases.

Fetal and neonatal effects

Fetal effects are the result of decreased systemic circulation or decreased oxygenation. If maternal circulation is compromised because of cardiac functional incapacities, uterine blood flow may be reduced severely. In early pregnancy, this can result in spontaneous abortion. If the uterine blood flow reduction occurs with advancing pregnancy, the fetus can suffer effects of deprivation ranging from growth retardation to central nervous system hypoxia. Preterm delivery may be necessary if maternal life is threatened, and the resultant neonatal morbidity associated with prematurity is high.

If maternal oxygenation is impaired, as in cyanotic heart disease or in acute pulmonary edema, fetal oxygenation is also impaired. Depending on the severity and the acuity or chronicity of decreased oxygenation, fetal central nervous system hypoxia can result in degrees of mental retardation, fetal distress, or even fetal death.

If either parent has a congenital cardiac defect, the fetus has an increased risk for having a congenital cardiac defect. This could be devastating to the neonate already compromised by hypoxia or prematurity.

MEDICAL DIAGNOSIS

Diagnosis of cardiac disease is made by the presentation of symptoms. Definition of the cardiac lesion, if unknown, is usually made by a cardiologist. An electrocardiogram, echocardiogram, series of laboratory tests including cardiac enzymes and electrolytes, and a chest x-ray film are the usual means, during pregnancy, for definition of the lesion.

USUAL MEDICAL MANAGEMENT

Usual medical management is accomplished with the obstetrician and cardiologist working together as a team involving the pregnant cardiac patient in the management of her care. Cardiac medications are usually adjusted to be compatible with pregnancy and dosages are adjusted when symptoms first present or worsen.

Early ultrasound of the fetus helps in accurate dating. Later, near 28 weeks, ultrasound can be used serially to document continued fetal growth and well-being. Fetal heart rate monitoring is also begun near 28 weeks with the contraction stress test being the test of choice.

Bed rest, or at least restricted activity, is necessary for women with Class III or IV heart disease throughout the last trimester. If symptoms present in women with Class I or II heart disease, limitations may be necessary for maternal comfort and well-being and also for adequate fetal oxygenation. The time of presentation of symptoms of cardiac decompensation is usually when maternal fluid volume expansion is greatest. This occurs during the pregnancy near 28 weeks and again in the postpartum period as unneeded volume is remobilized.

When cardiac disease is due to rheumatic fever, prophylactic antibiotic therapy should be instituted during labor and continue into the postpartum period. Penicillin is the antibiotic usually used.

Throughout pregnancy and labor, care is aimed at reduction of cardiac workload. During labor, pain relief is usually provided by regional anesthesia. Assistance with the delivery through the use of forceps in the second stage is often necessary. Vaginal delivery is preferred, if possible, because there are fewer hemodynamic disturbances. Some time after 36 weeks of gestation, a labor induction is usually planned after amniocentesis shows lung maturity. In addition to other monitoring, a Swan-Ganz line for hemodynamic monitoring of the mother will be necessary during labor and during the unstable postpartum period. Central venous pressure and pulmonary wedge pressure readings aid in controlling preload and afterload pressures. Careful titration of fluid volume can prevent pulmonary edema and cardiac overload. Oxygen at 5 to 6 liters/min may be needed if cyanotic cardiac disease is present. When decompensation of the cardiac disease occurs, placing the mother's life in jeopardy, termination of the pregnancy might be necessary. This can occur prior to fetal viability or can result in extreme prematurity of the neonate. Consideration should always be for the safety of the mother.

NURSING PROCESS
Prevention

Nursing measures must be directed toward prevention of complications. Nutrition should be adequate in iron and folic acid to prevent anemia, which would increase cardiac workload. Sodium restriction may be necessary but intake should not fall below 2.5 gm per day during pregnancy.

Plans should be made early in the pregnancy for restriction of activities and possible prolonged bed rest. Relief from emotional stress can be facilitated if family care can be prearranged. At all times during the pregnancy, attention must be directed at reducing and eliminating anxiety. Anxiety regarding her own well-being, fetal well-being, and her family's care in her absence is likely to cause increased cardiac workload. Sedation provides only a partial solution. Information that is realistic about risks and benefits for mother and fetus will facilitate adequate coping and reduce anxiety over uncertainties.

When pregnancy termination must occur for the mother's safety and well-being, consideration of her future childbearing is very important. Contraceptive means may be limited. Permanent surgical intervention is often not a safe procedure for a woman with class III or IV cardiac disease. Birth control pills also are often contraindicated because of thromboembolic potential. For the sexually active couple, consistent use of the diaphragm, condoms, or foam might be a problem. Careful counseling in the area of contraception must include a realistic examination of the hazards of subsequent pregnancy to the health of the woman. Ideally, her sexual partner should be included in the counseling.

Assessment

Maternal vital signs should include measurement of blood pressure and apical/radial pulse assessment at each visit. The woman should be questioned about palpitations, shortness of breath, increasing edema, and any increase in preexisting symptoms.

Symptoms of pulmonary edema should be assessed by listening to the chest for rales and diminished breath sounds. This is especially important in the hospitalized woman approaching week 28. Chest sounds should be assessed at least once every 8 hours. If the woman presents symptoms of pulmonary edema, hemodynamic monitoring will probably be instituted.

Nursing responsibilities for hemodynamic monitoring include some special assessments. As the line is being inserted, the ECG monitor should be observed for arrhythmias, especially premature ventricular contractions. Waveforms also need to be observed for changes indicating specific passage through the right atrium (low-amplitude waves), right ventricle (tall amplitude), and pulmonary wedge (smaller, lower pressures with diastolic and systolic waves). Continuous ECG monitoring for the cardiac rate is usual. The site of arterial catheter insertion should be inspected at least once each shift for signs of infection such as redness or drainage, and vital signs must include maternal temperature at least every 4 hours.

While the catheter is in place, waveform readings can be obtained for central venous pressure (CVP), pulmonary artery pressure (PAP), and pulmonary capillary wedge pressure (PCWP). Table 6-1 outlines normal readings for each and the significance of low or high readings.

Assessments for pressure reading will vary depending on the cardiac lesion and whether or not afterload or preload pressures are abnormal and require therapy.

Other observations for problems with circulating blood volume or effectiveness of myocardial contractions include measurement of daily weight and hourly intake and output during hemodynamic monitoring and assessment for dependent edema. Urinary output of at least 30 ml/hr is a sensitive measure of adequacy of circulating volume to other vital areas of the body.

If the maternal condition can be stabilized without inducing labor, fetal assessments must be made. Continuous fetal heart rate monitoring includes careful observation for signs of fetal hypoxia such as late decelerations and loss of variability. Fetal distress can also be exhibited by decreased fetal activity and

TABLE 6-1. *Hemodynamic pressure readings*

	Normal	Low	High
CVP (measures right ventricular end-diastolic pressure when the tricuspid valve is open and therefore the right atrium and ventricle are common chambers)	1 to 6 mm Hg	Reflects inadequate circulatory volume from Hemorrhage Third spacing Extreme vasodilation	Reflects Increased preload High pulmonary resistance such as pulmonary embolus Poor cardiac contractility
Systolic PAP (reflects the pressure in the pulmonary artery when the right ventricle is contracting and the pulmonic valve is open)	15 to 25 mm Hg	Reflects a decreased venous return to the heart from Hemorrhage Third spacing Extreme vasodilation	Reflects Increased blood volume Pulmonary arteriole constriction in response to increased pCO_2 and decreased pO_2 Increase with pulmonary disease such as embolus or edema
Diastolic PAP (reflects the left heart when the pulmonary valve is closed and left valves are open)	8 to 10 mm Hg		
PCWP (reflects only pressure from the left side of the heart)	10 to 15 mm Hg	Results from A low circulating volume Extreme vasodilation	Reflects Increased preload Poor contractility Increased afterload Increased pCO_2

Modified from Norris, D., and Klein, R.: What all those pressure readings mean and why, RN 44(10):41, 1981.

decreased growth. Assessments for more subtle signs can be made with fundal measurements and maternal daily reports of fetal activity.

Antepartum intervention

When pregnancy is first diagnosed in a woman with cardiac disease, the nurse should begin education of the woman and her family for whatever physical limitations the functional class of cardiac disease suggests. Information regarding special tests such as laboratory studies and cardiac evaluations and their significance aids in reducing anxiety and in planning financial resources.

Bed rest can be valuable in improving the maternal condition as well as fetal well-being. Total bed rest or bed rest with limited periods of physical activity should be suggested by 26 to 28 weeks of gestation for class II, III, or IV functional disease.

The woman needs education about early signs and symptoms of decreasing cardiovascular function and the necessity of reporting these. Medications may be new to her, and she will need instructions for reporting side effects.

If hypertension complicates the cardiac disease, daily blood pressure measurements might need to be monitored by a family member. How to do this and what to report must be clearly demonstrated and defined by the nurse.

Antepartum fetal monitoring, such as CST, should be arranged beginning at 26 to 28 weeks of gestation. Fetal activity charts should also be kept daily beginning at this gestational age. Instructions for fetal surveillance should be encouraged and reassurance provided.

Cardiac disease can pose obvious physical crises for the woman, but it must also be remembered that this high-risk event can also lead to psychologic crises for the woman and her family. Each person's concern for maternal well-being must be openly discussed. Realistic appraisal of risks to the mother's life will support the couple's ability to cope and make judgments in the best interest of both mother and fetus.

Concerns for fetal well-being can also cause undue anxiety. Explaining measures for assessing fetal well-being can reduce anxiety and prevent increased cardiac workload from chronic stimulation by adrenal epinephrine. Appropriate referrals may also be made to specialists (Burrows and Ferris, 1980).

1. Antepartum testing nurse
2. Social worker for financial evaluation and aid in home care arrangements
3. Perinatal nurse specialists
4. Clergyman for spiritual assistance
5. Home care coordinator for help in obtaining special equipment such as oxygen or a wheelchair for home use
6. Dietician for sodium restriction and adequate iron and folic acid intake
7. Prenatal childbirth educator

Intervention—drug therapy

Drug therapy will depend on the cardiac lesion. Consideration should be given to maternal benefits and fetal risks. Common drugs used in cardiac disease and pregnancy are heparin, furosemide (Lasix), digitalis, beta blockers such as propranolol (Inderal), antiarrhythmics such as quinidine, or disopyramide phosphate (Norpace).

When taking the history, the nurse should be aware of specific drugs commonly used in cardiac disease that are contraindicated in pregnancy and note the dosage, which may need to be changed. Women are usually very aware of potential fetal harm from any drug therapy and often have numerous questions that the nurse should be prepared to answer.

Heparin. Heparin is the only anticoagulant recommended during pregnancy. Warfarin crosses the placenta and may have teratogenic effects and cause bleeding in the fetus. Heparin, however, has no such problems associated with its use. Ideally, the pregnant woman on anticoagulation therapy should be placed on heparin prior to pregnancy or at the earliest possible time. This will usually necessitate instructional information such as giving injections, correctly drawing up the dose, and the importance of reporting side effects such as bleeding gums, nose bleeds, and easy bruising. The importance of taking the medication at the same time each day should be stressed. Prophylactic doses range from 5,000 to 7,500 U twice daily, 12 hours apart.

Special instructions in giving the injection should be carefully outlined for the patient. It is suggested that the patient be taught that:

1. The sites should be rotated in the fatty tissue of the thighs, hips, and the abdomen.
2. The area should be cleansed in a circular motion with alcohol and then iced for 1 min with an ice cube to reduce bruising.
3. The injection should be given in one motion without aspiration. A syringe with a short, 25-gauge needle should be used.
4. The area should not be rubbed after the injection.

A return demonstration of the technique can be provided with normal saline. At least three correctly executed injections should be demonstrated by the woman and also by one family member.

Furosemide (Lasix). Furosemide is a commonly used diuretic. Dosage can vary from 40 to 80 mg one to two times daily. Intravenous dosage is usually ordered by the single dose and is also 40 to 80 mg depending on the severity of fluid overload. Thiazides are rarely used because of the severe potassium deficiency that can result.

With any diuretic prescribed for home use, the woman should be instructed to reduce dietary intake of sodium. She should have special dietary instructions considering pregnancy needs. Foods high in potassium, such as bananas, citrus fruits, and whole grains, should be included in her diet.

Digitalis. Digitalis is a drug commonly utilized in cardiac disease for its improvement of myocardial contractility. Although it does cross the placental barrier, it does not affect fetal cardiac function. However, this can decrease maternal concentrations and require dosage adjustment. In addition, it must be kept in mind that, just as myocardial contractility is increased, so can uterine contractility be affected leading to preterm labor (Burrow and Ferris, 1980).

Tocolytics. The drugs ritodrine and terbutaline are contraindicated in the treatment of preterm labor for the woman with cardiac disease. Beta-sympathomimetics increase cardiac rate and workload and increase the potential for pulmonary edema. Magnesium sulfate decreases calcium levels and has a direct effect on myocardial contractility. If used to treat preterm labor, magnesium and calcium levels must be monitored frequently (Burrow and Ferris, 1980).

Propranolol (Inderal). Propranolol may be used to treat hypertension because of the decreased pulsating effect on the aorta, or it may be used as an antiarrhythmic. It can increase uterine tone and lead to preterm labor. Propranolol decreases cardiac output and therefore can reduce uterine blood flow. Other antiarrhythmics utilized during pregnancy include quinidine and disopyramide phosphate. Most antiarrhythmics have not been well studied for their fetal effects (Burrow and Ferris, 1980).

Quinidine. Quinidine is used as an antiarrhythmic because it depresses myocardial excitability, conductive velocity, and contractility. It has never been studied in animals for effects on the fetus. Therefore, as with most of the antiarrhythmics, it is given when the benefits outweigh the risks.

Disopyramide phosphate (Norpace). This is an antiarrhythmic drug with effects similar to those of quinidine. However, it is chemically unrelated to any of the other antiarrhythmics. It decreases the sinus node recovery period and lengthens the response time in the atrium. It has no effect on alpha- or beta-adrenergic receptors but has been reported to cause increased uterine contractility. Its use in pregnancy has been studied in animals and no fetal anomalies have been found.

Because most of the cardiac medications used in pregnancy are reported to increase uterine contractility, the woman with cardiac disease should be taught how to detect early signs of preterm labor and to report these promptly. She should also be taught the benefits of bed rest in reducing uterine irritability and improving uterine blood flow.

Intrapartum intervention

Intervention during labor focuses on pain relief and prevention of hemodynamic changes that would compromise cardiac output and efforts. Labor induction will usually be a planned and well-controlled event, with close monitoring of maternal and fetal vital signs.

The fetal monitor should be applied, first, using the external monitor. Later, after an amniotomy has been performed, the internal monitor should be used. Explanations to the woman and her coach regarding the purpose of the monitor will help to allay concern for the fetus.

Preparation must be made for insertion of a central monitoring line for hemodynamic monitoring of the mother. Explanations directed at reassuring the woman that her comfort will be attended to during the procedure are important before equipment is brought to the bedside. Because the insertion site is often above the clavicle, draping of the site will prevent the woman from observing people and events. This can reassure some women but frighten others. It is important for the nurse to explain this and to assure the woman that, throughout the procedure, someone will support and comfort her. The cardiac monitor should be in use prior to the procedure and baseline strips documented in the chart. Because the procedure is surgical in nature, gowns and masks will be worn by the physician and nurses and this, too, should be explained to the woman. Local anesthesia will be used near the insertion site.

Once the hemodynamic monitoring procedure is accomplished, preparation for labor induction should be initiated. An intravenous infusion should be started with an 18-gauge catheter for mainline fluid, and 10 U of oxytocin diluted in 1,000 ml of a salt-poor solution such as 0.45 normal saline should be administered via an infusion pump.

As soon as cervical changes begin, preparation for epidural or caudal anesthesia should be made. Adequate pain relief will reduce anxiety and cardiac workload. Regional anesthesia with an epidural or caudal block causes fewer hemodynamic changes and more relief than narcotics, which depress the entire central nervous system. The major risk to the mother during the epidural or caudal block is hypotension. The nurse should monitor the blood pressure closely.

The nursery should be notified of the induction and a brief maternal history outlined to the neonatologist. Preparation can then be made for care of the neonate, who might have problems associated with hypoxia or prematurity.

The woman should be coached by her significant other with the nurse's assistance so that the woman can exercise control and yet be provided adequate rest between contractions. A quiet atmosphere with lights dimmed and low voices should be provided despite the frequency of necessary intrusive assessment.

Hemodynamic monitoring should be done with the woman preferably on her left side to facilitate uterine blood flow and oxygenation to the fetus. This position will also provide better hemodynamic homeostasis in the mother.

Delivery is usually accomplished with forceps assistance. A choice of forceps should be made available in the instrument set-up of the delivery room. The nursery team should be notified so that they can be present and waiting for the neonate with resuscitation equipment ready.

Postpartum intervention

The first hours after delivery can be critical for maternal safety because of the remobilization of the large blood volume. Hemodynamic monitoring must therefore continue. Adequate relief of discomfort from the episiotomy and uterine contractions must be provided to reduce cardiac workload.

If the neonate is being cared for in the intensive care nursery, the mother is likely to be unable to have contact because of her physical limitations. Early close-up pictures of the neonate's face can be provided and can help allay unnecessary anxieties. Nursery personnel should be encouraged to give frequent information of a reassuring nature to the mother and the father. Early contact by the father will often aid the mother and should be encouraged.

If the neonate is well enough for visits to the mother's room, this should occur as soon and as often as the mother's condition allows. This contact, rather than causing too much activity for the mother, often reduces cardiac workload by decreasing unnecessary anxiety.

As the maternal cardiac condition stabilizes, plans for discharge should be made. Help at home should be provided, for several weeks, until the woman can gradually resume her previous activities.

Contraception is important for the woman; an early subsequent pregnancy would definitely be contraindicated. The choice of means may be limited because of the cardiac disease. Counseling regarding the limits must be included.

SUGGESTED PLAN

Cardiac disease and pregnancy

Potential patient problem	*Outcome criteria*
A. Potential increased cardiac workload related to: Anxiety Lack of adequate rest Pain during labor Increased blood volume	Exhibits no signs of anxiety such as depression, withdrawal, anger, or increased fear Obtains rest and is able to follow activity restrictions as recommended
B. Potential infection related to: Symptomatic murmur and previous rheumatic fever	No recurrence of rheumatic fever
C. Potential loss of current pregnancy/preterm delivery related to: Worsening maternal condition Fetal distress	Continuation of pregnancy to optimal maternal well-being and fetal viability Signs of emotional acceptance if pregnancy terminates before viability
D. Limited choices for contraception related to: Surgical risk for permanent maternal sterilization Increase risk of thromboembolism related to oral contraceptive pills	Selects a birth control method safe and effective for her cardiac lesion Seeks information and verbalizes understanding of need for birth control

Lactation increases the need for maternal rest and necessary iron and folic acid. Dietary instruction and supplements should be discussed prior to discharge. Discussion of ways to plan for adequate rest when the baby sleeps should also be stressed.

Evaluation

The primary goal of nursing care throughout pregnancy in a woman with cardiac disease is to provide a balance between cardiac functional deficiencies

O F   N U R S I N G   C A R E

Assessment and intervention

Dx.	Assess for signs of anxiety and lack of rest
Th.	Discuss anxieties and fears
	Prepare for epidural in labor
Ed.	Instruct in disease and maternal and fetal/neonatal outcome
	Explain benefits of bed rest
Ref.	Clergy
	Social service
	Parent support groups

Dx.	Assess for history of rheumatic fever if valvular disease
Th.	Administer antibiotics as ordered prophylactically during labor and postpartum

Dx.	Assess for signs that the cardiac condition is deteriorating and threatening maternal well-being
	Assess for anticipatory grief work, for couple's ability to cope with termination or preterm delivery
Th.	Support parental decision
Ed.	Reinforce realistic expectations of maternal and fetal outcome
Ref.	Clergy or grief counselor

Dx.	Assess for knowledge of birth control methods, efficacy, and proper use
Ed.	Give information regarding above
Ref.	Physician for selection of and prescription for method

Dx., diagnostic; Th., therapeutic; Ed., education; Ref., referral.

Continued.

Cardiac disease and pregnancy—cont'd

Potential patient problem	*Outcome criteria*
E. Potential congestive heart failure and pulmonary edema related to: Increased circulating volume Increased afterload Increased or decreased preload	No evidence of pulmonary edema (rales, frothy sputum, increased respiratory rate, retention of pCO_2, decreased pO_2, difficulty breathing) No generalized edema Normal values for CVP, PAP, PCWP if hemodynamic monitoring
F. Potential fetal distress related to: Hypoxia Poor maternal oxygenation Intrauterine growth retardation	No evidence of decreased variability or late decelerations Evidence of fetal activity daily Evidence of acceleration of FHR with activity Adequate growth for gestation No evidence of oligohydramnios on ultrasound examination and lack of variable decelerations on NSTs

Assessment and intervention

Dx. Assess lung sounds, respiratory rate, pulse rate, and blood pressure every 15
   min if pulmonary edema present or each 8 hr if not present
   Assess for palpitations
   Assess above each office visit
   Assess for other signs of edema such as increased weight gain and dependent
   pitting edema
   Refer to blood gases and laboratory studies
Th. Prepare for hemodynamic monitoring
   Daily weight if hospitalized
   Administer diuretics and digitalis as ordered intravenously or orally
   Sodium-restricted diet
   Administer oxygen as ordered
   Hourly intake and output
Ed. Teach early signs of congestive failure such as shortness of breath, cough, in-
   creased rapid weight gain, and generalized edema
Ref. Report to physician early signs of congestive heart failure or pulmonary
   edema
   Dietician regarding sodium restriction

Dx. Assess for at least four fetal movements in 1 hr of counting per day
   Assess all monitoring strips for late decelerations or decreased variability
   Assess for presence of accelerations with fetal activity and average variability
   Assess for variable decelerations with spontaneous contractions or fetal activ-
   ity
   Assess for fundal growth/cm/week after 20 weeks of gestation
Th. Continuous FHR monitoring if mother presents in congestive failure or dur-
   ing labor
   Do biweekly NSTs
   Prepare for ultrasound examinations during first trimester, at 28 and 35
   weeks of gestation, or any other time ordered
   Prepare for labor induction
   Labor on left side with oxygen by facemask at ordered liters/min
   Prepare for epidural anesthesia during induced labor and for delivery
   Salt-poor intravenous fluids as ordered for maternal hydration to run only at
   ordered rate via infusion pump
Ed. Encourage and explain benefits of maternal bed rest, left side lying, on fetal
   oxygenation and growth potential
Ref. Report to physician first signs of fetal distress
   Notify nursery personnel when delivery is planned
   Utilize visiting nurse or public health nurse services if home care is planned

Continued.

Cardiac disease and pregnancy—cont'd

Potential patient problem	*Outcome criteria*

G. Potential anxiety related to:
  Potential maternal effects
  Potential poor fetal/neonatal out-
  come
  Financial burdens
  Inability to care for family
  Separation from family or friends
	Overt expression of fears verbally
	Shares feelings reciprocally with partner or
	  other significant person
	Has satisfactory arrangements for care of
	  family if hospitalization is necessary
	Obtains adequate financial resources

H. Potential thromboembolic episode
  related to:
  Valvular defects
	No evidence of pulmonary or cerebral em-
	bolism

and cardiovascular adaptations during pregnancy. This is best accomplished by reducing physical and psychologic stressors in the antepartum period. Bed rest or restriction of activities, emotional support, and education regarding the disease process are necessary. During the intrapartum period, pain relief and provision of the quiet atmosphere, despite intrusive monitoring, can facilitate prevention of hemodynamic complications such as fetal hypoxia and maternal cardiac compromise. In the postpartum period, interventions are aimed at providing rest while encouraging parenthood tasks.

REFERENCES

Benedetti, T.J., and others: Hemodynamic observations in severe preeclampsia with a flow-directed pulmonary artery catheter, Am. J. Obstet. Gynecol. **136:**465, 1980.

Berkowitz, R.L., and Rafferty, T.D.: Invasive hemodynamic monitoring in critically ill pregnant patients: role of Swan-Ganz catheterization, Am. J. Obstet. Gynecol. **137:**127, 1980.

Berkowitz, R.L., and Rafferty, T.D.: Pulmonary artery flow-directed catheter use in the obstetric patient, Obstet. Gynecol. **55:**507, 1980.

Brinkman, C., and Meldrum, D.: Physiology and pathophysiology of maternal adjustments to pregnancy. In Aladjem, S., and others, editors: Clinical perinatology, St. Louis, 1980, The C.V. Mosby Co.

Assessment and intervention

Dx. Assess for signs of abnormal anxiety or fear such as
    depression
    withdrawal
    failure to communicate
    refusal to take medications, adhere to restrictions, fetal and maternal examination
    Determine arrangements for home help
Th. Initiate discussion of feeling, concerns, and fears
Ed. Instruct regarding realistic concerns versus nonrealistic
Ref. Social service
    Clergy
    Nursery personnel
    Parent support survices

Dx. Assess susceptible women for changes in mental acuity, chest pain, shortness of breath, paresthesias
Th. Prepare for heparin infusion via infusion pump for duration of pregnancy
Ed. Instruct in early signs
Ref. Physical therapy or respiratory therapy as ordered

Burrow, G., and Ferris, T.: Medical complications during pregnancy, Philadelphia, 1980, W.B. Saunders Co.

Cotton, D.B., and Henedetti, T.J.: Use of the Swan-Ganz catheter in obstetrics and gynecology, Obstet. Gynecol. **56**:641, 1980.

Cotton, D.B., and others: Hemodynamic observations in evacuation of molar pregnancy, Am. J. Obstet. Gynecol. **138**:6, 1980.

Hodgkinson, R., Husain, F.J., and Hayashi, R.H.: Systemic and pulmonary blood pressure during caesarean section in parturients with gestational hypertension, J. Can. Anaesth. Soc. **27**:389, 1980.

Keefer, J.R., and others: Noncardiogenic pulmonary edema and invasive cardiovascular monitoring, Obstet. Gynecol. **58**:46, 1981.

Kjeldsen, J.: Hemodynamic investigations during labour and delivery, Acta Obstet. Gynecol. Scand. **89**[Suppl]:1, 1979.

Larkin, H., and others: Cardiac and haemodynamic measurements in hypertensive pregnancy, Clin. Sci. **6**[Suppl]:357, 1980.

Norris, D., and Klein, R.: What all those pressure readings mean and why, RN **44**(10):41, 1981.

Rafferty, T.D., and Berkowitz, R.L.: Hemodynamics in patients with severe toxemia during labor and delivery, Am. J. Obstet. Gynecol. **138**:263, 1980.

Selzer, A.: The heart of pregnancy, Emergency Med. **8**(10):267, 1976.

Sinnenberg, R.J., Jr.: Pulmonary hypertension in pregnancy, South Med. J. **73**:1529, 1980.

Strauss, R.G., and others: Hemodynamic monitoring of cardiogenic pulmonary edema complicating toxemia of pregnancy, Obstet. Gynecol. **55:**170, 1980.

Ueland, K.: Intrapartum management of the cardiac patient. Clin. Perinatal. Med. **8:**155, 1980.

Van Dongen, P.W., and others: Postural blood pressure differences in pregnancy. A prospective study of blood pressure differences between supine and left lateral position as measured by ultrasound, Am. J. Obstet. Gynecol. **138:**1, 1980.

CHAPTER 7

Renal disease and pregnancy

During pregnancy, the kidneys undergo many changes that balance and counterbalance one another. These changes are both anatomic and physiologic. Renal disease can be present symptomatically or asymptomatically when conception occurs or it can be brought about by complications of pregnancy such as pregnancy-induced hypertension.

INCIDENCE

The incidence of renal disease in pregnancy varies with the form it takes. It is estimated that 4% to 6.9% of childbearing women have asymptomatic bacteriuria. Another 1% to 1.5% will develop bacteriuria later in pregnancy. Approximately 30% of women with untreated asymptomatic bacteriuria will develop pyelonephritis during pregnancy (Alvarez, 1976).

Renal calculi rarely occur in pregnancy. Less than 1 in 1,000 pregnancies will require surgery to correct this problem.

Lupus is exacerbated during pregnancy in 40% of women with the disease. Prior to the pregnancy many have renal involvement, which will deteriorate during or immediately after the pregnancy.

Acute glomerulonephritis during pregnancy is extremely rare, occurring in 1 out of 40,000 pregnancies. This is attributed to the usual failure to ovulate in women with the disease.

Diabetic renal disease can be seen more frequently now that better control can be established and it is known that pregnancy does not adversely affect diabetes. Kimmelstiel-Wilson disease is, however, rarely seen in pregnancy, probably due to the failure of ovulation associated with the disease.

Because polycystic kidney disease does not generally become evident until after the age of 40 years it is also rarely seen in pregnancy. It is associated with autosomal dominant genetic transmission. Therefore there is a 50% chance of it having been transmitted to each child born to a parent prior to the disease having become evident in that parent.

Pregnancy following a renal transplant has been reported infrequently. The University of Colorado Medical Center reported in 1975 (Alvarez, 1976) on 35 pregnancies following renal transplant. Of those, 22 resulted in live births and one in a stillbirth. None of the women had impairment of renal function attributable to the pregnancy although 32% had superimposed pregnancy-induced hypertension.

ETIOLOGY

Renal disease can be caused by a urinary tract infection prior to or during pregnancy, can be the result of other diseases such as diabetes, or can occur in pregnancy from complications such as pregnancy-induced hypertension.

The etiology of urinary tract infection is often bacteria from the gastrointestinal tract contaminating the perineal area. Often the organism implicated is *Escherichia coli*. It is more common when contaminants from the rectal area are brought forward across the urethral meatus during perineal hygiene. It can also occur from trauma to the meatus during sexual intercourse forcing perineal contaminants into the urethra. Bacteria may migrate from the urethra into the bladder and proliferate before the next urination. Bacteria may also pass into the dilated ureters during pregnancy and migrate into the kidney itself, causing inflammation of the tubules. Occasionally other perineal organisms such as yeast are introduced into the bladder and cause infection.

Staphylococcal or streptococcal bacteria can enter the blood in the kidney and result in renal tissue reaction to the organism or to its toxins. However, these organisms are rarely the cause of infection during pregnancy.

PHYSIOLOGY
Normal

The kidneys fulfill several functions essential for the body. They excrete water, electrolytes, and nitrogenous waste products. They perform a major function in acid-base balance and are active in the renin-angiotensin-aldosterone system.

The kidneys have the largest blood supply of any organ in the body. Renal blood flow accounts for 20% to 25% of the cardiac output. The blood supply to each kidney is supplied by a renal artery, which branches finally into the afferent arteriole leading into the glomerulus. From the glomerulus, the efferent arteriole leads out via branches into the renal vein.

The filtration of the blood through the glomerulus is the result of four forces acting on the capillaries. These are the permeability of the capillary walls, the hydrostatic pressure in the glomerular capillaries, the hydrostatic pressure in the glomerular capsule, and the osmotic pressure of the circulating plasma proteins. It is the pressure within the glomerular capillaries that determines the filtration rate. Glomerular filtration produces a protein-free filtrate of plasma. The glomeruli act as ultrafilters with microscopic pores. The microscopic pores do not normally allow the larger protein or glucose molecules through but rather send them along the circulatory route to the tubules. The major excretory product into urine is sodium.

The tubules act on the glomerular filtrate to produce urine. Substances are reabsorbed from the glomerular filtrate either actively or passively. Substances such as water passively follow sodium that is actively reabsorbed into the urine. Urea, a nitrogenous waste product, diffuses passively. Glucose is actively reabsorbed against the concentration gradient after being freely filtered in the glomerulus.

The tubule cells also secrete a number of substances, such as potassium, hydrogen, NH_4, and organic anions and cations. As the glomerular filtrate flows through the proximal tubule, sodium is actively reabsorbed and chloride follows passively. Water follows with the change in osmotic pressure. As it reaches the loop of Henle in the tubule, the fluid volume is reduced by 80%. As the fluid flows through the thin, descending loop of Henle, water is removed passively because of the hypertonicity of the interstitial tissues. As the fluid enters the distal convoluted tubules, it becomes hypotonic.

If circulating antidiuretic hormone is elevated, the distal tubule is permeable to water and the urinary fluid then becomes isotonic to the interstitial fluid. Chloride, sodium, and passive osmotic diffusion of water further reduce the urinary fluid volume as it enters the collecting duct, where it changes from an isotonic to a hypertonic fluid. The urinary fluid and sodium removed in the loop of Henle return to the general circulation.

If the antidiuretic hormone is low, the distal tubule is not permeable to water and the urinary fluid remains hypotonic. It loses its solutes and increases its hypotonicity. The ultimate outcome is that the urine is both dilute and increased in volume.

The kidney regulates acid-base balance by maintaining plasma bicarbonate between 26 and 28 mEq/liter in response to the respiratory system's maintenance of carbonic acid at 1.3 to 1.4 mEq/liter. Organic anions in the urine accept hydrogen ions producing carbonic acid, which is in turn broken down into water and carbon dioxide. Ammonia (a combination of nitrogen and three hydrogen ions) takes on another hydrogen ion and becomes ammonium (NH_4^+) and then is excreted in the urine. In this way the kidney serves as an efficient buffering mechanism.

During pregnancy, a number of alterations occur in renal function. Secondary to prostaglandin E_2, renal blood flow increases, vascular resistance decreases, and glomerular filtration rate increases 30% to 50% over that in the nonpregnant state. Because of this increased filtration rate, nitrogenous waste products such as creatinine, urea, and uric acid are cleared in greater quantities.

As the filtrate enters the tubules, considerable changes in the mechanisms controlling salt and water excretion occur. Progesterone normally causes increased salt loss. In pregnancy, this is countered by a rise in aldosterone to two to three times nonpregnant levels. As a result, sodium is actually retained in the tissues in larger amounts, thus aiding in the necessary volume expansion of pregnancy.

The healthy pregnant woman also excretes larger amounts of sugar in her urine. This is not related to the blood glucose levels but rather to an intermittent tubular failure to reabsorb glucose.

Amino acid excretion is known to be increased in pregnancy. This is thought to be due to a partial failure of the normal reabsorptive mechanisms. The increased excretion of amino acids is related to high levels of cortisol in pregnancy.

Water-soluble vitamins, such as ascorbic acid, nicotinic acid, and folates, are also excreted at higher levels in the urine. This increased excretion is due to failure of the tubules to reabsorb and can be serious when folate and protein intake is marginal.

Another important consideration of the high nutrient content of the urine is acknowledging its value as a culture medium for bacteria. Progesterone enhances the potential for urinary tract infection by relaxing the musculature of the bladder and the ureters. The dilation of the ureters, especially on the right side, is further compromised by the obstruction of the gravid uterus. All of these factors contribute to the likelihood of urinary stasis of a fluid rich in nutrients, which substantially increases the potential for ascending urinary tract infection.

The activity of the renin-angiotensin system is greatly increased in pregnancy. Progesterone stimulates the increased plasma level of the enzyme renin. It is generally assumed that the maternal kidney is primarily responsible for this increase, although it is believed that the uterus is also a source of renin (Alvarez, 1976).

Renin then acts to form angiotensin, which in turn increases the production of aldosterone. The aldosterone increase preserves sodium and facilitates blood volume expansion. The sensitivity to the pressor effects of renin-angiotensin is low during pregnancy, and normally the blood pressure does not rise.

Pathophysiology

When infection from urinary bacteria ascends the urinary tract, the renal tubules can become inflamed. The inflammatory process leads to a decrease in tubular function. Reabsorption of sodium into the urinary fluid and secretion of buffering substances are affected adversely if large localized areas become inflamed. Sodium will then be retained in body tissues and water will remain compartmentalized in tissues or in the intravascular space, which can cause edema or increased cardiac afterload.

Secretion of buffering substances may also be reduced. When buffering substances such as potasssium, ammonia, and organic ions are deficient in quantity, free hydrogen ions cannot be absorbed. The blood pH will reflect the increased carbonic acid with a tendency toward acidemia. Concurrent conditions such as diabetes can complicate potential acidemia because of nephropathy or metabolic failures inherent in the disease.

Renal disease reflected as hypertensive renal disease, diabetic nephropathy, pregnancy-induced hypertension, and glomerulonephritis can be differentiated by the specific histology of the lesion in the kidneys. Basically, lesions can be either in the glomeruli or in the tubules. Some affect the vasculature surrounding or comprising the glomeruli and tubules; others affect the cells within the glomeruli or tubules.

When the vasculature of the renal tissues is damaged, and blood supply to the kidneys is compromised, renin activity increases and blood pressure rises. Pregnancy sometimes initially improves the blood pressure because of the vasodilating effect of progesterone. However, this may be counteracted by a continuation of sensitivity to the pressor effect, and preeclampsia may become superimposed.

If the glomeruli are damaged, filtration rate cannot increase to meet the demands of pregnancy. Nitrogenous waste cannot be removed from the bloodstream in sufficient quantities and build up in abnormal amounts in the bloodstream. Creatinine, uric acid, and urea levels rise in the serum and fall in the urine.

Increased excretion of nitrogenous waste into the sweat and saliva can produce a characteristic ammonia odor. This can also cause itching and irritation of the skin.

If tubular cells or the surrounding vasculature are damaged, the primary tubular functions are affected. Because the tubules serve as the major sodium pump, it is this function that is dramatically decreased. Sodium cannot be pulled into the urine fluid in the proximal tubule, and therefore water cannot follow. Urine output will then reflect this in a reduced volume with sodium remaining elevated in the blood and water increasing in the intravascular space. Sodium and water will therefore be increased in the tissues and result in edema.

If proteins are lost into the glomerular filtrate because of damage to the micropores, osmotic pressure changes and fluid is lost from the intravascular space into the tissue more readily. Because pregnancy favors increased spillage of protein, a marginal kidney function can cause greater likelihood of spillage of large quantities of protein into the urine.

As renal blood flow diminishes, increased renin activity occurs. The usual pregnancy vasodilation may no longer offset the pressor effects of renin-angiotensin and blood pressure will rise rapidly.

Signs and symptoms

Women with an acute renal infection exhibit specific symptoms of bladder infection or kidney infection. Bladder infection may be heralded by frequency, dysuria, and urgency of urination, suprapubic pain, or low back pain. Pyelonephritis is usually present when fever, chills, nausea, vomiting, malaise, and flank pain occur.

Chronic renal disease from other origins can be associated with generalized edema, proteinuria, increased blood pressure, and decreased urinary volume. These symptoms rarely worsen during pregnancy unless pregnancy-induced hypertension is superimposed on an impaired renal function.

Symptoms of increased nitrogenous waste products in the bloodstream include mental confusion, apathy, and itching of the skin. The quantity of urinary output may be diminished and the specific gravity will be low.

Signs of electrolyte imbalance, especially potassium, sodium, and calcium excess or deficits can appear. Signs of potassium excess include the following.
1. Plasma potassium above 5.6 mEq/liter
2. Electrocardiogram changes with a high T wave and depressed ST segment
3. Oliguria, intestinal colic, or diarrhea

Signs of potassium deficit include the following.
1. Plasma potassium below 4 mEq/liter
2. Heart block
3. Anorexia, gaseous distension of the intestine, or soft muscles

Signs of sodium excess include the following.
1. Plasma sodium greater than 147 mEq/liter
2. Specific gravity of urine above 1.030
3. Excitement, mania, convulsions, dry sticky mucous membranes, oliguria, or firm tissue turgor

Sodium deficit does not occur. Signs of calcium excess are listed below.
1. Plasma calcium above 5.8 mEq/liter
2. Heart block
3. Relaxed muscles, flank pain, or deep thigh pain

Signs of calcium deficit including the following.
1. Plasma calcium below 4.5 mEq/liter
2. Electrocardiogram changes in T wave and ST segments as in potassium excess
3. Convulsions, tingling of fingers, muscle cramps, tetany

Primary base bicarbonate deficit can occur because of the inability of the tubules to secrete buffers. Below are listed signs of metabolic acidosis.

1. Urine pH below 6.0
2. Plasma pH below 7.35
3. Disorientation, shortness of breath, or deep rapid breathing

If renal tissues are severely damaged from hypertensive lesions, diabetic nephropathic lesions, or infectious processes, the loss of intravascular osmotic pressure can produce systemic edema and pulmonary edema. Signs and symptoms of pulmonary edema are sudden in onset and include shortness of breath, rales, frothy sputum, and decreased pO_2.

Other signs of severe renal damage include serum potassium excess, which can lead to cardiac arrhythmias, dilation of the myocardium, and cardiac arrest. Serum calcium levels may also be low, with similar cardiac effects. Loss of buffering can lead to signs of metabolic acidosis including compensatory increase in respiratory rate.

Maternal effects

Infection in the urinary tract may predispose the woman to preterm labor. The exact mechanism is not clear and the cause and effect relationship is controversial (Alvarez, 1976). Certainly repeated urinary tract infection increases the likelihood of the same organisms infecting the fetal membranes.

Severe chronic renal impairment usually causes infertility, so it is rarely seen in pregnant women. Chronic renal impairment does not usually deteriorate during pregnancy unless severe preeclampsia or eclampsia is superimposed on the disease. If that occurs, lesions in the kidneys caused by preeclampsia or eclampsia can compromise what function is left and precipitate total renal failure (Alvarez, 1976).

Fetal and neonatal effects

Because of the loss of water from the plasma volume, circulation to the uterus can be diminished. The fetus can suffer nutritionally from the resultant deficiency. Intrauterine growth retardation is common in the fetus of a woman with renal disease. If hypertension is also present, arterial resistance to blood flow into the intervillous space can cause chronic hypoxemia of the fetus. Depending on the severity and chronicity of hypoxia, the fetus can suffer central nervous system damage and faces potential demise.

MEDICAL DIAGNOSIS

The diagnosis of asymptomatic or symptomatic bacteriuria is made by obtaining a clean-catch urine specimen and doing a quantitative urine culture. Bacteria of the same species greater than 10^5/ml of urine is significant. A presumptive diagnosis can be made on urinalysis with bacteria greater than 20 in centrifuged urine or white blood cells greater than 5 to 10 on HPF when symptoms are present. All pregnant women should be screened for asymptomatic bacteriuria with a quantitative urine culture early in their prenatal care.

Significant bacteriuria may represent either bladder or kidney infection. The differentiation is made by the symptoms presented. However, asymptomatic pyelonephritis can occur, just as bladder infection can be asymptomatic. Asymptomatic pyelonephritis should be suspected when urine cultures detect recurrent or persistent infection despite antibiotic therapy. It is for this reason that urine cultures should be repeated after a course of antibiotic therapy.

When disease or complications of pregnancy exist and there is renal impairment, renal function studies are usually done to ascertain the degree of impairment. It is therefore common to do renal function studies for baseline data in pregnant women who have class D or greater diabetes, have systemic lupus, have a history of chronic renal disease or chronic hypertension, or who develop pregnancy-induced hypertension. Such laboratory studies include 24-hour urine collection for creatinine clearance, serum creatinine, serum uric acid, blood urea nitrogen (BUN), and total urinary protein. Laboratory values differ in pregnancy beginning as early as 8 to 10 weeks of gestation. This should be considered when interpreting the results. Table 7-1 describes differences between nonpregnant and pregnant normal values.

Renal biopsy for diagnosis of a specific renal lesion is contraindicated during pregnancy because of the increased blood flow to the kidney. Increases in capillary pressures predispose the kidney to greater potential for hemorrhage, which can lead to further kidney damage.

The differentiation of chronic hypertension versus pregnancy-induced hypertension is made on the basis of persistent hypertension before 20 weeks of gestation. If preeclampsia does not develop, the differentiation can be made based on the existence or absence of generalized edema and proteinuria. Con-

TABLE 7-1. *Renal function studies*

Study	Nonpregnant normal value	Pregnant normal value
BUN	10 to 16 mg/100 ml	8.7 ± 1.5 mg/100 ml
Serum creatinine	0.67 to 0.17 mg/100 ml	0.46 to 0.6 mg/100 ml
Uric acid	4.2 ± 1.2 mg/100 ml	3 ± 0.17 mg/100 ml
Urinary creatinine clearance	100 mg/100 ml	140 mg/100 ml
24 hr urinary protein	Not different	Not greater than 300 mg/24 hr

Modified from Alvarez, R.: The kidney in pregnancy, New York, 1976, John Wiley and Sons, Inc., and Good Samaritan Medical Center Laboratory Manual, Phoenix, 1983.

current hypertension is not manifested by generalized edema nor often by proteinuria (Willis, 1982, and see Chapter 13).

Other diagnostic studies, such as renal ultrasound, can aid in the diagnosis of obstruction of the ureters or pyelonephritis. Radiographic studies, such as intravenous pyelogram, have rarely been used in pregnancy since the advent of sophisticated ultrasonic examinations.

USUAL MEDICAL MANAGEMENT

Treatment for renal disease in pregnancy depends on the nature of the disease. Urinary tract infection is treated with antibiotics. Asymptomatic and symptomatic bacteriuria are treated primarily with ampicillin because *Escherichia coli* is usually the causative organism. Antibiotic therapy must be continued in maximum doses for 10 to 14 days. High doses are required during pregnancy because of increased excretion due to greater renal blood flow. If reculture demonstrates continued bacterial growth, the course of antibiotics must be reinstituted for 6 weeks. Reculture is again done and, if positive, an antimicrobial such as nitrofurantoin can be continued for the duration of the pregnancy (Alvarez, 1976). If infection has been recurrent during the pregnancy or if acute pyelonephritis occurs, a postpartum intravenous pyelogram is often done to rule out an obstruction in the urinary tract.

The treatment for hypertensive renal disease is more complicated. The hypertension requires control with an antihypertensive drug. The urinary output and fluid intake must be closely monitored to prevent fluid overload. Salt solutions must be administered with great caution because of the inability to excrete large quantities of salt and the potential for overwhelming edema, especially in the lungs. Diuretics can be used to aid in excretion of retained fluid, and electrolyte balance must then be closely monitored. If acidosis occurs, lack of an adequate buffering system in the kidneys can create further problems when salt solutions must be administered for their alkalinizing effects.

The effects of hypertension, loss of protein, and retention of sodium and water can create a life-threatening situation for the mother. If the fetus has little chance of surviving, the choice for termination of the pregnancy should be offered to the mother. If the maternal condition is likely to deteriorate, the risks and benefits of continuing the pregnancy should be discussed with the woman and her significant other. Acute renal failure, which is rarely seen in pregnancy except with sepsis, dictates the termination of the pregnancy if the mother's life is to be saved.

For the pregnancy that continues, fetal evaluation will be ordered. Ultrasound examinations may be done every 2 weeks from 24 weeks on. Stress tests are usually ordered weekly after 26 weeks. Daily fetal activity charts should also be kept.

NURSING PROCESS
Prevention

Prevention of symptomatic urinary tract infections is greatly aided by nursing interventions. Pregnant women should be educated to practice correct perineal hygiene and to report any indication of vaginitis or a urinary tract infection.

Routine evaluation of the urine should be carried out at each office visit. The voided specimen should be fresh, not saved from home, and should be evaluated for protein and nitrites, which are produced in increased amounts when bacterial growth is significant. If protein is 1 + or more in the absence of pregnancy-induced hypertension or nitrites are evident, a clean-catch or sterile catheterized specimen should be obtained for urinalysis, culture, and sensitivity studies. The pregnant woman should be encouraged to drink at least 3,000 ml of fluid every 24 hours.

Prevention of complications from existing renal disease is also important. A careful history should include questions regarding repeated urinary tract infections, hypertension when not pregnant, and renal function studies if hypertension, diabetes, or collagen vascular diseases have been previously diagnosed. This information will help in screening those women at risk for complications such as preeclampsia, pulmonary edema, uteroplacental insufficiency, and progression of existing renal disease.

ASSESSMENT

Assessment by history and evaluation of the urine aids in the preventive aspects of renal disease in pregnancy. Women with persistent renal disease should be assessed for evidence of complications and signs of progression of the disease.

Blood pressure readings should be determined in the same arm and same position each visit. Elevations of greater than 10 to 15 mm Hg, both systolic and diastolic, are significant when taken 15 minutes apart or on two visits. Assessment for increased fluid retention should be made at each office visit. A weight gain of greater than 3 pounds in 1 week can be considered significant. In the hospitalized patient, weight should be assessed daily and a gain of 1 pound or more per day is significant.

For the hospitalized woman, careful assessment of fluid intake and output should be made. If intravenous fluids are given, hourly assessments of intake should be made. Output of less than 5,000 ml/24 hours is oliguria and less than 100 ml/24 hours is anuria.

Assessment for sodium excess, potassium excess or deficit, calcium excess or deficit, and metabolic acidosis must also be made in the hospitalized woman with marginal renal function. These assessments are made based on the symptoms that are presented.

Antepartum intervention

Interventions for the antepartum woman at risk for urinary tract infection are primarily directed at education in the preventive aspects. Proper perineal hygiene should be taught. The pregnant woman should be taught that cleansing of the perineal area should always be from the vulvar area to the rectal area, tissues should not be reused for subsequent cleansing, and soap and water cleansing should be practiced at least once each day.

Fluid intake should exceed 1,500 ml of liquids other than at mealtimes to help prevent infection. Because of other nutritional concerns, liquids providing calories without other nutrients should be avoided. High-acid fluid, such as coffee and tea, should also be avoided; the acid is converted and predisposes to alkaline urine, which favors bacterial growth. If a urinary tract infection is evident, these instructions are particularly important to prevent reflux of bacterial growth.

The woman with pyelonephritis will be initially treated with intravenous antibiotics. A mainline IV line is usually necessary to provide adequate fluid intake, especially if high fever accompanies the infection. Once symptoms improve, the intravenous antibiotic can be given through a heparin lock. Pain relief should also be provided with analgesics. If high fever has been present, nutritional supplements high in calories might be needed during recovery, and dietary consultation should be sought.

If marginal renal function is part of other disease processes, interventions are directed at prevention of complications such as fluid overload, retention, and pulmonary edema. Accurate titration of all intravenous fluids is extremely important. Left side lying should be encouraged to prevent vena cava compression and improve uterine blood flow.

If nitrogenous waste cannot be eliminated by the kidneys, skin care and adequate oral hygiene are important to prevent skin and mucous membrane ulcerations. Edema and bed rest reduce circulation to extremities and inspection and cleansing daily are important.

For the woman whose fetus is in jeopardy, concern is often directed at fetal well-being when emotional support is offered. However, if renal function is impaired, the woman might have considerable fear and concern for her own well-being. These concerns should be addressed and emotional support provided. Decisions regarding continuation versus termination of the pregnancy can result in frustration and conflict over the woman's desire for a child and her fear for her own life if the pregnancy continues. Couples need to be provided with time together and need to receive support from the nursing staff in their decisions for continuation or termination of the pregnancy. Spiritual assistance may be desired at this time as well.

For the woman with renal disease, especially when hypertension is part of the disease, fetal surveillance should be instituted by 26 weeks of gestation.

The pregnant woman should have the purpose and frequency of the tests explained. Fetal activity charts should be started daily.

The woman with hypertension may not require hospitalization in the early part of her pregnancy if a family member can be taught how to monitor her blood pressure daily at home. A record should be kept and brought on each office visit. Consistent changes of 10 to 15 mm Hg or greater should be reported. Counseling should include the probability of home bed rest and the necessity of eventual hospitalization before delivery. Signs of disease progression, such as headache, vision changes, rapid weight gain, epigastric pain, and decreased urinary output, should be reported.

If the woman must be hospitalized, assistance may be needed in arranging for the care of her family. Financial concerns may also worry the family, and social service consultation should be obtained. When hospitalization can be anticipated, consultation should be sought before hospitalization.

Referral to a dietician will supplement other care. Dietary intake may require adjustments of sodium intake, potassium replacement, protein supplements, and adequate caloric intake to protect from increased protein catabolism. Because the kidney forms an enzyme favoring red blood cell formation, women with kidney damage may have a reduced capacity to increase red blood cell mass. Iron and folate supplements must therefore be provided.

Intervention—drug therapy

The hypertensive pregnant woman with renal disease is treated with antihypertensives and diuretics. The antihypertensives of choice are usually methyldopa (Aldomet) or hydralazine. Home instruction should include information about possible side effects such as light-headedness or extreme lethargy. Both of the drugs should be taken at the same times each day.

Diuretics are often used if fluid retention is contributing to hypertension. They also help to prevent pulmonary edema. Any diuretic can cause electrolyte imbalance. The pregnant woman should be instructed especially to report signs of potassium deficit and to help prevent this condition with an increased dietary intake of potassium. Bananas and citrus fruits are high in potassium.

Antimicrobials will be prescribed for urinary tract infections. It is important, for maintenance of blood levels, to administer them at evenly spaced intervals. The woman should be instructed to ingest increased fluids and to take the entire prescription. In the hospital setting, when antimicrobials are given intravenously, there should be inspection of the site for an inflammatory reaction. The site should also be changed every 48 hours to prevent phlebitis.

Tetracyclines are contraindicated for use in pregnancy because of rare maternal acute fatty liver necrosis. In addition, they bind with calcium orthophosphates and cause a permanent yellow staining of the fetal dentition. Chloramphenicol is not used in pregnancy because of the fatal gray syndrome that occurs in infants born of mothers receiving the drug. Sulfonamides and nitrofurantoin are contraindicated somewhat in the last trimester because of their potential for increasing levels of fetal bilirubin.

Intrapartum intervention

Intrapartum intervention for the care of the mother with renal impairment includes cardiac monitoring, hemodynamic monitoring, and careful regulation of fluid infusion. If intravenous oxytocin is used, the concurrent stimulation of the antidiuretic hormone increases the potential for fluid retention.

The laboring woman should be positioned on her left side to provide optimal renal blood flow and optimal blood flow to the fetus. Continuous fetal monitoring is important to detect early signs of fetal distress such as late decelerations. Oxygen may be administered to the woman at 10 liters/min by tight facemask to improve oxygenation to the fetus. If the fetus is growth retarded, oligohydramnios can predispose the fetus to cord compression. Variable decelerations should be responded to by changing maternal position and observing for tachycardia or loss of variability.

If the baby is to be delivered by cesarean section, preparations should be made for regional anesthesia. In the presence of renal impairment, most general anesthesia is contraindicated. The nurse must remember that a fluid load cannot be given prior to regional anesthesia in the presence of kidney involvement.

Because of intrusive monitoring of the mother, necessitating frequent assessments by more than one member of the health care team, provision must be made for a quiet atmosphere. The birth experience allows for few choices, but inclusion of the significant other should be encouraged.

The nursery personnel should be notified well in advance of the delivery so that preparations for neonatal support and resuscitation can be made. The infant may be extremely premature, and parents may desire the presence of clergy for early blessing or baptism.

Postpartum intervention

If urinary tract infection was present prior to delivery, postpartum lochia provides an excellent medium for relapse. Frequent perineal care, at least every 2 hours during the first 12 hours, should be instituted. Fluids should be encouraged to at least 200 ml/hr.

When hypertension remains severe (BP greater than 160/110), invasive maternal monitoring must continue until the blood pressure is stabilized. This will result in separation from the neonate, especially the extremely premature neonate. Therefore the significant other should be encouraged to visit, take pictures, and keep the mother informed to facilitate the development of parenting bonds.

If renal disease has progressed during the pregnancy, the woman may need to be transferred to a renal dialysis intensive care setting. This move can further strain the tasks of parenthood.

EVALUATION

It is of paramount importance during pregnancy to prevent a urinary tract infection whether asymptomatic or symptomatic bacteriuria is present. Education in preventive measures is essential. Instruction as to the importance of reporting any developing symptoms should also be included.

SUGGESTED PLAN

Renal disease and pregnancy

Potential patient problem	Outcome criteria
A. Potential asymptomatic urinary tract infection related to: Asymptomatic bacteriuria	Normal urinalysis as indicated by Bacteriuria less than 10^5/ml or urine Proteinuria less than 1 + Negative nitrites
B. Potential symptomatic urinary tract infection related to: Symptomatic bacteriuria Increased urinary stasis during pregnancy Increased excretion of nutrients in urine	Normal urinalysis No evidence of bladder or kidney infection such as fever malaise painful urination flank pain

Symptomatic infections require care to prevent complications that may ensue such as permanent scarring of renal tissue and impairment of function. Early reporting of symptoms and administration of antimicrobials should accomplish this.

If renal function is impaired, the goal of therapy should include maintenance of electrolyte, fluid, and acid-base balance along with prevention of fetal distress and further maternal morbidity.

Neonatal outcome may have to be compromised if maternal renal function is impaired. The goal then is to provide support for decision making and coping mechanisms.

O F   N U R S I N G   C A R E

Assessment and intervention

Dx. Check urine for nitrites and protein each office visit and each day for the hospitalized patient

Th. Collect a clean-catch for catheterized specimen for culture and sensitivity if either of the above are positive

Prepare for antibiotic therapy for 2 weeks

Ed. Teach correct perineal hygiene, such as cleaning from front to back and not rewiping, using soap and water at least each day

Teach to report signs of vaginitis so early treatment can be instituted

Fluid intake of 3,000 ml/day

Ref. Report to physician signs of asymptomatic bacterium

Dx. Refer to clean-catch or catheterized specimen of urine for bacteriuria of same species of 10^5/ml urine

Check centrifuged urine specimen for greater than 20 bacteria or more than 5 to 10 on HPF microscope

Assess for relief of symptoms

Th. Administer antibiotics as ordered for 2 weeks

Reculture urine after 1 month

Administer analgesic as ordered

Ed. Instruct to increase fluid intake, especially water, to 3,000 ml/24 hr

Ref. Report to physician a fever greater than 100.4° F

Dietary assistance with increased fluid needs

Dx., diagnostic; Th., therapeutic; Ed., education; Ref., referral.   *Continued.*

Renal disease and pregnancy—cont'd

Potential patient problem	Outcome criteria

C. Potential hypertension related to:
    Continued sensitivity to increased renin
    Superimposed renal disease
    Superimposed preeclampsia or eclampsia
	Maintenance of BP between 110/70 and 130/90

D. Potential fetal distress related to:
    Hypertension
    Intrauterine growth retardation
    Uteroplacental insufficiency
	Continued fetal well-being as evidenced by adequate growth and normal fetal survey on ultrasound
	reactive negative CST
	at least four fetal movements in 1 hr each day

E. Potential renal failure related to:
    Preexisting marginal renal function
	Urinary output of greater than 30 ml/hr or 120 ml/4 hr
	Renal function studies normal
	  BUN—8.7 ± 1.5 mg/100 ml
	  Serum creatinine—0.46 to 0.6 mg/100 ml
	  Uric acid—3 ± 0.17 mg/100 ml
	  Urinary creatinine not less than 140 mg/100 ml
	  24 hr urinary protein not greater than 300 mg/24 hr

F. Potential fluid overload related to:
    Renal failure
    Loss of protein
    Retention of Na
    Retention of water
	No evidence of pulmonary edema or excessive generalized edema

Assessment and intervention

Dx. Check BP each office visit or each 8 hr if hospitalized
Th. Administer antihypertensive and diuretic as prescribed
Encourage bed rest with BRP
Ed. Instruct in side effects of antihypertensive such as light-headedness
Instruct in dietary intake of increased potassium and decreased sodium (not less than 2.5 gm/day)
Instruct in side effects of decreased potassium such as muscle weakness
Instruct in home monitoring of own BP
Instruct in need for modified bed rest
Ref. Dietician for decreased sodium (2.5 to 4 gm daily) and increased potassium
Report to physician BP greater than 140/90

Dx. Observe all fetal monitor strips for normal baseline FHR, average variability, absence of late decelerations
Th. Begin antepartum FHR testing by 26 weeks
Begin fetal activity chart record at 26 weeks
Facilitate uterine blood flow by encouraging left side lying and bed rest except for bathroom privileges
Prepare for ultrasound examinations at ordered times
Prepare for emergency cesarean delivery after 26 weeks if ominous signs of fetal distress are present
Ed. Explain all testing
Ref. Report immediately to physician decreased fetal activity
Report to physician FHR signs of fetal distress

Dx. Refer to laboratory data for deviation from normals
Accurate observation of intake and output
Observe for signs of renal failure such as less than 30 ml urine every hour, electrolyte imbalance, mental confusion, or apathy
Th. Careful titration of IV fluids
Prepare for Na restriction
Prepare for infusion of salt poor plasma to replace protein loss
Prepare for pregnancy termination
Ed. Explain all tests and procedures
Ref. Renal dialysis team if appropriate

Dx. Listen to chest for rales
Check daily weight
Assess for pitting dependent edema
Th. Use salt-poor IV fluids if IV fluid is ordered
Increase protein intake as ordered
Prepare for hemodynamic monitoring
Ref. Report to physician weight gain of greater than 2 pounds per day
Report to physician signs of pulmonary edema

Continued.

Renal disease and pregnancy—cont'd

Potential patient problem	*Outcome criteria*

G. Potential anxiety or fear related to:
    Maternal effects
    Fetal/neonatal effects
	Verbalizes feelings
	Seeks support of significant others
	Seeks early contact with neonate if viable

REFERENCES

Alvarez, R.: The kidney in pregnancy, New York, 1976, John Wiley & Sons, Inc.

Chesley, L.: Disorders of kidney, fluids and electrolytes. In Assali, N., editor: Pathophysiology of gestation, vol. 1, New York, 1972, Academic Press, Inc.

Clark, A., and Alfonso, D.: Childbearing: a nursing perspective, Philadelphia, 1979, F.A. Davis Co.

Danforth, D.: Obstetrics and gynecology, ed. 3, Hagerstown, Md., 1977, Harper & Row, Inc.

Davison, J.: Physiological adjustments in pregnancy. In Hytten, E.F., editor: Clinics in obstetrics and gynecology, Philadelphia, 1975, W.B. Saunders Co.

Hytten, F., and Leitch, I.: The physiology of human pregnancy, Oxford, 1971, Blackwell Scientific Publications.

Jensen, M., Benson, R., and Bobak, J.: Maternity and gynecologic care: the nurse and the family, St. Louis, 1985, The C.V. Mosby Co.

Assessment and intervention

Dx. Assess coping and adaptive behaviors of both parents
Assess attachment behaviors of parents
Th. Encourage discussion of feelings
Encourage frequent and prolonged visitation with significant others if hospitalized
Ed. Maintain free flow of information about neonate if in intensive care
Ref. To support services such as social service, clergy, grief counselor
Neonatal intensive care personnel

Kelly, M., and Mongiello, R.: Hypertension in pregnancy: labor, delivery, and postpartum, AJN **82**:83, 1982.

Niswander, K.: Manual of obstetrics, Boston, 1980, Little, Brown & Co.

Olds, S., and others: Obstetric nursing, Menlo Park, Calif., 1980, Addison-Wesley Publishing Co.

Perez, R.: Protocols for perinatal nursing practice, St. Louis, 1981, The C.V. Mosby Co.

Pritchard, J., and MacDonald, P.: Williams' obstetrics, New York, 1980, Appleton-Century-Crofts, Inc.

Quinn, E., and Kass, E.: Biology of pyelonephritis, Boston, 1960, Little, Brown & Co.

Reeder, S., Mastroianni, L., and Martin, L.: Maternity nursing, Philadelphia, 1980, J.B. Lippincott Co.

Willis, S.: Hypertension in pregnancy: pathophysiology, AJN **82**:793, 1982.

Willis, S., and Sharp, E.: Hypertension in pregnancy: prenatal detection and management, AJN **82**:798, 1982.

UNIT IV

COMPLICATIONS
IN PREGNANCY

Various complications can develop during the course of a pregnancy that can affect the health and well-being of the mother and fetus and the outcome of the pregnancy. With early recognition and the advanced technology of today, the incidence of maternal and perinatal mortality and morbidity resulting from these complications is declining. However, the current maternal mortality is still 6.9 per 100,000 live births. Hemorrhage is the number one cause of maternal mortality. Infections, anesthesia, and pregnancy-induced hypertension are other causes. In order to continue to reduce the maternal mortality and further decrease maternal morbidity related to these complications, the maternity nurse needs an in-depth understanding of these complications of pregnancy.

The next nine chapters present a physiologic and pathologic basis of the most common complications of pregnancy and outline appropriate nursing care that can provide a basis for early recognition and effective management.

CHAPTER 8

Spontaneous abortion

A spontaneous abortion is a natural termination of pregnancy before the fetus has reached viability. According to the World Health Organization, a fetus of less than 20 weeks of gestation and weighing less than 500 gm is not considered viable. They further divide abortions into "early" and "late." An early abortion occurs before 12 weeks of gestation, and a late abortion occurs between 12 and 20 weeks of gestation. A spontaneous abortion is commonly referred to as a *miscarriage* and this term is preferred in talking with patients because the word abortion is frequently associated with induced abortions.

INCIDENCE

It is difficult to determine how many pregnancies end in spontaneous abortion; many are thought to be a delayed menstrual period. In these cases, the state of pregnancy is not identified. Therefore spontaneous abortion has commonly been quoted to occur in 10% to 20% of all pregnancies. Boue and Boue (1978) report statistically that the mean incidence of spontaneous abortion is 15%, but according to Roberts and Lowe (1975) at least 75% of all human conceptions are aborted.

ETIOLOGY

Early abortions are likely to be caused by a nonrecurring genetic abnormality of the embryo or fetus (Poland and Yuen, 1978). Several studies substantiate the fact that 50% to 60% of most early abortions before 12 weeks of gestation have a chromosome abnormality (Boue and Boue, 1978). The majority of these chromosomal abnormalities are related to numerical error occurring during meiotic cell division of the ovum or sperm or early mitotic cell division of the zygote or blastocyst. If two sperm penetrate one ovum, this can also lead to a chromosomal abnormality. The chromosomal makeup of both parents is usually normal (Pritchard and MacDonald, 1980). Abnormal development of the placenta can also lead to an early spontaneous abortion.

Late abortions are usually related to maternal or external factors and the fetus is often chromosomally healthy (Poland and Yuen, 1978). Maternal factors that can contribute to an abortion are exposure to or contact with such teratogenic agents as radiation, chemicals, drugs, viruses, alcohol, smoking, poor nutrition, and uterine disorders. Viruses that are known to cause congenital malformations and stimulate abortions are rubella, cytomegalovirus (CMV), active herpes, and toxoplasmosis if contracted during pregnancy. Occasionally, acute pneumonia or influenza has caused an abortion. It is not known whether the organism itself or the toxins liberated by the organism cause the fetal death. Systemic diseases that are not well controlled such as diabetes, sickle cell anemia, hypertensive cardiovascular disease, and thyroid imbalance can cause abortion. Uterine disorders that may elicit an abortion include the following.

1. An abnormal uterine environment that interferes with implantation and nourishment of the blastocyst
2. Structural uterine defects that interfere with the growth and development of the embryo or fetus
3. A weak cervix that dilates before term

There is no proven relationship between external physical trauma or emotional stress and an increased risk of abortion.

Guerrero and Rojas (1975) noted in their study of spontaneous abortions that the postmature gamete, sperm or ovum, increased the chance of abortion. The more time the gamete spent in the fallopian tube before fertilization the greater the risk of abortion.

A small number of spontaneous abortions are related to an immunologic factor. This occurs when the mother and father are genetically similar and share a significant number of major antigens but are different enough to arouse the mother's immune system defenses. Then the mother's immune system fails to produce the IgG-blocking antibody that protects the embryo and fetus against maternal lymphocytes.

Another small number of spontaneous abortions are related to a luteal phase defect. This occurs when the corpus luteum fails to secrete significant amounts of progesterone and estrogen to maintain the endometrial lining of the uterus and the pregnancy.

PHYSIOLOGY
Normal

The gametes, sperm and ovum, undergo developmental changes prior to fertilization. During the maturation process, the number of chromosomes is reduced to 23, which is half the original number. This process is called *meiosis*. When fertilization takes place and a mature sperm enters the mature ovum, the 23 chromosomes from each gamete pair up to form a new cell with 46 chromosomes called the *zygote*. This new cell begins mitotic cell division. When the zygote has developed into a solid ball of cells, it is called a *morula*. As maturation continues, the morula develops into a *blastocyst*. At this stage, there is an outer layer of cells called the *trophoblast,* which will form the placenta and fetal membranes, and an inner cluster of cells called the *embryoblast,* which will form the embryo. On approximately the sixth day following fertilization, the blastocyst is ready to implant into the endometrium of the uterus. This is accomplished as the trophoblast cells begin to secrete a proteolytic enzyme that digests an opening a few cells wide and burrows its way into the uterine lining. A small amount of blood may be lost at this time, which can cause mild vaginal spotting. The opening is closed by a blood clot at first and then regenerated epithelium. After the blastocyst is implanted into the endometrium of the uterus, the endometrium is called the *decidua*. The decidua is usually divided into three parts. The part of the decidua lying directly beneath the implanted blastocyst is called *decidua basalis*. This is where the placenta will primarily grow. The part of the decidua that covers the buried blastocyst is called *decidua capsularis,* and the remainder of the decidua that is not in direct contact with the blastocyst is called *decidua vera.*

Following ovulation, when the mature ovum is released from the ovary, the ovary enters its luteal phase. During this time it excretes high levels of progesterone and some estrogen to prepare and maintain the endometrium for the fertilized ovum. Both hormones stimulate the glandular cells of the endometrium to secrete mucus and glycogen and increase the blood supply to the endometrium to facilitate an adequate nutritional environment for the implanted blastocyst/embryo/fetus. These hormones also facilitate the maintenance of pregnancy by keeping the myometrium quiet so that implantation can take place. For the corpus luteum to continue its production of progesterone and estrogen, the trophoblastic tissue must secrete human chorionic gonadotropin (HCG) until the placenta is mature enough to take over the production of hormones. This hormone maintains the corpus luteum for approximately the first 8 weeks of gestation.

Why the mother's body does not reject the blastocyst remains a mystery. On the surface of all body cells there are structural antigens. The lymphocyte white blood cells are able to identify these antigens as either familiar or unfamiliar/foreign and manufacture antibodies to destroy them if they are identified as foreign. Because the antigens are determined genetically, half the antigens on fetal cells come from each parent. Therefore half the antigens should be foreign to the mother's body.

Currently it is unknown what mechanism or mechanisms prevent the rejection of the fetus. Several theories are being considered. First, the blood supply of the fetus and mother is kept fairly separate. Secondly, the embryo or fetus is surrounded by trophoblastic tissue. This tissue prevents fetal lymphocytes from entering the maternal system freely. However sensitized, T cells capable of destroying the embryo or fetus have been identified in the pregnant woman's bloodstream (Scott, 1982). Therefore these two theories cannot totally explain the immunology of pregnancy. Some of the latest research is beginning to indicate that when the mother's lymphocytes identify the foreign paternal antigens on the products of conception her immunologic system produces an IgG-blocking antibody that prevents further recognition of these foreign antigens (Beer, 1981). This decreases the immune response of the mother toward the embryo or fetus.

Another important structure that also facilitates the maintenance of pregnancy is the cervix. The cervix must resist the forces of gravity and intrauterine pressure for 9 months of pregnancy and then become soft and distensible, allowing the fetus to pass through. Therefore the cervix undergoes extensive changes during pregnancy. The composition of the cervix allows for these. The cervix is composed primarily of connective tissue and elastin, with some scattered smooth muscle fibers (Leppert et al., 1982). The connective tissue is composed of collagen fibers and a ground substance (Norstrom, 1982). The collagen fibers give the cervix elasticity and make it resistant to tears; the elastin and ground substance allow it to stretch and retract. Numerous cervical glands line the cervical canal. The cervical canal contains a sphincter at both ends called the *internal os* and the *external os*. During pregnancy, hypertrophy and hyperplasia of the cervical glands occur, ground substance and elastin are increased, and the number of collagen fibers is decreased (Liggins, 1978).

Pathophysiology

Death of the embryo or failure of the embryo or placenta to develop normally is usually the first step in the sequence of events that leads to a spontaneous abortion. Hemorrhage into the decidua basalis results, which causes necrotic changes at the site of implantation. Infiltration of leukocytes follows. Because of the absence of a functioning fetal circulation, the chorionic villi often become edematous and resemble a hydatidiform mole. At the same time, hormonal levels of progesterone and estrogen drop, causing decidual sloughing, which results in vaginal bleeding. The uterus becomes irritable and uterine contractions result.

In the presence of an incompetent cervix, the sphincter control of the cervix has been lost and with increased intrauterine pressure the cervix begins to dilate and efface. This allows the amniotic sac to begin to bulge into the vagina, which causes it to rupture or allows it to become infected.

Signs and symptoms

The classical sign of a spontaneous abortion is vaginal bleeding. Initially it is usually dark spotting related to the decreased hormonal levels of progesterone and estrogen that causes the decidua (endometrium) to begin to slough. It may progress to frank, bright red bleeding as the products of conception begin to separate, opening up uterine blood vessels.

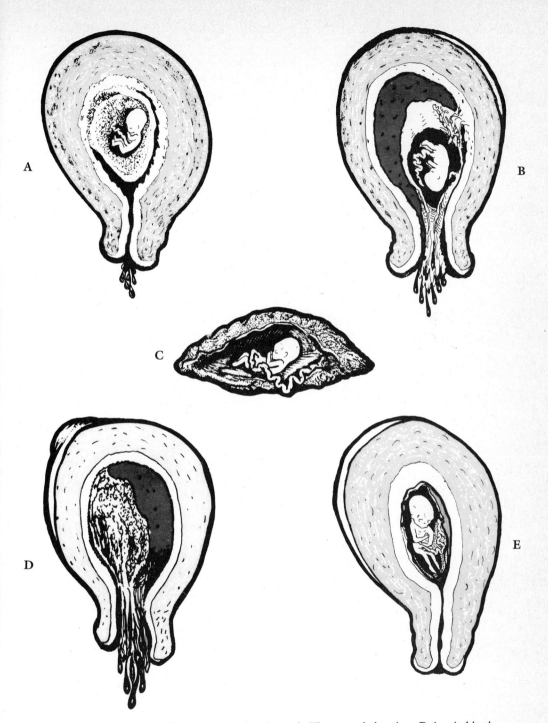

FIG. 8-1. Types of spontaneous abortions. **A,** Threatened abortion; **B,** inevitable abortion; **C,** complete abortion; **D,** incomplete abortion; **E,** missed abortion. (Illustration by Vincenza Genovese, Phoenix, Ariz. Modified from Netter, F.: Ciba collection of medical illustrations, Vol. 2, reproductive system, Summit, N.J., 1965, Ciba Pharmaceutical Co.)

TABLE 8-1. *Clinical classification of spontaneous abortions*

Classification	Definition	Manifestations
Threatened	A condition in which the continuation of the pregnancy is in doubt	Vaginal bleeding or spotting, which may or may not be associated with mild cramps of the back and lower abdomen A closed cervix A uterus that is soft, nontender, and enlarged appropriate to gestational age
Inevitable	A condition in which termination of the pregnancy is in progress	Cervical dilatation is present Membranes may or may not be ruptured Vaginal bleeding Mild to painful uterine contractions
Complete	A condition in which the passage of the products of conception is totally expelled from the uterus	
Incomplete	A condition in which fragments of the products of conception are expelled and part are retained in the uterus	Profuse bleeding because the retained tissue parts interfere with myometrial contractions
Missed	A condition in which the embryo or fetus dies during the first 20 weeks of gestation but is retained in the uterus for 4 weeks or more afterwards	Amenorrhea or intermittent vaginal bleeding, spotting, or brownish discharge No uterine growth No fetal movement felt Regression of breast changes
Septic	A condition in which the products of conception become infected during the abortion process	An elevated temperature of 100.4° F (38° C) or greater Foul-smelling vaginal discharge
Habitual	A condition in which two or more successive pregnancies have ended in a spontaneous abortion	

Spontaneous abortions are classified into seven clinical types: threatened, inevitable, complete, incomplete, missed, septic, and habitual (Fig. 8-1). Signs and symptoms manifested by each type are outlined in Table 8-1.

Maternal effects

According to Selik, Cates, and Tyler (1981), the major causes that contribute to a maternal death surrounding a spontaneous abortion are the following.
1. Hemorrhage related to a delay of the patient in seeking medical treatment or perforation of the uterus during surgical treatment
2. Infection related to a delay in diagnosing a septic abortion or inappropriate use of antibiotics

However, the actual incidence is very small.

The largest maternal effect is the risk of a subsequent abortion. Poland and associates (1977) found the risk of a subsequent abortion to be 46%. Warburton and Fraser (1961) report the risk to be 24% after one abortion, 26% after two, and 32% after three. The risk appears to be less if the woman has carried a prior pregnancy to term (Schoenbaum et al., 1980). The significant increase is in women who have had consecutive abortions with identifiable abnormalities. They have a 50% chance of a subsequent abortion.

Fetal and neonatal effects

Death of the fetus always occurs as the result of a spontaneous abortion, or it is the actual cause of the abortion.

MEDICAL DIAGNOSIS

When vaginal bleeding occurs during the first 20 weeks of pregnancy, careful evaluation must be made to determine whether it is a threatened abortion or the bleeding is related to another cause. About 20% of all patients experience some vaginal bleeding during the first trimester and only about half of these actually abort (Cavanagh and Comas, 1977). Therefore consideration must be given to other possible causes of vaginal bleeding which can be related to one of the following.

1. Lesions of the cervix or vagina or cervical polyps that bleed due to increase vascularity of the vagina and cervix during pregnancy
2. A hydatidiform mole
3. An ectopic pregnancy
4. Carcinoma of the cervix
5. Normal implantation of the blastocyst into the endometrium

The evaluation to differentiate between the various possible causes of vaginal bleeding usually includes inspecting the vagina and cervix by a speculum examination to rule out vaginal or cervical lesions or cervical polyps and a Pap smear to rule out carcinoma. Ultrasound examination is usually done to determine if there is an intrauterine gestational sac. This rules out an ectopic pregnancy. A gestational sac, if present, should be identifiable with ultrasound by 6 weeks from the last menstrual period. Serial ultrasounds can be used to document lack of fetal growth, which indicates fetal death. Serial radioimmunoassay tests for human chorionic gonadatropin (HCG) can also be done to determine whether the HCG levels continue to rise rapidly or drop prior to 100 days of gestation. (HCG normally begins to drop after approximately 100 days of gestation.) If the HCG levels drop significantly or become negative prior to this time, this indicates fetal death. However, a positive HCG does not indicate a live embryo or fetus; trophoblastic tissue can continue to produce HCG for as long as 2 weeks following fetal death.

If the patient presents with signs of an inevitable abortion, tests are not usually necessary to make the diagnosis. Any patient with a history of cervical trauma or painless second trimester abortion should be examined weekly during the second trimester for an incompetent cervix.

USUAL MEDICAL MANAGEMENT

Most often, when vaginal bleeding is definitely related to a spontaneous abortion, treatment centers around determining the cause, if possible, keeping the couple informed, and providing emotional support instead of attempting to sustain the pregnancy. This protocol is based on the following factors.
1. In an early threatened abortion, the embryo or fetus is usually dead before the bleeding begins.
2. Approximately 60% of all early abortions are associated with chromosomal anomalies and are nature's way of preventing the birth of a genetically defective child.
3. In late abortions, after 12 weeks of gestation, maternal factors are usually the cause and death does not usually precede the vaginal bleeding. However, if the pregnancy is maintained, studies indicate that the bleeding itself can increase perinatal mortality or the risk of developing congenital abnormalities (South and Naldrett, 1973).
4. Controlled studies have also failed to prove that bed rest, hormones such as progesterone, or sedatives have any effect on the outcome of a threatened abortion.
5. Administration of medications during organogenesis (weeks 3 to 8) exposes the embryo to possible teratogenic effects.

Threatened abortion

When a threatened abortion is diagnosed, an assessment is done to determine the probable outcome. Prompt evacuation of the uterus must be carried out if any of the following findings is present.
1. Bleeding has become excessive
2. Any part of the products of conception have been lost
3. The cervix shows signs of dilatation
4. There are signs and symptoms of an intrauterine infection
5. There is a definite diagnosis of a dead fetus

To assess for the presence of one of these negative findings, a medical workup is done that usually includes the following.
1. A pelvic examination to determine signs of dilatation
2. A blood count for red blood cells, hemoglobin, and hematocrit to aid in the determination of the amount of blood lost and the presence or absence of anemia
3. A blood count for white blood cells (WBC) to determine whether or not an infection is present

If the assessment does not reveal a negative finding, then the patient is usually managed as an outpatient with frequent physician's visits and instructed to limit her activity and abstain from intercourse. If an IUD is in place, it is usually removed. Hormonal therapy with estrogen and progesterone is not usually recommended when signs of possible abortion are present. Further treatment depends on the signs and symptoms that develop.

Inevitable, complete, or incomplete abortion

Once the cervix begins to dilate, there is no hope for the pregnancy and an abortion becomes inevitable. If part of the products of conception are lost, then the abortion becomes incomplete, and, if all the products of conception are lost, then the abortion is complete.

From the time an abortion becomes inevitable until it becomes complete, naturally or with surgical intervention, there is a high risk for complications such as hemorrhage or an infection. The risk of hemorrhage usually correlates with the gestational age of the pregnancy. For the first 6 weeks, the placenta is very tentatively attached to the decidua of the uterus. Therefore, if a spontaneous abortion occurs prior to 6 weeks of gestation, the bleeding usually takes the form of a heavy menstrual period. Between 6 and 12 weeks of gestation, the chorionic villi of the placenta begin to grow into the myometrium of the uterus, and, by week 12 or shortly after, the chorionic villi have deeply penetrated into the myometrium. If a spontaneous abortion occurs after the placenta has completed its penetration process (week 12), the fetus is usually expelled prior to placental separation. Bleeding is usually held in check by the placenta until it is separated and then by uterine contractions if the separation is complete. Therefore the most severe bleeding is seen between 6 and 12 weeks of gestation because the placenta can detach prior to expulsion of the fetus, or severe bleeding can result after 12 weeks of gestation if the placenta does not separate completely and parts are retained. Thus, if the gestational age is known, the risk of bleeding can be more easily estimated.

The risk of infection usually depends on many factors, such as the nutritional state of the patient, perineal hygiene, and whether or not anything, except a sterile speculum, entered the vagina after dilatation had begun to take place.

Prompt evacuation of the uterus is the focus of treatment to prevent these complications. This is usually carried out by either curettage, vacuum aspiration, or injection of oxytocin intravenously followed by curettage. If vacuum aspiration is used to remove the products of conception, a vacuum aspirator suction curet is inserted through the dilated cervix after the patient is anesthetized. The vacuum aspirator is moved gently over the surface of the uterine wall in a systematic pattern so as to cover all of the uterine cavity and the products of conception are collected in a vacuum container. When curettage is done, a sharp curet, a spoon-shaped instrument, is gently moved in downward strokes over the uterine wall in order to remove the products of conception and the necrotic decidua.

These procedures can be done in an outpatient setting or in the hospital. The woman is usually hospitalized if gestational age is 12 weeks or greater or if severe bleeding or signs of infection are present. If time permits, a history and physical examination are usually performed and a complete blood count is done. A tube of blood is usually held for typing and cross matching in case a transfusion becomes necessary. A dilute solution of intravenous oxytocin is often started prior to the surgery to reduce blood loss and decrease the risk of uterine perforation by causing the uterus to contract and thicken. A preoperative medication of 5 to 10 mg of diazepam (Valium) may be ordered. The procedure can be done with a paracervical block, especially if an outpatient setting is used, or under a light general anesthesia. If done under a local, the patient may experience some cramping sensations during the procedure.

If the bleeding is severe, the patient's vital signs must be stabilized prior to surgery. This is usually accomplished by transfusing whole blood or administering Ringer's lactate intravenously with 30 U of oxytocin per 1,000 ml. If Ringer's lactate with oxytocin is used, the IV infusion is usually set to infuse at 200 ml/hr or more. This large dose of oxytocin is needed during the first half of pregnancy because the uterus is less sensitive to oxytocin at this time due to the low levels of estrogen present to potentiate its effect. If signs of infection are present or develop, antibiotic therapy is usually initiated.

If the cervix is not partially dilated, dilatation is usually accomplished slowly by placing a laminaria tent or prostaglandin suppository or gel in the cervix prior to the evacuation procedure. A laminaria is a seaweed, the stems of which have been peeled, dried, and sterilized. It is placed in the entire length of the cervical canal and absorbs the cervical secretions, which causes it to swell to about five times its dry size, thereby dilating the cervix (Fig. 8-2). The patient may experience cramping, which is easily controlled with a mild analgesic. Then at the time of surgery or prior to the evacuation procedure the laminaria is removed. Serial applications of prostaglandin gel or vaginal suppositories placed in the cervix can accomplish the same result. According to Laversen and associates (1982), prostaglandin E_2 suppositories are the most effective and cause the fewest side effects. Because both methods dilate the cervix slowly, they decrease the risk of cervical trauma, which can occur with mechanical dilators.

If all the embryonic or fetal and placental tissue can be identified and there are no signs of bleeding or an infection, the abortion is complete and no surgical intervention is necessary. However, some physicians believe that all abor-

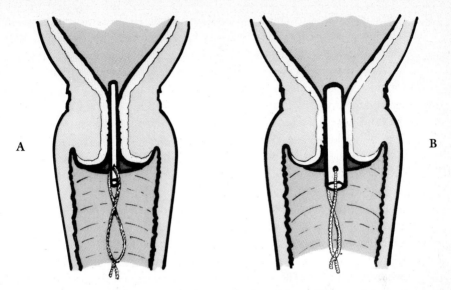

FIG. 8-2. A, Properly inserted laminaria. **B,** Laminaria after 18 hours of absorbing cervical fluid causing it to swell and dilate the cervix gradually. (Illustration by Vincenza Genovese, Phoenix, Ariz. Modified from Pritchard, J., and MacDonald, P.: Williams' obstetrics, ed. 16, New York, 1980, Appleton-Century-Crofts, Inc.)

tions should be considered incomplete until curettage is performed in order to remove the necrotic decidual tissue. Therefore some physicians routinely do curettage after all abortions.

Missed abortion

In the past, missed abortions were left untreated until the patient spontaneously expelled the products of conception and then a uterine curettage was performed. Today, when a fetus is known to be dead, the physician usually evacuates the uterus as soon as possible because of the following potential problems.

1. Psychologic stress related to carrying a dead fetus
2. Sepsis
3. Disseminated intravascular coagulation (DIC), a coagulation defect with hypofibrinogenemia, increased fibrin, and decreased platelets; this occurs because the dead products of conception release thromboplastin into the maternal circulation stimulating this process (see Chapter 12).

The techniques used for the evacuation usually depend on the length of pregnancy. Pregnancies up to 12 weeks of gestation are usually terminated by dilatation and evacuation by curettage or vacuum aspiration. Vacuum aspiration is preferable to curettage during the first 10 weeks of gestation; there is less chance of perforation, bleeding, or infection. After 12 weeks, the likelihood of uterine perforation, cervical lacerations, hemorrhage, incomplete removal of the products of conception, and infection are the usual reasons given for not using curettage or vacuum aspiration. However, many obstetricians advocate the use of dilatation and evacuation by curettage or vacuum aspiration and have found it effective without undue risks up to 16 weeks of gestation (Cadesky et al., 1981; Grimes and Gates, 1978; Hodari et al., 1977). Therefore the method to be used between 12 and 16 weeks gestation is in obstetrical controversy. Suction curettage may be used. Serial intramuscular injections of prostaglandin are quite successful, but intraamniotic instillations are not yet effective. Various prostaglandin preparations are being used from 16 to 20 weeks of gestation.

Prostaglandins can be administered orally, parenterally, into the amniotic sac, or as a vaginal suppository. The oral method is not used because of the extreme uncomfortable side effects, such as severe GI distress. All other routes are being used in order to induce contractions and cause the uterus to expel the products of conception. Abortion occurs within 24 hours in over 56% of cases and within 48 hours in 93% of cases (Brenner, 1975). Side effects that the patient may experience are nausea, vomiting, diarrhea, fever, dizziness, headache, and hypertension. Rare side effects are bronchospasm, cardiac arrhythmias, chest pain, and hyperventilation.

Intraamniotic injection of hypotonic saline is rarely used because of the reduced volume of amniotic fluid, which makes the procedure too difficult. The hypertonic saline solution can also further increase the risk of developing a coagulation defect.

Dilatation of the cervix should take place prior to any of these methods of evacuation. A laminaria tent or intravaginal prostaglandins are usually the choice of treatment to dilate the cervix without risk of its injury.

All patients carrying a dead fetus are at risk for developing disseminated intravascular coagulation (DIC). A good indicator of this condition is fibrinogen levels below 150 mg/100 ml. Delivery is the only cure for DIC; this stops the release of thromboplastic material into the maternal bloodstream from the dead products of conception. However, this coagulation defect may need to be treated prior to evacuation of the uterus to prevent hemorrhage. If the circulatory system is intact, indicated by no signs or symptoms of bleeding, then intravenous infusion of heparin can be administered to block the pathologic consumption of fibrinogen (see Chapter 12). This treatment must be stopped prior to evacuation of the uterus or hemorrhage results due to the heparin treatment. If bleeding is present when the fibrinogen levels are less than 150 mg/100 ml, heparin is contraindicated and the administration of fluids, blood products, and cryoprecipitate is the treatment of choice (Pritchard and MacDonald, 1980). Steps to promote delivery should follow promptly.

Habitual abortion

Some habitual abortions occur by chance; others are related to a maternal or paternal cause.
1. Incompetent cervix
2. Chromosomal disorder
3. Uterine defect
4. A luteal phase defect
5. An immunologic factor

If the patient has painless cervical dilatation after 16 weeks of gestation, the cause is usually related to an incompetent cervix. Cervical dilatation related to an incompetent cervix rarely occurs before week 16 because the products of conception are not heavy enough to cause dilatation. An incompetent cervix can result from any of the following.
1. A congenital defect
2. Mechanical trauma such as excessive dilatation for curettage or cervical biopsy
3. Cervical lacerations acquired during a previous delivery

Treatment is usually cerclage, a surgical procedure in which a pursestring suture is placed around the cervix to reinforce it. This procedure is usually performed around 14 to 16 weeks of gestation before cervical dilatation or effacement takes place and any bleeding or cramping is present.

When a couple repeatedly loses an embryo or fetus early in gestation, a chromosomal disorder of the father or mother may be the cause. A genetic history should be taken, karyotyping is recommended, and genetic counseling should follow as indicated.

Uterine defects are occasionally the cause of late habitual spontaneous abortions. During curettage for a spontaneous abortion, the uterine cavity should be closely examined for any abnormalities.

If no structural defects of the cervix or uterus or chromosomal abnormality can be found, the woman should be tested for a luteal defect or immunologic cause. When an endometrial biopsy done late in the menstrual cycle indicates inadequate production of progesterone by the corpus luteum, a luteal defect may be the cause, and supplemental natural progesterone suppositories can be beneficial. The usual dose is 25 to 100 mg twice per day. To be most effective, the progesterone should be started at the time of ovulation and continued until week 16 of gestation (Stenchever, 1983). Some, however, have found it effective when started as soon as pregnancy is suspected.

Following two or three spontaneous abortions for which no cause can be determined, the couple should be tissue typed to identify the antigens on the white blood cells (called *human leukocyte antigen typing* or *HLA typing*). If the couple is found to share a significant number of antigens, it is currently thought that the mother's body might not be stimulated to make a blocking antibody and is rejecting the products of conception. Taylor and Faulk (1981) have been successful in the treatment of three women found to have this problem by giving them transfusions of white blood cells that contain the potential father's antigens. They concluded that it tricked the mother's body into producing the blocking antibodies. Beer (1981) treated four pregnant patients in this same manner and the results were similar.

NURSING PROCESS
Prevention

Recent research clearly demonstrates that alcohol causes damage to the growing fetus in the form of growth deficiency, microcephaly, and mental deficiency. The damage can be severe enough to cause fetal death and lead to an abortion (Robinson, 1977). In order to prevent fetal anomalies as well as abortion from alcohol, medical personnel should increase the public's awareness of the effects of alcohol on the fetus through education programs. On the first prenatal visit, the nurse should include in the history the amount of alcohol used by the patient. Research indicates that there is no "safe" level of alcohol consumption during pregnancy (Dunn et al., 1979). Therefore the nurse must initiate appropriate measures depending on why the patient drinks. If the patient drinks only for social reasons usually an explanation of the risk of alcohol and a word of encouragement to abstain during pregnancy is enough. For the psychologically or physiologically dependent patient, the hazards of alcohol can be clearly explained, but, because of her complex problems, it might be necessary to refer her to a professional counselor or to a psychiatrist.

Like alcohol, smoking has negative effects on a growing fetus. Nicotine increases the heart rate and cardiac output, causes vasoconstriction of the umbilical blood vessels, decreases the oxygen-carrying capacity of the blood, and interferes with the assimilation of various essential vitamins and minerals (McKay, 1980; Deibel, 1980). Therefore smoking reduces the blood supply and nutrients to the fetus increasing fetal risk of death and a spontaneous abortion and causing babies to be small for gestational age or children to have impaired physical and intellectual development.

To promote preventive care, the nurse has a responsibility to assess the woman's smoking habits on the initial prenatal visit. The nurse must determine in a nonthreatening manner whether or not the woman smokes, how long she has smoked, approximately how many cigarettes she smokes daily, and for what reasons. The pregnant patient should then be instructed concerning the potential damaging effects of smoking on her baby. The fetal damage appears to be dose-related (Crockett, 1977). With this information, the patient can make an informed decision as to whether she will stop smoking, decrease her habit, smoke low tar or low nicotine cigarettes, or continue her habit and take chances on the consequences. The nurse must then support and assist the patient in her decision. If the patient chooses to stop smoking, a referral to a local stop smoking program can be beneficial.

Does routine prenatal care include education on the effects of smoking and alcohol? Davidson (1981) conducted a survey and found that only 57% of the women surveyed were given any information about the effects of alcohol on a growing fetus. Of those who received advice, only 35% were encouraged to quit, and 64% were told that social drinking was acceptable. One woman was advised of its benefits. As for smoking, 68% of the women surveyed were instructed regarding its harmful effects and 90% of these women were instructed not to smoke. With this research data, it appears that nurses can improve their patient education performance.

Because teratogenic agents increase the risk of a spontaneous abortion, preventive measures should be taken to avoid this risk. These measures should be instituted prior to pregnancy by encouraging all women of childbearing age to receive available immunizations against infectious diseases. When pregnancy is diagnosed, instructions given to expectant mothers should include ways they can decrease their chance of contracting an infection, such as eating nutritionally, avoiding fatigue, and avoiding people with infections. They should also be instructed if they eat meat to cook it well and if they have a pet cat or bird to leave the cleaning of the litter area to someone else in order to avoid contact with the toxoplasmosis virus. When pregnancy is diagnosed, instructions should be given regarding the avoidance of x-rays and medications, especially nonprescription ones unless ordered by their obstetrician, and to report any signs of vaginal bleeding immediately.

Assessment

When a patient calls and states that she is pregnant and experiencing vaginal bleeding or spotting, which may or may not be associated with mild cramps, the nurse should assess the following.
1. How many weeks of gestation is the pregnancy?
2. What were the onset, duration, intensity, and type of bleeding (dark or bright red)?
3. Is there any tissue or amniotic fluid accompanying the bleeding?

4. Are there any other symptoms present such as cramps or abdominal pain?

5. What has the patient done regarding the bleeding?

With this information, the physician will decide if the woman should be seen in the office or hospital.

Upon admission, further evaluation should include an assessment of the vaginal bleeding noting the color and the actual amount present on the pads and if any clots or tissue have been passed. Blood pressure, pulse, and respiration should be appraised and the red blood cell, hemoglobin, and hematocrit levels should be evaluated. Because infection, anemia, and disseminated intravascular coagulation (DIC) are complications that can develop in the presence of a spontaneous abortion, the nurse should assess for their presence. Signs indicating an infection are listed below.

1. Foul-smelling vaginal discharge
2. Elevated temperature greater than 100.4° F (38° C) (elevation less than 100.4° F may indicate dehydration)
3. A white blood cell count (WBC) greater than 16,000 because the white blood cells normally increase during pregnancy

Anemia is usually indicated by low hematocrit or hemoglobin. Signs of disseminated intravascular coagulation (DIC) are bleeding from the nose, gums, or sites of slight trauma. The mother's blood type and Rh factor should be identified if not already known to determine whether or not Rh immune globulin should be given in the event of an actual abortion.

The patient's psychological response should be assessed as to how she feels about the possible loss of pregnancy, sad, frightened, or relieved, and her coping strategies. An evaluation of the parent's level of understanding regarding the cause should be made, noting any expressions of self-blame or guilt.

Antepartum intervention

If the diagnosis of a threatened abortion is made, the patient should be instructed to limit her activity for 24 to 48 hours. Complete bed rest is not usually considered necessary. The patient should also be instructed not to strain with bowel movements and not to use a cathartic. She should be encouraged to continue to take her prenatal vitamins and to eat foods high in iron to prevent the development of anemia. In order to decrease the risk of infection, the patient should be instructed not to use tampons or douche and to abstain from sexual intercourse for up to 2 weeks after the bleeding stops. She should be instructed to report any increase in vaginal bleeding greater than a menstrual flow, cramping, or passage of tissue, which indicates an inevitable abortion, and report an elevated temperature or abdominal tenderness, which indicate the possible development of an infection. She should save any tissue or clots passed for examination and return for further evaluation in 1 or 2 days.

To help allay psychological stress, the nurse should allow the patient and her significant other time to express their concerns about what this bleeding episode means to them and what could have possibly caused the bleeding. The nurse should be very cautious about answering questions regarding the possible outcome of the pregnancy and should not be unduly optimistic. In an early threatened abortion without cramping there is about a 50% or greater chance of the pregnancy continuing. If cramping accompanies the bleeding, the chances are much lower.

If cervical dilatation occurs or fetal death is identified, then a spontaneous abortion becomes certain and the patient must be prepared for the evacuation of the uterus. An intravenous infusion is usually ordered and should be started with an 18-gauge intravenous catheter to allow administration of blood if needed. The nurse should acquaint the patient with the treatment plan. If a dilatation and curettage or vacuum aspiration is going to be done, the nurse should explain the procedure to the patient. If the cervix is not dilated sufficiently, the nurse should be prepared to assist the physician with some form of cervical dilatation to minimize potential cervical injury if mechanical dilatation is done at the time of surgery. If a laminaria tent is used, cervical dilatation usually takes place in 6 to 12 hours. During this time the patient should be assessed for side effects such as feelings of anxiety, nausea, respiratory distress, and uterine cramping. A mild antiemetic or analgesic should be administered as ordered to control the discomfort. If prostaglandin E_2 vaginal suppositories or gel is used, cervical dilatation usually takes place in 4 to 5 hours. The patient should be assessed for side effects such as nausea, vomiting, diarrhea, and hypotension. An antiemetic should be administered as ordered to control the nausea and vomiting. Oxytocin should never be administered if prostaglandins are being used. Together they can lead to hyperstimulation, cervical trauma, or uterine rupture (Sasso, 1983). Just prior to the procedure, the patient should empty her bladder. The nurse should also explain what sensations she may experience during the procedure such as mild cramping if it is to be done under a local anesthetic. If some form of prostaglandins is to be used in order to induce uterine contractions, the patient should be acquainted with the route of administration and told when the contractions should start. If intraamniotic prostaglandins (PGF_{2a} and PGE_2) are to be used, the nurse should prepare for and assist with amniocentesis. If prostaglandin vaginal suppositories or gel is used, the nurse should be prepared to assist with vaginal insertion every 4 hours until adequate contractions are stimulated. The nurse should then assess for any side effects such as nausea, vomiting, diarrhea, or hypertension if PGF_{2a} is used, or hypotension if PGE_2 is used.

Uterine contractions should be monitored routinely for any patient receiving a labor stimulant. The patient should be made as comfortable as possible by having someone stay with her, providing the same comfort measures that are used with women in labor and administering an antiemetic or analgesic as ordered. The family members also need support. After the fetus is aborted, the couple might have questions about the sex of the fetus and what it looked like. The nurse should spend time answering these questions. The couple may even wish to see the fetus. The nurse should also ask and carry out the wishes of the couple as to the need for baptism.

Postoperative intervention

Following any of the medical or surgical interventions that are used to treat a spontaneous abortion, the patient should be closely observed for 2 to 6 hours. Close observation for hemorrhage is important because if any of the placental tissue remains attached the myometrial muscle is unable to contract and close off the opened blood vessels on the uterine wall and hemorrhage will result. The amount of vaginal bleeding should be assessed by counting the number of perineal pads saturated, and by taking the pulse, respirations, and blood pressure. The vaginal bleeding should also be checked for the presence of clots and tissue. On discharge, the patient should be instructed to report to her physician if bleeding becomes excessive or persists or if cramps are severe or persist. She should also be instructed to eat foods high in iron and protein to aid the body in its repair and replacement of blood that was lost. Her usual activities can be resumed as soon as she feels up to it. She can be advised that, if she chooses, pregnancy can be attempted again after two normal menstrual periods.

Until the uterine wall heals, where the placenta was attached, there is a potential for an infection. As long as the cervix is dilated to any degree, an entrance for infection is present. Therefore close observations for signs of an infection should be included in the nursing care along with measures to decrease the risk. Signs of an infection usually include an elevated temperature or foul-smelling vaginal discharge. The patient's bed should be kept clean and dry and her perineal pads changed often to decrease this risk. The patient should be instructed in ways to decrease the risk of an infection.

1. Cleaning the perineum from front to back
2. Not taking tub baths until the cervix is closed, which is usually 2 weeks following surgery
3. Not using tampons, douching, or having sexual intercourse for 2 weeks
4. Changing her perineal pads often

On discharge the patient should be instructed to report to her physician if she develops signs of an infection such as a foul-smelling vaginal discharge, a fever, or an achy feeling.

When oxytocin is used, fluid intake and output must be monitored carefully because of the antidiuretic effect of oxytocin, which can lead to fluid retention. The patient's vital signs also should be monitored closely for signs of hypotention; this is also a potential side effect of oxytocin. The Rh-negative woman should be treated with Rh immune globulin. The usual dose of Rh immune globulin is 50 μg for a gestation of 12 weeks or less and 300 μg if the gestation age is greater than 12 weeks.

One of the main needs of the patient will be emotional support. Allow her time to express her feelings. Many women feel that they did something to cause the abortion or that they are inadequate physically to bear children. Deal with their feelings in an objective manner. Do not give false reassurance. Discuss with the couple the cause, if known, or otherwise explain possible reasons for a spontaneous abortion. The couple should be provided time to be alone so that they can communicate with and support each other. If the nurse perceives an abnormal psychologic reaction, the patient should be referred to an appropriate health care professional. If the couple asks, discuss the prognosis of future pregnancies. If this is their second or third spontaneous abortion, they should be encouraged to have a diagnostic and genetic workup so that an attempt to determine the cause can be made.

Prior to discharge, discuss with the couple the advantage of waiting 3 months or more before trying pregnancy again. This is best because the body needs to adjust to a normal, nonpregnant state prior to another pregnancy; also, there is the need for a period of grief. If they choose to wait before they attempt pregnancy again, they should be instructed to use contraceptive measures, because about 85% will ovulate before their first menstrual period (Boue and Boue, 1978).

Evaluation

Many times a spontaneous abortion is nature's way of eliminating a chromosomally defective fetus. These defects can be caused by an unpreventable, nonrecurring genetic abnormality or by a preventable teratogenic agent. The nurse can have an impact on lowering the incidence of spontaneous abortion by implementing an education program. This program should include the effects of alcohol, smoking, infections, x-rays, and other teratogenic agents on the developing fetus. In these and the other cases in which the cause is unpreventable, the nurse should provide adequate emotional support so the parents will not be left with scars due to anxiety or guilt over their failure to maintain the pregnancy to term.

In a few cases the cause is related to a maternal defect. The nurse should work with the health care team in recognizing these cases and then make appropriate referrals to facilitate treatment so that habitual abortions will not occur.

S U G G E S T E D   P L A N

Spontaneous abortion

Potential patient problem	*Outcome criteria*
Antepartum care **A.** Potential hypovolemia related to: Partially detached placenta	Vital signs stable Blood loss will not exceed 500 ml Urine output greater than 300 ml/hr or 1,200 ml/4 hr Hematocrit maintained between 30% and 45%

OF NURSING CARE

Assessment and intervention

Dx. Obtain history of onset, duration, amount, color, and consistency of bleeding
Obtain history regarding associated symptoms, prior bleeding episodes, and activity at onset of bleeding
Record visual blood loss by pad count (1 pad = 30 ml) or weight saturated pads, Chuxs, or linen (1 gm = 1 ml)
Record BP, P, and R as indicated (depends on severity)
Observe for signs of shock
Keep an accurate record of intake and output
Refer to such lab data as hemoglobin, hematocrit, and red blood cell count
Determine gestational age by EDC

Th. Save all tissue and clots expelled for examination
If bleeding is severe or hemoglobin or hematocrit low:
start an IV with an 18-gauge intracatheter and normal saline
start another IV to administer a lactated Ringer's solution or solution ordered until blood is available
prepare for type and cross match
prepare for administration of blood as ordered
have oxytocin available (usual dose 30 ml to 1000 ml at 200 ml/hr)

Ref. Notify physician if
BP drops, pulse or respirations increase
saturates more than one pad in 1 hr
urinary output drops below 30 ml/hr or 120 ml/4 hr
hematocrit less than 30%

Dx., diagnostic; Th., therapeutic; Ed., education; Ref., referral. *Continued.*

Spontaneous abortion—cont'd

Potential patient problem	Outcome criteria
B. Potential termination of pregnancy related to: Inevitable, incomplete, or missed abortion	No cervical dilatation No uterine contractions White blood count between 10,000 and 16,000 mm^3 Temperature normal No vaginal discharge odor

Dx. Observe for passage of tissue
Check amount of cervical dilatation
Observe for signs of an infection by:
    checking temperature every 4 hr
    referring to such lab work as a WBC
    assessing vaginal discharge for an odor
Assess for uterine contractions

Th. Assist with diagnostic procedures such as serial HCG levels and ultrasound
If no signs of an inevitable, incomplete, or missed abortion are found:
    instruct patient regarding the importance of limiting her activity, abstaining from intercourse, and returning for her reevaluation appointment
    instruct patient to notify physician immediately if bleeding becomes more than a period or persists, if cramps develop, or if a fever occurs
    encourage patient to continue to take her prenatal vitamins and eat foods high in protein, iron, and fiber
If signs of an inevitable, incomplete, or missed abortion are present:
    prepare for surgical or medical intervention as applicable
    explain procedure to patient
    surgically prepare patient
If curettage or vacuum aspiration is used:
    have patient empty bladder prior to procedure
    be prepared to start an IV so that oxytocin can be administered to facilitate uterine contractions during or after the procedure
    if cervix is not dilated, be prepared to assist with some form of cervical dilatation
    administer an antiemetic or analgesic as ordered
    explain sensations that may be experienced during the procedure
If prostaglandins are used:
    Observe for side effects such as
        nausea/vomiting
        diarrhea
        drug-related fever
        hypotension if PGE_2 is used
        hypertension if PGF_{2a} is used
If intraamniotic prostaglandins are used:
    prepare for and assist with amniocentesis
    if prostaglandin vaginal suppositories or gel is used be prepared to assist with vaginal insertion every 4 hr until adequate contractions
    assess uterine contractions
    provide comfort measures
    if patient is Rh-negative, be prepared to administer RhoGAM to prevent a future blood incompatibility

Ref. Notify physician if:
    WBC is greater than 16,000 mm^3
    foul-smelling vaginal discharge develops
    an elevated temperature greater than 38° C (100.4° F)

Continued.

Spontaneous abortion—cont'd

Potential patient problem	*Outcome criteria*

C. Potential anxiety or guilt related to:
  Cause of abortion
  Loss of a pregnancy
	Verbalizes fears and concerns

D. Potential DIC related to: Retention of a dead fetus	Clotting factors within normal limits

Postoperative care
A. Potential hypovolemia related to:
  Retained placental parts
  Cervical tears
	Vital signs stable for patient
	No excessive bleeding (no more than one saturated pad in 1 hr for the first 6 hr, then less)

B. Potential anemia related to: Blood loss	Hemoglobin between 12 and 14 gm/100 ml

Assessment and intervention

Dx. Assess level of anxiety
Evaluate level of understanding regarding cause, presence of self-blame

Th. Encourage parent(s) to express feelings related to loss of pregnancy
Provide emotional support
Avoid false reassurance and statements such as "you can have another child"
Promote open communication between the couple by providing time for them to be alone

Ed. Explain the cause, if known; otherwise, discuss possible reasons for a spontaneous abortion

Ref. Notify chaplain at parent(s) request

Dx. Observe for nose or gum bleeds, oozing from IV sites, or petechia
Refer to such laboratory data as fibrinogen, platelets, partial thromboplastin time, and clotting time

Th. If DIC develops (see DIC Suggested Plan of Nursing Care)

Dx. Check pulse, respirations, and blood pressure every 15 min eight times, every 30 min two times, every 1 hr two times, every 4 hr two times, then routine
note the presence of clots or tissue
refer to such lab data as hemoglobin, hematocrit, and red blood cell counts

Th. Maintain oxytocin and parenteral fluids as ordered

Ed. Discharge instructions should include
notify physician if bleeding increases or persists
resume routine activity as soon as one feels up to it
have patient arrange for a follow-up appointment as ordered (usually in 2 weeks)

Ref. Report to physician if:
excessive bleeding is noted
vital signs unstable
hemoglobin less than 11 gm

Dx. Refer to laboratory data such as hemoglobin
Note level of fatigue

Ed. Discharge instructions should include:
eat foods high in iron and protein
notify physician if feeling of fatigue persists beyond 2 weeks

Continued.

Spontaneous abortion—cont'd

Potential patient problem	Outcome criteria
C. Potential infection related to: Open uterine blood vessels Dilatated cervix	Temperature below 38° C (100.4° F) Absence of foul-smelling vaginal discharge White blood cell count between 4,500 and 10,000 mm^3
D. Potential pain related to: Surgical intervention	Verbalize relief from discomfort with ordered analgesia
E. Potential fluid retention and hypotension related to: Oxytocin	Urinary output greater than 30 ml/hr or 120 ml/4 hr Blood pressure stable for patient
F. Potential anxiety related to: Future childbearing	Verbalize fears and concerns

Assessment and intervention

Dx. Check temperature every 4 hr for 48 hr
Check vaginal discharge for foul odor every shift
Refer to laboratory data such as white cell count

Th. Perineal care every shift
Keep bed linen clean and dry
Encourage patient to change perineal pads often
If signs of infection develop be prepared to administer antibiotics as ordered

Ed. Discharge instruction should include:
    appropriate perineal care
    shower only for first 2 weeks
    do not use tampons, douche, or have sexual intercourse for 2 weeks
    notify physician if an elevated temperature develops over 38° C (100.4° F)

Ref. Notify physician if
    elevated temperature over 38° C (100.4° F)
    foul-smelling vaginal discharge

Dx. Observe for restlessness and discomfort at least two times per shift

Th. Administer analgesia as needed
Position in the most comfortable position

Ed. Instruct patient to report to nurse when uncomfortable

Ref. Notify physician if ordered analgesic is ineffective

Dx. Keep an accurate intake and output record
Check blood pressure every 4 hr

Ref. Notify physician if:
    urinary output is less than 30 ml/hr or 120 ml/4 hr
    blood pressure drops below 90/60

Dx. Assess level of anxiety
Evaluate level of understanding regarding future effect on childbearing

Th. Allow time for the parent(s) to express feelings
Answer questions parent(s) have regarding the fetus
If fetus is aborted intact, provide an opportunity for viewing

Ed. Discuss with the couple the advantage of waiting 3 months or more before
    trying pregnancy again
Discuss with couple the prognosis of future pregnancies
Discuss with couple the need to use a contraceptive method until they are
    ready for another pregnancy

Ref. If notice an abnormal psychologic reaction, refer to an appropriate health
    care professional
If this is their second or third abortion, encourage a diagnostic workup

REFERENCES

Abaci, F., and Aterman, K.: Changes of the placenta and embryo in early spontaneous abortions, Am. J. Obstet. Gynecol. **102**:252, 1968.

Beer, A.: Genetic compatibility may explain recurrent spontaneous abortions, JAMA **246**:315, 1981.

Boue, A., and Boue, J.: Chromosomal anomalies associated with fetal malformations. In Scringeous, J.B., editor: Toward the prevention of fetal malformation, Edinburgh, 1978, Edinburgh University Press.

Brenner, W.E.: The current status of prostaglandins as abortifacients, Am. J. Obstet. Gynecol. **123**:306, 1975.

Cadesky, K.I., Ravinsky, E., and Lyons, E.R.: Dilation and evacuation: a preferred network of midtrimester abortion, Am. J. Obstet. Gynecol. **139**:329, 1981.

Cavanagh, D., and Comas, M.: Spontaneous abortion. In Danforth, D., editor: Obstetrics and gynecology, ed. 3, New York, 1977, Harper & Row, Inc.

Cousins, L.: Cervical incompetence, 1980: a time for reappraisal, Clin. Obstet. Gynecol. **23**:467, 1980.

Crockett, E.: How to help the pregnant patient who smokes, Female Patient **2**:4, 1977.

Davidson, S.: Smoking and alcohol consumption, JOGN Nursing **10**(4):256, 1981.

Deibel, P.: Effects of cigarette smoking on maternal nutrition and the fetus, JOGN Nursing **9**(6):333, 1980.

Dunn, P.M., Steward, B., and Peel, R.: Metronidazole and the fetal alcohol syndrome, Lancet **2**:144, 1979.

Fabricant, J.D., Boue, J., and Boue, A.: Genetic studies on spontaneous abortion, Contemp. Obstet. Gynecol. **11**:73, 1978.

Grimes, D., and Gates, W.: Gestational age limit of 12 weeks for abortion by curettage, Am. J. Obstet. Gynecol. **132**:207, 1978.

Guerrero, R., and Rojas, O.I.: Spontaneous abortion and aging of human ova and spermatozoa, N. Engl. J. Med. **293**:573, 1975.

Hodari, A.A., and others: Dilatation and curettage for second trimester abortions, Am. J. Obstet. Gynecol. **127**:850, 1977.

Laversen, N.H., and others: Cervical priming prior to dilatation and evacuation: a comparison of methods, Am. J. Obstet. Gynecol. **144**:890, 1982.

Leppert, P.C., and others: Conclusive evidence for the presence of elastin in human and monkey cervix. Am. J. Obstet. Gynecol. **142**:179, 1982.

Liggins, G.C.: Ripening of the cervix, Sem. Perinatol. **2**:261, 1978.

Luke, B.: Maternal alcoholism and fetal alcohol syndromes, AJN **12**:1924, 1977.

McKay, S.: Smoking during the childbearing years, MCN **5**(1):49, 1980.

Moghissi, K.S.: What causes habitual abortion? Contemp. Obstet. Gynecol. **20**(5):45, 1982.

Netter, F.: The Ciba collection of medical illustrations: Vol. 2, reproductive system, Summit, N.J., 1965, Ciba Pharmaceutical Co.

Norstrom, A.: Influence of prostaglandin E_2 on the biosynthesis of connective tissue constituents in the pregnant human cervix, Prostaglandins **23**:361, 1982.

Ornoy, A., and others: Placental findings in spontaneous abortion and stillbirths, Teratology **24**:243, 1981.

Pantelakis, S.N., Papadimitrions, G.C., and Doxiadis, S.A.: Influence of induced and spontaneous abortion on the outcome of subsequent pregnancies, Am. J. Obstet. Gynecol. **116**:799, 1973.

Poland, B.J., and others: Reproductive counseling in patients who have had spontaneous abortion, Am. J. Obstet. Gynecol. **127:**685, 1977.

Poland, B., and Yuen, B.H.: Embryonic development in consecutive specimens from
recurrent spontaneous abortions, Am. J. Obstet. Gynecol. **130:**512, 1978.

Pritchard, J., and MacDonald, P.: Williams' obstetrics, ed. 16, New York, 1980, Appleton-Century-Crofts, Inc.

Roberts, C.J., and Lowe, C.R.: Where have all the conceptions gone? Lancet **25:**498,
1975.

Robinson, R.: Fetal alcohol syndrome, Dev. Med. Child Neurol. **19:**538, 1977.

Rocklin, R.E., and others: Maternal fetal relation: absence of an immunologic blocking
factor from the serum of women with chronic abortions, N. Engl. J. Med.
295:1209, 1976.

Sasso, S.: Prostaglandins for ob/gyn, MCN **8**(2):107, 1983.

Schoenbaum, S.C., and others: Outcome of the delivery following an induced or spontaneous abortion, Am. J. Obstet. Gynecol. **136:**19, 1980.

Scott, J.R.: Immunobiologic aspects of obstetrics and gynecology. In Danforth, D.N.,
editor: Obstetrics and gynecology, ed. 4, Hagerstown, Md., 1982, Harper & Row,
Inc.

Selik, R.M., Cates, W., and Tyler, C.W.: Behavioral factors contributing to abortion
deaths: a new approach to mortality studies, Obstet. Gynecol. **58:**631, 1981.

South, J., and Naldrett, J.: The effect of vaginal bleeding in early pregnancy on the
infant born after the 28th week of pregnancy, J. Obstet. Gynecol. Br. Commonwealth **80:**236, 1973.

Stenchever, M.A.: Habitual abortion, Contemp. Ob/Gyn **21**(1):162, 1983.

Taylor, C., and Faulk, W.P.: Prevention of recurrent abortion with leucocyte transfusion, Lancet **2:**68, 1981.

Wallner, H.J.: The fate of the child after threatened abortion, J. Perinatal Med. **2:**54,
1974.

Warburton, D., and Fraser, F.D.: On the probability that a woman who has had a
spontaneous abortion will abort in subsequent pregnancies, J. Obstet. Gynecol. Br.
Commonwealth **68:**784, 1961.

Wetzel, S.K.: Are we ignoring the needs of the woman with a spontaneous abortion?
MCN **7**(4): 1982.

CHAPTER 9

Ectopic pregnancy

An ectopic pregnancy develops as the result of the blastocyst implanting somewhere other than in the endometrium of the uterus. Primary sites of an ectopic pregnancy are the fallopian tube, ovary, cervix, or abdominal cavity (Fig. 9-1). The majority of ectopic pregnancies (95% to 98%) are located in the fallopian tube, with less than 1% locating on the ovary, less than 1% on the cervix, and 1% in the abdominal cavity (Table 9-1).

Of all tubal ectopic pregnancies, 55% are located in the ampullar or largest portion of the tube. Two percent are located in the interstitial or muscular portion of the tube adjacent to the uterine cavity. Twenty-five percent are located in the isthmus or the narrow part of the tube that connects the interstitial to the ampullar portion, and 17% locate in the fimbria or terminal end of the tube (Droegemueller, 1982). The outcome and gestational length of the ectopic pregnancy will be influenced by its location in the fallopian tube.

INCIDENCE

The incidence of ectopic pregnancies varies from $\frac{1}{28}$ to $\frac{1}{280}$ deliveries, depending on the sample population (Helvacioglu et al., 1979). Kitchin and associates (1979) found the overall incidence in the 16 years prior to 1978 to be $\frac{1}{126}$, with an increased incidence of $\frac{1}{60}$ for the 3 years prior to 1978. The increased incidence is felt to be related to *(1)* limiting of family size, *(2)* the use of an IUD which limits intrauterine but not ectopic pregnancies, and *(3)* the increased incidence of pelvic infections.

ETIOLOGY

Several researchers (Halpin, 1970; Panayotou et al., 1972; Brenner et al., 1980) have studied hundreds of patients who had ectopic pregnancies. They agree on the following general causes.

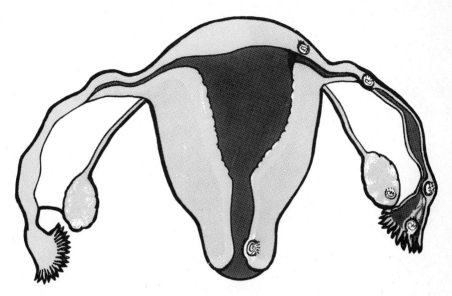

FIG. 9-1. Common sites for an ectopic pregnancy. (Illustration by Vincenza Genovese, Phoenix, Ariz. Modified from Netter, F.: Ciba collection of medical illustrations, Vol. 2, reproductive system, Summit, N.J., 1965, Ciba Pharmaceutical Co.)

TABLE 9-1. *Common ectopic sites with percent of occurrence*

Site	Incidence
Fallopian tube	95% to 98%
Ampullar	55%
Isthmus	25%
Interstitial	2%
Fimbria	17%
Ovary	Less than 1%
Cervix	Less than 1%
Abdominal	1%

Data from Droegemueller, W.: Ectopic pregnancy. In Danforth, D.N., editor: Obstetrics and gynecology, ed. 4, Hagerstown, Md., 1982, Harper & Row.

1. Tubal adhesions resulting from previous pelvic infections, such as salpingitis, postpartum endometritis, and postabortal uterine infections
2. Tubal adhesions resulting from the irritation of blood at the time of an abdominal pelvic surgery, especially a surgery involving the fallopian tubes (Salpingectomy for previous ectopic pregnancy or for treatment of an inflammatory process or salpingoplasty for infertility or previous ectopic pregnancy are the surgeries that most frequently cause tubal adhesions. Occasionally irritation results from an appendectomy.)
3. Transperitoneal migration of the ovum (When an ovum migrates from an ovary to the opposite tube, this delays fertilization. Then trophoblastic tissue is present on the blastocyst prior to its reaching the uterine cavity and implants itself on the wall of the fallopian tube.)
4. The presence of endometrial tissue located outside of the uterine cavity (which increases the receptivity of the fertilized ovum to implantation)

Therefore it appears that an ectopic pregnancy is frequently associated with a fallopian tube defect. A cervical ectopic pregnancy, however, is usually associated with a uterine defect that causes rapid migration of the fertilized ovum.

An ectopic pregnancy should not be ruled out even after a hysterectomy or tubal ligation or when an IUD is in place. An ectopic pregnancy can occur after a hysterectomy, although the incidence is rare. After reviewing 21 cases of ectopic pregnancy following a total hysterectomy, Niebyl (1974) found that it can be the result of a fertilizated ovum being present in the fallopian tube at the time of the surgery or it can occur months or years following the surgery if a fistula develops between the vagina and the peritoneal cavity.

When an IUD or low-dose progesterone oral contraceptive is used, an ectopic pregnancy can occur. An IUD only prevents a fertilized ovum from implanting itself in the uterine cavity but does not prevent the ovum from implanting itself outside of the uterine cavity.

PHYSIOLOGY
Normal

The fallopian tubes extend from the fundal portion of the uterus to the ovaries and provide the pathway for the ovum to reach the uterine cavity. They are approximately 8 to 14 cm long and 0.5 to 1 cm in diameter. Each fallopian tube is divided into four anatomic parts. Starting at the uterine side, they are referred to as *interstitial, isthmus, ampullar,* and *fimbria.*

Fertilization normally takes place in the distal third or ampullar area of the fallopian tube, and then the fertilized ovum starts moving slowly toward the uterine cavity by peristaltic and ciliated activity of the fallopian tube. It should reach the uterine cavity in 6 to 7 days, just about the time the trophoblast cells begin to secrete the proteolytic enzyme and start to develop the threadlike projections called *chorionic villi* that initiate the implantation process.

The uterus is normally prepared by estrogen and progesterone to accept the fertilized ovum, now called a *blastocyst*. As the chorionic villi invades the endometrium it is held in check by a fibrinoid zone. The myometrium is capable of enlarging as the embryo or fetus grows. The uterus is also supplied with an increased blood supply capable of nourishing the products of conception.

Pathophysiology

Tubal ectopic pregnancy. Because most ectopic pregnancies initially implant in a fallopian tube, the pathophysiology will focus on tubal ectopic pregnancies. The blastocyst burrows into the tubal endometrium and invades the tissue, tapping blood vessels, by the same process as normal implantation into the uterine endometrium. However, the environment of the tube is quite different because of the following factors.

1. There is a decreased resistance to the invading trophoblastic tissue by the fallopian tube.
2. There is a decreased muscle mass lining the fallopian tubes; therefore their distensibility is greatly limited.
3. The blood pressure is much higher in the tubal arteries than in the uterine arteries.

It is because of these characteristic factors that termination of a tubal pregnancy occurs gestationally early by either an abortion or rupture, depending on the location of the implantation (Table 9-2). Usually an ampulla or fimbriated tubal pregnancy ends in an abortion and an isthmic or interstitial pregnancy ends in a rupture.

A tubal abortion (Fig. 9-2) usually results because of separation of all or part of the placenta caused by the pressure exerted by the tapped blood vessels.

TABLE 9-2. *Tubular pregnancy*

Type	Duration	Usual method of termination
Ampullar	6 to 12 weeks	Tubal abortion
Fimbria	6 to 12 weeks	Tubal abortion
Isthmus	6 to 8 weeks	Tubal rupture
Interstitial	6 to 20 weeks	Tubal rupture

Data from Droegemueller, W.: Ectopic pregnancy. In Danforth, D.N., editor: Obstetrics and gynecology, ed. 4, Hagerstown, Md., 1982, Harper & Row.

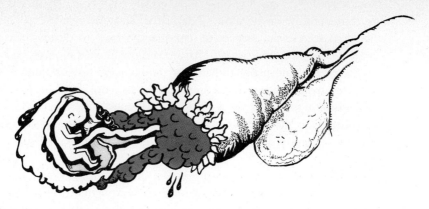

FIG. 9-2. Tubal abortion. (Illustration by Vincenza Genovese, Phoenix, Ariz. Modified from Netter, F.: Ciba collection of medical illustrations, Vol. 2, reproductive system, Summit, N.J., 1965, Ciba Pharmaceutical Co.)

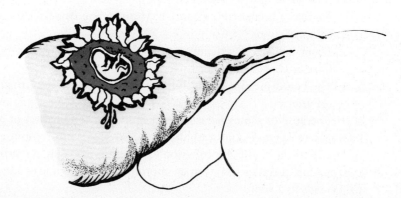

FIG. 9-3. Tubal rupture. (Illustration by Vincenza Genovese, Phoenix, Ariz. Modified from Netter, F.: Ciba collection of medical illustrations, Vol. 2, reproductive system, Summit, N.J., 1965, Ciba Pharmaceutical Co.)

With complete separation, the products of conception are expelled into the abdominal cavity by way of the fimbriated end of the fallopian tube and, unless there is an injured blood vessel, the bleeding stops. With an incomplete separation, bleeding usually continues until complete separation takes place, and the blood flows into the abdominal cavity collecting in the rectouterine cul-de-sac of Douglas.

Tubal rupture (Fig. 9-3) usually results from the uninterrupted invasion of the trophoblastic tissue or tearing of the extremely stretched tissue. In either case, the products of conception are completely or incompletely expelled into the abdominal cavity or between the folds of the broad ligaments by way of the torn tube.

The duration of the tubal pregnancy depends on the location of the implanted embryo or fetus and the distensibility of that part of the fallopian tube. For instance, if the implantation is located in the narrow isthmic portion of the tube, it will rupture very early, usually within 6 to 8 weeks; the distensible interstitial portion may be able to retain the pregnancy up to 4 months. An ampulla or fimbria tubal pregnancy is usually lost between 6 and 12 weeks of gestation.

The outcome of the pregnancy at the time of the interruption depends on the age of the embryo or fetus and whether the rupture is complete or incomplete. In rare cases, when the abortion occurs very early in the pregnancy and the placenta is initially separated completely from the tubal wall, the trophoblastic tissue will reimplant in the abdominal cavity and the placenta and embryo or fetus will continue to grow. This leads to the development of a secondary abdominal pregnancy. Only a small amount of blood is usually lost at this time. If the rupture is incomplete, in rare cases, the ruptured part of the placenta will reattach to some surrounding abdominal tissue. This leads to the development of a tuboabdominal, tuboovarian, or a broad ligament pregnancy. In most instances, however, the embryo or fetus dies at the time of the abortion or rupture. If not surgically removed, it can be absorbed if small or, if too large to be absorbed, it can mummify or calcify. When the bleeding is slight, no problems result. However, in most cases blood vessels are torn open and bleeding is profuse. This blood and the lost products of conception collect in the cul-de-sac of Douglas, causing severe pain and hypovolemia. A real emergency is present, which can end in maternal death if the bleeding is not quickly stopped.

Abdominal ectopic pregnancy. Occasionally the fertilized ovum will not enter the fallopian tube and implants itself initially on some abdominal structure. This leads to a primary abdominal pregnancy. Because the invading trophoblastic tissue is not held in check, it can erode major blood vessels at any time and cause severe bleeding. Fetal movements are also very painful because they are not cushioned by the myometrium.

Cervical ectopic pregnancy. In very rare cases, the fertilized ovum bypasses the uterine endometrium and implants itself in the cervical mucosa. Painless bleeding usually results shortly after implantation, and surgical termination is usually required prior to the twentieth week of gestation.

Signs and symptoms

Early in an ectopic pregnancy there are usually no signs or symptoms present. The woman may experience some signs of pregnancy because the uterus enlarges and the decidua develops as in a normal pregnancy in response to ovarian and placental hormones. However, these signs can be confused; the woman may experience slight vaginal bleeding or spotting due to constriction of the spiral arteries, which results from the lower hormonal levels associated with an ectopic pregnancy.

The first sign of an ectopic pregnancy is usually pain of varying degrees ranging from a dull, aching pain to a sudden, excruciating pain in the pelvic area. The second classic sign is related to the amount of blood lost; this can be a gradual oozing or a frank hemorrhage. The gradual oozing of blood will be demonstrated by anemia, pallor, and fatigue, whereas frank hemorrhage would be demonstrated by signs of shock. The amount of vaginal bleeding does not indicate the actual amount of blood being lost; the products of conception and the blood lost at the time of the rupture or abortion are expelled into the pelvic cavity rather than the uterine cavity. The vaginal bleeding is the result of sloughing of the endometrium. Because of the circulatory changes during pregnancy, hemoglobin and hematocrit levels and blood pressure and pulse are not good indicators of the amount of blood lost unless it is a rapid and continuous loss (Kitchin et al., 1979).

Other signs and symptoms that can be manifested in the presence of an

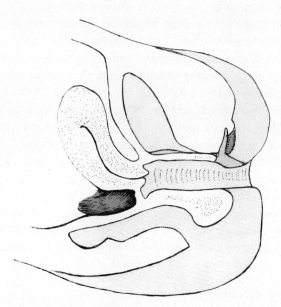

FIG. 9-4. Cul-de-sac of Douglas. (Illustration by Vincenza Genovese, Phoenix, Ariz.)

ectopic pregnancy, according to Helvacioglu and associates (1979) and Brenner and associates (1980), are the following.

1. Uterine enlargement
2. Palpable unilateral mass lateral to the uterus
3. Palpable mass in the cul-de-sac at vaginal examination (Fig. 9-4)
4. Signs of syncope
5. Occasional pain radiating to shoulder due to irritation of the diaphragm by blood
6. Pain experienced when the cervix is moved slightly

Maternal effects

According to Brenner and associates (1980), ectopic pregnancies account for the major portion of first trimester maternal deaths. Helvacioglu and associates (1979) identify ectopic pregnancy as one of the top three causes of maternal death along with pregnancy-induced hypertension and sepsis. The actual risk of maternal death related to hemorrhage from ectopic pregnancy is about 1 in every 800 ectopic pregnancies, and it is the cause of 6% to 11% of all maternal mortality. The high mortality rate can be related to the difficulty in diagnosing an ectopic pregnancy prior to an abortion or rupture of the pregnancy because the signs and symptoms mimic other abdominal diseases. Table 9-3 shows the comparison of diseases that are frequently confused with an ectopic pregnancy.

Fetal neonatal effects

Death is almost certain for the fetus in an ectopic pregnancy. Stafford and Ragan (1977), after reviewing the cases of ectopic pregnancy from the past 40 years, found only one infant who had survived an abdominal pregnancy. Rahman and associates (1982) reported from Saudi Arabia that 5 out of 10 cases of abdominal pregnancies ended with a live fetus. However, they do not recommend the continuation of an abdominal pregnancy if diagnosed early because of the extreme risk of hemorrhage at any time during the pregnancy. The risk of fetal deformity is also high. According to Tan and associates (1971), 20% to 40% will have such deformities as facial asymmetry, severe neck webbing, joint deformities, and hypoplastic limbs. These are pressure deformities caused by oligohydramnios. Augensen (1983) reports one unruptured tubal pregnancy ending in a viable fetus. However, this is extremely rare.

MEDICAL DIAGNOSIS

Early diagnosis prior to extrauterine rupture or abortion can decrease maternal mortality from hemorrhage and simplify the management of an ectopic

TABLE 9-3. *Comparison of frequently confused diseases*

	Salpingitis	Ectopic pregnancy	Spontaneous abortion	Appendicitis
Vaginal bleeding	Normal periods	History of missed period followed by vaginal bleeding, usually brownish red or scanty last menstrual period Signs of shock not related to obvious bleeding	Usually more profuse than a normal period and bright red except in threatened abortion; it can then be spotty dark red in color Signs of shock equal to obvious bleeding	Normal periods
Pain	Bilateral pelvic pain	Before rupture: Colicky abdominal/pelvic pain After rupture: Sudden sharp abdominal pelvic pain Abdominal tenderness Cervical motion pain	Rhythmic cramplike abdominal pain No abdominal tenderness No cervical motion pain	Before rupture: Generalized abdominal tenderness or localized over McBurney's point (right lower quadrant) After rupture: Abdominal rigidity Little to no cervical motion pain
Palpable mass		If palpable: Unilateral adnexal mass After rupture: cul-de-sac mass	None felt	
Vital signs	Elevated temperature greater than 38° C	Decreased BP and pulse if bleeding is continuous and rapid		Elevated temperature greater than 38° C
Other signs	History of recurrent attacks of pelvic pain Uterus not enlarged or cervix not softened	Uterus enlargement Cervix softened After rupture: Bulging cul-de-sac Shoulder referred pain related to diaphragmatic irritation Nausea and vomiting Fainting episodes	Uterine enlargement Cervix softened and may be dilating	Nausea and vomiting
Laboratory work	Increased WBC	Culdocentesis positive for nonclotting blood Pregnancy test positive in 50% of cases Decreased Hgb/Hct levels Increased WBC to 15,000 mm^3		Increased WBC

pregnancy. However, because this condition mimics other diseases and not one diagnostic tool is specific for detecting an early ectopic gestation, early diagnosis is difficult. Currently there are a large number of diagnostic procedures being used such as physical exam, human chorionic gonadotropin radioimmunoassay, ultrasound, culdocentesis, and laparoscopy.

Radioimmunoassay tests that are specific for human chorionic gonadotropin (HCG) hormone must be used to confirm pregnancy if an ectopic gestation is suspected. Urinary pregnancy tests have only a 50% to 60% accuracy in confirming a pregnancy that is ectopic. These tests react to the hormones HCG and luteinizing hormone. Therefore the sensitivity of the test has to be adjusted to levels that are high enough to exclude the preovulatory LH surge. Because an ectopically implanted placenta secretes less HCG than an intrauterine placenta, the HCG levels may be too low for these tests to detect. Radioimmunoassay tests are able to detect minute amounts of HCG and have proven to be very accurate in detecting ectopic pregnancy (Rasor, 1977).

The usefulness of ultrasound is improving continuously. In the past, it was only useful in diagnosing an intrauterine pregnancy which would rule out an ectopic pregnancy. One exception was in the case of an advanced abdominal pregnancy. In these cases, it would show a fetal head outside of the uterus. With the more sophisticated real-time equipment and an expert technician, Gleicher and associates (1983) were able to correctly diagnose unruptured ectopic gestations with 94% accuracy in a small group of patients. Nyberg and associates (1983) found that ultrasound could demonstrate an ectopic pregnancy with the following criteria: *(1)* abnormal uterine echoes without a gestational sac by 3 weeks or without embryonic echoes by 5 to 6 weeks of gestation, *(2)* an adnexal mass (a mass on the appendages of the uterus), and *(3)* fluid in the cul-de-sac.

Currently, when a patient presents with suspected signs of an early ectopic pregnancy such as lower abdominal pain, with or without mild vaginal bleeding, a diagnostic workup includes the following.

1. A pelvic examination to determine the state of the cervix
2. Abdominal palpation to determine whether or not the uterus is enlarged
3. Ultrasound to rule out an intrauterine pregnancy and attempt to visualize other characteristic signs of an ectopic gestation

If the pelvic exam portrays a closed cervix with cervical motion pain and an enlarged uterus, a radioimmunoassay pregnancy test and ultrasound are ordered. If the pregnancy test is positive, and no intrauterine pregnancy is found with ultrasound, or abnormal extrauterine findings are found with ultrasound, then a laparoscopy is usually performed to verify the suspected diagnosis. A laparoscopy is a surgical procedure done under a general anesthesia in which a small abdominal incision is made to visualize the peritoneal cavity and organs by way of a laparoscope.

If signs and symptoms indicate a ruptured or tubal aborted ectopic pregnancy without signs of shock, then a culdocentesis can be done in the doctor's office or emergency room to verify the diagnosis. Culdocentesis is a procedure done under local anesthesia in which a small needle puncture is made through the cul-de-sac of Douglas in order to aspirate fluid from the peritoneal cavity. According to Brenner and associates (1980), nonclotted blood will be withdrawn in the presence of about 95% of all ruptured ectopic pregnancies. When this test is positive, a laparotomy is performed in order to confirm and treat the disorder.

USUAL MEDICAL TREATMENT

Treatment consists of early diagnosis, adequate blood replacement, and surgical management. The type of surgical management is dependent on the location and cause of the ectopic pregnancy, the extent of tissue involvement, and the patient's wishes for future fertility.

The choice of treatment for an unruptured tubal pregnancy is a salpingotomy, in which a longitudinal incision is made over the pregnancy site and the products of conception are removed. Segmental resection and subsequent end-to-end anastomosis after the swelling and infection have subsided may be necessary if the ectopic pregnancy was located in the proximal isthmus portion of the tube. This is because of the high risk of scarring due to its narrow lumen. Tubal patency is restored in about 80% of these patients (Novy, 1983). Following a ruptured tubal pregnancy, a salpingectomy (removal of the affected fallopian tube) is the most common surgical treatment. Occasionally a salpingo-oophorectomy (removal of the affected fallopian tube and adjacent ovary) is performed if the blood supply to the ovary is affected or the ectopic pregnancy involved the ovary. Otherwise, conservation of the ovary is recommended. If the couple does not wish to have more children, then a hysterectomy may be done if the woman's condition is stable.

For an abdominal pregnancy, hemorrhage is a serious possibility because the placenta can separate from its attachment site at any time. Abdominal surgery to remove the embryo or fetus is usually done as soon as an abdominal pregnancy is diagnosed. Unless the placenta is attached to abdominal structures that can be removed, such as the ovary or uterus, or the vessels that supply blood to the placenta can be ligated, the placenta is left without being disturbed (Clark, 1978). If the placenta was removed, large blood vessels would be opened and there would not be a constricting muscle such as the uterus to apply a sealing pressure. If left intact, the placenta is usually absorbed by the body.

In the case of a cervical pregnancy, the risk of hemorrhage is as great as in any other type of ectopic pregnancy. A vaginal delivery should be attempted if the gestational age is less than 12 weeks (Gitstein et al., 1979). The cervix is then packed or sutured in an attempt to curtail the bleeding from the opened blood vessels after the removal of the placenta. If this does not stop the bleeding, amputation of the cervix or a hysterectomy must be done. After 12 weeks of gestation, or if the couple does not wish to have any more children, an abdominal hysterectomy is generally the method of treatment.

NURSING PROCESS
Prevention

Because an ectopic pregnancy is closely associated with a previous pelvic infection or a previous elective abortion, education regarding contraception can reduce the abortion rate. Education regarding the importance of treating a vaginal or pelvic infection early would also decrease the incidence. If an elective abortion is desired, it should always be carried out only by medically prepared people. These measures should decrease the chance of tubal defects and thereby decrease the incidence of ectopic pregnancy.

Assessment

Because of the high maternal mortality rate if an ectopic pregnancy goes undiagnosed until after rupture or tubal abortion, it is very important for nurses to be alert to signs and symptoms of this complication of pregnancy. Therefore, any woman during her childbearing years who experiences irregular vaginal spotting associated with a dull, aching pelvic pain, with or without signs of pregnancy, should be evaluated for a possible ectopic pregnancy. A history of any pelvic inflammatory disease, previous ectopic pregnancies, elective abortions, or a history of infertility disorders should be determined; they can increase the patient's risk for a tubal defect.

If an ectopic pregnancy is suspected, a detailed history should include questions regarding type of abdominal pain, amount of vaginal bleeding, menstrual history, and presence of any signs of syncope. The pain caused by an unruptured ectopic pregnancy can be a unilateral, cramplike pain related to tubal distension by the enlarging embryo or fetus. At the time of tubal rupture many patients experience a sudden, sharp, stabbing pain in the lower abdomen. Blood in the peritoneum can cause a dull aching or severe generalized pain. If the blood touches the diaphragm, it usually causes referred shoulder pain. Many times movement of the body will aggravate the pain.

Vaginal bleeding is usually related to the sloughing of the endometrial lining related to lowering progesterone and estrogen levels and can present as a continuous or intermittent vaginal bleeding in small or large quantity. It is usually

different from the patient's normal period. When an ectopic pregnancy ruptures or aborts, blood is lost into the peritoneal cavity. At this time the patient
can experience a feeling of faintness or weakness related to hypovolemia. If the
bleeding is not continuous, the depleted blood volume is restored to near normal in a day or two by hemodilution and the faint or weak feeling subsides. If
the bleeding is profuse, the patient can go into shock quickly. Pad counts
should be kept to determine the amount of vaginal bleeding. In order to assess
the amount of intraperitoneal blood loss, the patient's vital signs should be
checked as frequently as the situation indicates. Any change in the amount or
type of pain the patient is experiencing should be noted. The hemoglobin and
hematocrit levels should be determined as well.

The nurse should then be prepared to assist the physician with diagnostic
tests such as abdominal and pelvic examinations, ultrasound, a pregnancy test
if pregnancy has not been confirmed, or a culdocentesis.

A woman who is diagnosed with an ectopic pregnancy will experience psychologic stress as well. She will not only grieve over the loss of a child but
must face surgery. The nurse must assess the level of her anxiety and knowledge regarding the condition.

Antepartum intervention

If the patient is diagnosed with an unruptured ectopic pregnancy, she
should be prepared for surgery by starting an intravenous infusion with an 18-
gauge intravenous catheter, typing and cross matching two to four units of
blood as ordered, and carrying out preoperative protocol. No enemas should
be given; this could stimulate a tubal ectopic pregnancy to rupture. The patient and her significant other should be allowed time to express their fears
about what is happening and what this means to them. The type of surgery
should be explained to them. The patient should be taught postoperative exercises such as turning, coughing and deep breathing, and abdominal tightening to decrease postoperative complications such as respiratory infection, abdominal distension, or paralytic ileus.

If the patient is exhibiting signs and symptoms of shock, she should be
prepared for emergency surgery by starting an intravenous infusion with an
18-gauge intracatheter in preparation for a blood transfusion and by obtaining
laboratory data such as a complete blood count, type, and cross match as ordered. Then, preoperative protocol should be carried out. Oxygen by mask
might be needed. Vital signs, intake and output, amount of vaginal bleeding,
and signs of shock should be carefully monitored. The patient should not be
left alone, and she should be kept informed of what is happening.

The patient is usually very uncomfortable. Therefore the patient should be
kept quiet and helped to maintain a position most comfortable for her. Sitting

or standing usually intensifies rectal pain, and lying can intensify shoulder pain if blood is in the abdomen.

Postoperative intervention

Hemorrhage is the most common complication postoperatively. Therefore the patient's blood pressure, pulse, and respiration should be checked according to postoperative protocol. The surgical dressing should be assessed every hour for the first 4 hours for bleeding and the hemoglobin and hematocrit values noted. The amount of vaginal bleeding should be determined by a pad count.

Blood is very irritating to the peritoneum and is an ideal medium for bacterial growth. Therefore patients who experience rupture of an ectopic pregnancy have an increased risk of pelvic infection and a paralytic ileus. These patients are usually given prophylactic antibiotics.

Any patient is at risk following abdominal surgery for abdominal distension, pneumonia, and urinary tract infection; therefore all patients following surgery should be observed for signs of an infection by checking their temperature every 4 hours; inspecting the surgical incisions for redness, swelling, and drainage on every shift; auscultating the lung fields at every shift for rales; and asking the patient if she experiences any burning or pain on urination. The abdomen should be palpated for distension, bowel sounds auscultated, and the patient asked to report the passage of flatus. In order to decrease the risk of these complications, the patient should be instructed to turn and breathe deeply every 2 hours and use an inspiratory incentive spirometer. To decrease the risk of abdominal distension, she should be given nothing by mouth until bowel sounds are present and instructed to do abdominal tightening exercises every hour while awake. Leg exercises while in bed and early ambulation should be encouraged; they will facilitate the body's normal processes, which are slowed by anesthesia.

Once the gastrointestinal tract resumes normal function, adequate nutrition is important. High protein intake is essential in the body's repair of injured tissue, and iron is needed to correct anemia. Drinking six to eight glasses of fluid per day will increase the body's natural resistance to infection.

Patients that develop shock prior to or during surgery have a greater potential for developing pulmonary edema. These patients should have careful monitoring of intravenous fluid therapy by pulmonary wedge or central venous pressure (see Chapter 6).

Rh isoimmunization can result from an ectopic pregnancy. Therefore all Rh-negative women should receive Rh immune globulin within 72 hours of the termination of the ectopic pregnancy.

If time was not available preoperatively to explain to the patient and her significant other what was happening, time should be taken now to answer any questions and to allow them to express their fears and concerns. Parents who desire to have more children are frequently concerned about infertility problems and the risk of a recurrent ectopic pregnancy. False reassurance should not be given. The nurse's counseling should be based on statistics.

According to Novy (1983), there is a 30% to 60% chance of infertility following any form of treatment for an ectopic pregnancy, with a 28% to 50% chance following a salpingotomy. DeCherney and Kase (1979) reported a

---

SUGGESTED   PLAN

Ectopic pregnancy

Potential patient problem	*Outcome criteria*
Antepartum care	
A. Potential hypovolemia related to: Ectopic rupture or abortion	Blood loss will not exceed 500 ml Vital signs stable for patient
B. Potential pain related to: Stretching of tube Blood in abdomen	Verbal or nonverbal expression of reasonable comfort

52% chance of infertility and Kitchin and associates (1979) found a 66% chance of infertility. In regard to the risk of a repeat ectopic pregnancy, Hallatt (1975) and DeCherney and Kase (1979) both found about a 10% chance; Kitchin and associates (1979) reported a 24% chance. Following a salpingotomy, Novy (1983) found up to a 12% chance of a recurrent ectopic pregnancy. The reason the risk is so great for infertility and a repeat ectopic pregnancy is that the condition that caused the first ectopic pregnancy is still present and usually involves both tubes.

O F   N U R S I N G   C A R E

Assessment and intervention

Dx. Check vital signs as indicated (depending on severity)
Collect an in-depth history as to:
    amount and character of vaginal bleeding
    last menstrual period
    signs and symptoms of syncope
    method of contraception use
    history of ectopic pregnancies, elective abortions, infertility problems, and
        pelvic infections
Pad count
Keep an accurate intake and output record
Refer to hemoglobin and hematocrit
Th. Assist with the diagnostic procedures such as ultrasound, culdocentesis, laparoscopy, and abdominal and pelvic examination
Ed. Instruct patient regarding diagnostic procedures

Dx. Assess the type and location of pain
Th. Maintain position of comfort
Limit movement and support patient
Provide reassurance
Ed. Instruct regarding use of relaxation and breathing to reduce pain if pain
    medication cannot be administered

Dx., diagnostic; Th., therapeutic; Ed., education; Ref., referral.

Continued.

Ectopic pregnancy—cont'd

Potential patient problem	*Outcome criteria*
Preoperative care	
A. Potential hypovolemia related to: Ectopic rupture or abortion	Vital signs stable for patient Skin warm and dry Urine output greater than 30 ml/hr
B. Preoperative fear or anxiety related to: Lack of knowledge concerning surgery	Verbalizes fear and concerns Demonstrates ability to do postoperative exercises and explain reasons

Assessment and intervention

Dx. Check vital signs as indicated (depending on severity)
Check amount of vaginal bleeding
Check for signs of shock
Check state of mental acuity
Keep an accurate record of intake and output

Th. Start intravenous infusion with 18-gauge intracatheter as ordered
Type and crossmatch two to four units of blood as ordered
Administer oxygen by mask if ordered
Carry out preoperative protocol:
nothing by mouth
give *no* enemas or cathartics
be prepared to insert Foley catheter as ordered
get permit signed for surgery

Dx. Assess level of anxiety
Evaluate level of understanding

Th. Allow patient to express fears of what is happening
Keep patient informed of each procedure that is ordered

Ed. Teach patient need to do turn, cough, deep breathing, and abdominal tightening exercises postoperatively
Explain ectopic pregnancy and reason for surgery

Continued.

Ectopic pregnancy—cont'd

Potential patient problem	*Outcome criteria*

Postoperative care
A. Potential postoperative complications such as:
    Paralytic ileus
    Urinary tract infection
    Pneumonia
    Pelvic abscess
    Anemia
    Pulmonary edema
    Hemorrhage
	No signs of any postoperative complications

B. Potential anxiety related to: Possible fear of infertility	Verbalize any fear of infertility

Assessment and intervention

Dx. Check BP, P, and R every 15 min eight times, every 30 min two times, every 1 hr two times, every 4 hr two times, then routine
Assess vaginal bleeding by pad count
Check dressing every 1 hr four times, every 2 hr four times, then every shift for bleeding
Refer to laboratory work such as hemoglobin and hematocrit
Assess for cyanosis
Observe for signs of infection by:
    checking temperature every 4 hr
    referring to the WBC count
    checking incision for redness, swelling, drainage every shift
    assessing for burning or urination
    auscultating lung fields every shift for rales
    observing for coughing/dyspnea
Auscultate bowel sounds every shift
Assess abdomen for hard, boardlikeness
Assess for passage of flatus

Th. Turn, cough, deep breath every 2 hr
Use Triflow every 1 hr
NPO until bowel sounds present
Intake and output record
Carefully administer intravenous fluids as ordered
Leg exercises every 1 hr while awake
Abdominal tightening every 1 hr while awake
Encourage ambulation as soon as ordered
If Rh-negative, be prepared to administer RhoGAM

Ed. Instruct regarding:
    importance of a high-protein and high-iron diet for body repair
    importance of six to eight glasses of fluid per day
    importance of early exercise and ambulation

Ref. Notify physician if BP less than 90 systolic or P greater than 120/min, abdominal distension develops, temperature 38° C, signs of infection or anemia are present

Dx. Assess level of anxiety regarding future childbearing
Th. Answer questions regarding chances of recurrence and infertility problems

Evaluation

The ultimate goal for nursing intervention is prevention of complications that can cause tubal or uterine defects. These set the stage for an ectopic pregnancy. If an ectopic pregnancy develops, the goal is to prevent complications during the treatment. Therefore efforts are best directed at prevention of future impairment of fertility through patient education. Education should include information for self-detection of signs of infections contributing to ectopic pregnancy. Efforts should also be directed at detecting and reporting early signs of an ectopic pregnancy so diagnosis prior to a rupture or abortion can be made. Thus the complication of hemorrhage, which is the major cause of maternal death, could be prevented.

REFERENCES

Augensen, K.: Unruptured tubal pregnancy at term with survival of mother and child, Obstet. Gynecol. **61:**259, 1983.

Brenner, P.F., Roy, S., and Mishell, D.R.: Ectopic pregnancy: a study of 300 consecutive surgically treated cases, JAMA **243:**673, 1980.

Clark, J.F.: Preventing maternal death in advanced abdominal pregnancy, Contemp. Ob/Gyn **12**(9):137, 1978.

Clark, J.F., and Jones, S.A.: Advanced ectopic pregnancy, J. Reprod. Med. **14:**30, 1975.

DeCherney, A., and Kase, W.: The conservative surgical management of unruptured ectopic pregnancy, Obstet. Gynecol. **54:**451, 1979.

Droegemueller, W.: Ectopic pregnancy. In Danforth, D.N., editor: Obstetrics and gynecology, ed. 4, Hagerstown, Md., 1982, Harper & Row, Inc.

Gitstein, S., and others: Early cervical pregnancy, ultrasonic diagnosis and conservative treatment, Obstet. Gynecol. **54:**758, 1979.

Gleicher, N., and others: Direct diagnosis of unruptured ectopic pregnancy by real time ultrasonography, Obstet. Gynecol. **61:**425, 1983.

Hallatt, J.G.: Repeat ectopic pregnancy: a study of 123 consecutive cases, Am. J. Obstet. Gynecol. **122:**520, 1975.

Halpin, T.F.: Ectopic pregnancy: the problem of diagnosis, Am. J. Obstet. Gynecol. **106:**227, 1970.

Helvacioglu, A., Long, E.M. Jr., and Yang, S.: Ectopic pregnancy: an eight-year review, J. Reprod. Med. **22:**87, 1979.

Hughes, G.J.: The early diagnosis of ectopic pregnancy, Br. J. Surg. **66:**789, 1979.

Kellett, R.J.: Primary abdominal (peritoneal) pregnancy, J. Obstet. Gynecol. Br. Commonwealth **80**(12):1102, 1973.

Kitchin, J.D., and others: Ectopic pregnancy: current clinical trends, Am. J. Obstet. Gynecol. **134:**870, 1979.

Lucas, C., and Hassim, A.M.: Place of culdocentesis in the diagnosis of ectopic pregnancy, Br. Med. J. **1:**200, 1970.

McGovern, C.S.: Recognizing a tubal pregnancy, MCN **3**(5):303, 1978.

Maklad, N.F., and Wright, C.H.: Grey scale ultrasonography in the diagnosis of ectopic pregnancy, Radiology **126:**221, 1978.

Niebyl, J.: Pregnancy following total hysterectomy, Am. J. Obstet. Gynecol. **119:**512, 1974.

Novy, M.J.: Surgical alternatives for ectopics: is conservative treatment best? Contemp. Ob/Gyn **21:**91, 1983.

Nyberg, D.A., and others: Ultrasonographic differentiation of the gestational sac of early intrauterine pregnancy from the pseudogestational sac of ectopic pregnancy, Radiology **146:**755, 1983.

Panayotou, P.P., and others: Induced abortion and ectopic pregnancy, Am. J. Obstet. Gynecol. **114:**507, 1972.

Pritchard, J., and MacDonald, P.: Williams' obstetrics, ed. 6, New York, 1980, Appleton-Century-Crofts, Inc.

Rahman, M.S., and others: Advanced abdominal pregnancy—observations in 10 cases, Obstet. Gynecol. **59:**366, 1982.

Rasor, J., and Braunstein, G.: A rapid modification of the beta HCG radioimmunoassay, Obstet. Gynecol. **50:**553, 1977.

Rothe, D.J., and Birnbaum, S.J.: Cervical pregnancy: diagnosis and management, Obstet. Gynecol. **42:**675, 1973.

Schneider, J., Berger, C.J., and Cattell, C.: Maternal mortality due to ectopic pregnancy: a review of 102 deaths, Obstet. Gynecol. **49:**557, 1977.

Schoenbaum, S., and others: Gray-scale ultrasound in tubal pregnancy, Radiology **127:**757, 1978.

Stafford, J.C., and Ragan, W.: Abdominal pregnancy: review of current management, Obstet. Gynecol. **50:**548, 1977.

Tan, K.L., Goon, S.M., and Wee, J.H.: The pediatric aspects of advanced abdominal pregnancy, J. Obstet. Gynaecol. Br. Commonwealth **78:**1044, 1971.

Yaffe, H., Navot, D., and Laufer, N.: Pitfalls in early detection of ectopic pregnancy, Lancet **2:**272, 1979.

CHAPTER 10

Gestational trophoblastic disease

There are three categories of gestational trophoblastic disease: hydatidiform mole, invasive mole or chorioadenoma destruens, and choriocarcinoma. An invasive mole and choriocarcinoma are often referred to as *proliferative trophoblastic diseases*.

A hydatidiform mole (Fig. 10-1) is a benign degenerative process of the placenta in which the chorionic villi degenerate into edematous, cystic, avascular, transparent vesicles that hang in a grapelike cluster. There may or may not be an embryo present An invasive mole or chorioadenoma destruens occupies an intermediate position between the benign hydatidiform mole and the highly malignant choriocarcinoma. It occurs when the trophoblastic tissue continues to grow and locally invades the uterine myometrium, pelvic blood vessels, and occasionally the vagina or lungs. It lacks the widespread metastatic characteristics of choriocarcinoma, which proliferates profusely into body structures such as the lungs, brains, liver, kidneys, intestines, spleen, or vagina. Choriocarcinoma is not always preceded by a hydatidiform mole. Forty percent follow a spontaneous abortion, 20% a normal delivery, and only 40% a hydatidiform mole (Pritchard and MacDonald, 1980).

INCIDENCE

In the United States, the incidence of a hydatidiform mole is between 1 in 1,500 and 1 in 2,000 pregnancies, with a relatively higher incidence among women over 45 (McDonald and Ruffolo, 1983). In many other countries the incidence is much higher. There is four to five times greater risk associated with a repeat hydatidiform mole (DiSaia et al., 1975) and a ten times greater risk associated with a maternal age over 45 years (Martin, 1978). Following a hydatidiform mole, 20% of patients develop a proliferative trophoblastic disorder (Curry et al., 1975).

ETIOLOGY

The cause of a hydatidiform mole is unknown, but it is theorized that malnutrition, chromosomal anomalies, or hormonal imbalance contribute to its development (Novak and Woodruff, 1974). Protein and folic acid may be the

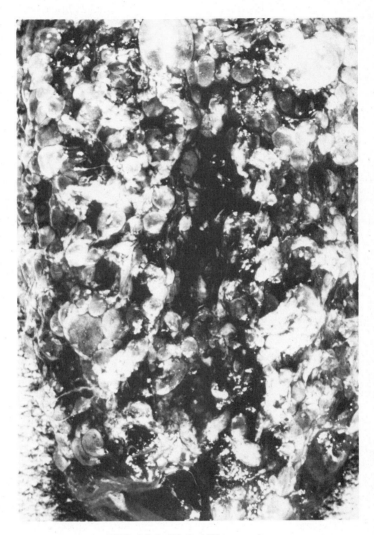

FIG. 10-1. Hydatidiform mole.

two main dietary factors because they are essential for rapid cellular metabolism. LaVecchia and associates (1982) suggest that a hydatidiform mole might result from a genetically defective ovum, lacking a nuclei, that is fertilized. It has also been noted that women receiving clomiphene citrate (Clomid) to induce ovulation have a higher incidence of hydatidiform mole. This might be related to a hormonal imbalance.

PHYSIOLOGY
Normal

Normally one sperm fertilizes one ovum and each contributes 23 chromosomes to form a new cell called a *zygote*. The zygote begins to grow immediately by undergoing a series of rapid mitotic cell divisions to form a solid mass of cells called a *morula*. As cellular activity continues, fluid begins to form in the center of the morula and causes the cells to rearrange until there is one single layer of cells lining the periphery and an inner cluster of cells. The single layer of cells called the *trophoblast* will grow and develop into the placenta and the inner cluster of cells called the *embryoblast* will develop into a fetus. The umbilical cord will eventually connect the two structures.

The placenta is formed by the trophoblast cells sending out threadlike projections termed *chorionic villi* into the endometrium of the uterus. As the chorionic villi grow, they erode areas of the endometrium, forming intervillous spaces that fill with maternal blood. Invasion is normally held in check by the endometrium. Inside the chorionic villi blood vessels and connective tissue begin forming. These blood vessels will connect with the blood vessels inside the umbilical cord.

Pathophysiology

What actually causes the degeneration of the placenta to occur is unknown. In any case the trophoblastic tissue absorbs fluid from the maternal blood. Fluid then begins to accumulate in the chorionic villi because of inadequate or the lack of fetal circulation. As the pooling of fluid continues, vesicles are formed out of the chorionic villi.

There are two categories of a hydatidiform mole: complete or classical and partial moles. The complete moles are characterized thus.

1. Generalized areas of the choronic villi that become hyperplastic, edematous, and avascular
2. Lack of an embryo or fetus and amniotic sac
3. A karyotype of 46XX chromosomes of paternal origin (The 23 sperm chromosomes duplicate instead of joining with the 23 chromosomes of the ovum [Szulman and Surti, 1982; Kajii and Ohama, 1977].)

The partial moles are characterized thus.

1. Localized areas of chorionic villi that become hyperplastic, edematous, and avascular
2. The presence of an embryo or fetus and amnionic sac usually with multiple congenital anomalies
3. A karyotype of 69XXY chromosomes; one set of chromosomes of maternal origin and two sets of paternal origin

Signs and symptoms

Characteristic symptoms of a hydatidiform mole are:

1. Abnormal uterine bleeding, which is intermittent or continuous, usually not profuse, and often brownish in color, occurs in approximately 90% of cases. This is usually related to the lack of circulatory integrity of molar tissue.
2. A uterus larger than expected for the estimated gestational age occurs in approximately 50% of the cases, and in approximately 40% of the cases the uterus will be small for dates (Curry et al., 1975).
3. Bilateral ovarian enlargement or cysts occur in 15% to 40% of cases. This is usually related to the elevated levels of HCG (DiSaia et al., 1975).
4. Hyperemesis gravidarum occurs in approximately 14% to 30% of cases.
5. Signs and symptoms of preeclampsia such as proteinurea, hypertension, and edema developing prior to week 24 of gestation occur in approximately 30% of cases. This is probably related to the rapid enlargement of the uterus (McDonald and Ruffolo, 1983).
6. Passage of grapelike vesicles occurs in approximately 50% of patients.
7. Lack of fetal movement and inability to palpate fetal parts or detect a fetal heart tone (Jones and Lauersen, 1975) are common findings.
8. Signs and symptoms of hyperthyroidism such as tachycardia, goiter, sweating, intolerance to heat, and elevated T_3 and T_4 levels occur in about 3% of cases. This is related to the binding of the elevated levels of HCG to the thyroid-stimulating hormone (TSH) receptor sites (Hershman and Higgins, 1978).

Maternal effects

A pregnant woman carrying a hydatidiform mole has approximately a 30% risk of developing pregnancy-induced hypertension before 24 weeks of gestation (McDonald and Ruffolo, 1983). Other complications frequently associated with a hydatidiform mole are first trimester bleeding, hyperemesis gravidarum, and emotional trauma. Following surgical evacuation of the mole, the woman has a 20% risk of developing some type of proliferative trophoblastic disease, of which 80% is for an invasive mole and 20% for choriocarcino-ma (Curry and associates, 1975). The patient who has had a complete hyda-tidiform mole is at a greater risk of developing a proliferative trophoblastic disease compared to the patient who had a partial mole. However, this form of cancer is 100% curable if diagnosed early and treated with chemotherapy (Lewis, 1980).

Fetal effects

The embryoblastic tissue of the complete hydatidiform mole never develops into a fetus. The embryoblastic tissue of the partial hydatidiform mole is al-ways abnormal and never matures. Suzuki and associates (1980) did report from their review of the literature that approximately 20 living children have been delivered from a hydatidiform molar pregnancy. However, in these cases there were twin gestations and only one of the gestational sacs was affected by the molar changes.

MEDICAL DIAGNOSIS

Diagnostic tests used to validate a hydatidiform mole can include the fol-lowing.
1. Ultrasound. This is the most accurate tool for diagnosing the presence of a mole. A characteristic pattern of multiple diffuse echoes is shown in place of, or along with, an embryo or fetus.
2. Serial HCG titers. In a normal pregnancy human chorionic gonadotro-pin (HCG) levels gradually increase until around day 100 of pregnancy and then drop sharply with no one normal level for any given time. Therefore, repeated assays, which fail to show a decline in HCG after day 100 of pregnancy, are suggestive of abnormal trophoblastic growth. A multiple gestation can have higher levels of HCG normally; therefore care should be taken to exclude a pregnancy with multiple fetuses.
3. Amniography. Radiopaque dye is injected transabdominally into the uterine cavity. In the presence of a hydatidiform mole, x-ray films would show a "honeycomb" pattern in place of or along with an embryo or fetus.

USUAL MEDICAL TREATMENT

Treatment consists of two parts: immediate evacuation of the uterus and a follow-up program to detect early the development of a proliferative tropho-blastic disease.

The uterus is usually emptied by suction curettage unless the patient is no longer interested in childbearing; then an abdominal hysterectomy might be done. Even if the ovaries are enlarged or cystic, they do not have to be removed; they usually regress spontaneously with the reduction of HCG.

Dilatation of the cervix is usually accomplished under general anesthesia unless the cervix is long and closed; then a laminaria might be used to dilate the cervix. If used, it is usually inserted 6 to 12 hours prior to surgery. It is a dried seaweed that expands by absorbing moisture from the endocervix and thereby dilating the cervix slowly and without trauma.

All patients who have had a hydatidiform mole should be followed closely for at least 1 year, because 20% of these patients will develop proliferative trophoblastic disease in which the trophoblastic tissue continues to live following removal of the mole (Curry et al., 1975). Of this group, 15% will develop an invasive mole and 5% choriocarcinoma (Delfs, 1957).

The follow-up program usually includes the following.

1. A baseline HCG level and chest x-ray film
2. Weekly serum radioimmunoassay for HCG until the HCG level drops to normal and remains normal for 2 to 3 consecutive weeks, then monthly for 6 months and bimonthly for 6 more months
3. Regular pelvic examinations to assess uterine and ovarian regression and to observe changes in the vagina that would indicate proliferative trophoblastic disease

The most specific indicators of proliferative trophoblastic disease are the HCG levels. Several laboratory tests are available to determine the HCG levels, such as biologic or immunologic pregnancy tests and bioassay or radioimmunoassay tests. Biologic and immunologic tests should not be used in the follow-up program because 1,000 or more IU/liter of HCG have to be present to give a positive reading. In trophoblastic disease, HCG levels can be lower than 1,000 IU/liter (Goldstein et al., 1975).

Treatment for proliferative trophoblastic disease with chemotherapy is instituted whenever the serum level of HCG rises or plateaus for more than 2 consecutive weeks, or if signs of metastasis are detected during a pelvic examination or on x-ray films. When an invasive mole or choriocarcinoma of limited metastases develops, a single-agent chemotherapy regimen is usually instituted. This consists of administering methotrexate or actinomycin D for 5 days. The response to chemotherapy is excellent and most patients will achieve a 100% cure (Horlacher, 1981). If metastasis has occurred beyond the lungs and pelvis, combination chemotherapy is usually instituted. A 90% recovery rate has been achieved in these patients (Surwit and Hammond, 1980).

Some obstetricians recommend the use of prophylactic chemotherapy; its use is controversial, however. According to Goldstein and associates (1979) it appears to be the best approach only if the patient is at high risk for developing a proliferative trophoblastic disease and the probability of the patient adhering to the follow-up program is poor. Indications of high risk are the presence of a complete mole, bilateral ovarian enlargement, a large for date uterus, or repeated molar gestations.

NURSING PROCESS
Prevention

Because the cause of a hydatidiform mole is unknown, there is no known prevention. However, malnutrition might play a part in influencing its development; therefore instructions should be given to all patients planning a pregnancy regarding the importance of a balanced diet high in protein and folic acid.

Assessment

To detect a hydatidiform mole early, the nurse should observe for signs of a mole at each prenatal visit during the first 20 weeks of gestation. Such signs as uterine bleeding, uterine size small or large for dates, hyperemesis gravidarum, signs of preeclampsia prior to 24 weeks of gestation, passage of grapelike vesicles, or inability to detect fetal heart rate with a Doppler after 10 to 12 weeks of gestation should be brought to the attention of the obstetrician immediately.

When a patient is admitted to the hospital with a tentative diagnosis of a hydatidiform mole, the nurse should monitor closely for signs of hemorrhage. Hemorrhage results from invasion of the trophoblasts into the myometrium, which ruptures pelvic blood vessels. Blood pressure, pulse, and respiration should be taken every 4 hours and the patient should be asked to report any pelvic pain. It should be kept in mind that abdominal pain may also be related to an ovarian cyst, with commonly develops with a hydatidiform mole.

These patients should also be assessed for signs of grief due to loss of the pregnancy and fear of a malignancy. In addition to determining what this loss means to the patient, the nurse should also determine how much the patient knows about this condition. She may be most concerned as to whether or not she can ever have children again and might have fears concerning what she did to cause this to happen.

Antepartum intervention

The patient should be prepared for the various diagnostic procedures, such as ultrasound and serum HCG determinations. When a hydatidiform mole is confirmed, the nurse should explain to the patient what it is and prepare the patient for surgery. An intravenous infusion should be started with an 18-

gauge intracatheter, and two to four units of blood should be typed and cross matched because of the risk of hemorrhage during surgery.

During the preparation for surgery, the nurse should maintain an unhurried manner if possible and allow the patient time to express her fears and grief related to the loss of an expected baby and a defective pregnancy. Spiritual assistance might help the parents to work through their grief.

Postoperative intervention

Hemorrhage, perforation of the uterus, and infection are the three primary complications of surgery and should be watched for during the immediate postoperative period. Oxytocin is usually added to the intravenous infusion during surgery in order to promote myometrial contractions, which will decrease bleeding and thicken the uterine wall to reduce the risk of perforation of the uterus. Intravenous infusions with oxytocin added are usually continued during the initial postoperative period to facilitate uterine contractions and decrease uterine bleeding. If the ovaries are enlarged, vigorous uterine massage can cause ovarian rupture and should be avoided. Because of the antidiuretic effect of oxytocin, urinary output should be closely observed.

With the increased risk of uterine infection, the nurse should carefully watch for signs and symptoms such as an elevated temperature, foul-smelling vaginal discharge, and elevated white blood cell count. Antibiotics are administered at the first sign of an infection.

Rh-negative women may become sensitized following the evacuation of a hydatidiform mole. Therefore they should receive Rh immune globulin within 72 hours following the surgery to prevent Rh isoimmunization.

Because of the existing risk of a proliferative trophoblastic disease developing, these patients should be assessed for such symptoms as dyspnea, cough, and pleuritic pain; these signs may indicate pulmonary metastasis. A dull headache, behavioral change, or dizzy spells may indicate cerebral metastasis. Right upper quadrant pain or jaundice may indicate liver metastasis, and vaginal bleeding may indicate vaginal metastasis. These patients should be instructed regarding the importance of a follow-up program that consists of weekly serum HCG levels until the HCG drops to normal and remains normal for 2 to 3 consecutive weeks. Then HCG levels should be drawn monthly for 6 months and bimonthly for 6 more months. There should also be regular chest x-ray films to detect pulmonary metastasis and regular pelvic examinations to assess uterine and ovarian metastasis. When the patient adheres to this type of follow-up program, early detection is possible and treatment is more effective. The patient should be advised not to become pregnant during the follow-up program, which usually lasts for about 1 year since the HCG of the prolifera-

Gestational trophoblastic disease

Potential patient problem	Outcome criteria

Antepartum care
A. Potential hemorrhage related to:
    Trophoblastic invasion of the
      myometrium
	Minimal to no bleeding
	Vital signs stable
	No abdominal pain

B. Anxiety related to:
    Loss of pregnancy
    Fear of a malignancy
    Concern regarding outcome of
      future pregnancies
    Fear of surgery
	Parent(s) will express fears and anxieties
	Parent(s) will participate in decisions re-
	    garding care

Postoperative care
A. Potential hemorrhage related to:
    Invasive qualities of a hydatidi-
      form mole
    Surgical intervention
	Minimal to no bleeding
	Vital signs stable
	Fundus firm

B. Potential infection related to:
    Invasive qualities of a hydatidi-
      form mole
    Surgical intervention
	Temperature below 38° C (100.4° F)
	Absence of four-smelling vaginal discharge
	White blood cell count between 4,500 and
	    10,000 mm^3

C. Potential urinary retention re-
    lated to:
      Oxytocin
	Urinary output greater than 120 ml/4 hr

O F   N U R S I N G   C A R E

Assessment and intervention

Dx. Check vital signs every 4 hr
 Assess for signs of abdominal pain
 Assess amount of vaginal bleeding
Th. Start intravenous infusion with 18-gauge intracatheter
 Prepare for surgery:
  according to preoperative protocol
  type and cross match two to four units of blood as ordered
Ed. Instruct regarding possible cause of bleeding
Ref. Notify physician at first signs of bleeding

Dx. Assess parent(s) knowledge of the disease
 Assess parent(s) fears surrounding this event, family resources, and coping
  abilities
Th. Allow parent(s) to ventilate and grieve
Ed. Explain the disease and plan of treatment
Ref. Notify chaplain on parent(s) request

Dx. Check BP, P, and R every 15 min four times, every 30 min two times, every
  1 hr four times, then every 4 hr if stable
 Assess amount of vaginal bleeding
 Assess for signs of abdominal pain
 Assess state of uterus
Th. Maintain IV fluids with oxytocin as ordered
 No uterine massage if ovaries are enlarged
Ref. Notify physician first signs of bleeding

Dx. Check temperature every 4 hr
 Assess vaginal discharge for foul odor
 Refer to laboratory work such as white blood count
Th. Administer pericare every shift
Ed. Instruct in pericare
Ref. Notify physician if temperature is greater than 38° C or if foul-smelling vagi-
  nal discharge develops

Dx. Keep an accurate intake and output record
Ref. Notify physician if urinary output is less than 120/ml 4 hr

Dx., diagnostic; Th., therapeutic; Ed., education; Ref., referral.   *Continued.*

Gestational trophoblastic disease—cont'd

Potential patient problem	Outcome criteria
D. Potential proliferative trophoblastic disease related to: Trophoblastic metastasis	HCG levels gradually decrease to 0

Assessment and intervention

Dx. Refer to HCG levels and chest x-ray film
Assess for signs of pulmonary metastasis such as
dyspnea
cough
pleuristic pain
Assess for signs of cerebral metastasis such as
dull headache
behavioral changes
dizzy spells
Assess for signs of liver metastasis such as
right upper quadrant pain
jaundice
Assess for signs of vagina metastasis such as
continued vaginal bleeding
Th. Assist physician in carrying out follow-up program
Assist parent(s) in decision of type of contraceptive to be used during the 1-year follow-up
Ed. Instruct as to importance of the follow-up in order to detect early proliferative trophoblastic disease
Instruct as to what will be involved in the follow-up program
Instruct regarding the importance of not getting pregnant during the follow-up care to prevent masking the HCG levels
Instruct regarding only a 20% risk to developing a proliferative trophoblastic disease
Instruct regarding treatment program if proliferative trophoblastic disease develops
Instruct that early detection followed by immediate treatment leads to a 100% cure
Instruct regarding risk of recurrence of a hydatidiform mole
Ref. Notify physician if any signs of metastasis are present

Continued.

tive trophoblastic disease cannot be distinguished from the HCG of pregnancy. Any effective contraceptive method may be used including estrogen/progestin oral contraceptives if no other contraindications are present.

Even though these patients must be instructed regarding the potential risk of proliferative trophoblastic disease, they should be informed that it is only a 20% risk. Reassurance that with early diagnosis treatment is 100% effective with chemotherapy should help. Even following chemotherapy, there is usually little difficulty in carrying a subsequent normal pregnancy to term (Curry et al., 1975). Pastorfide and Goldstein (1973) found similar results with only a slight increased risk of spontaneous abortion.

Evaluation

The goals of the nurse in treating patients who have had a hydatidiform mole are twofold. First, the nurse must impress them with the importance of the follow-up program. To determine if a proliferative trophoblastic disease is

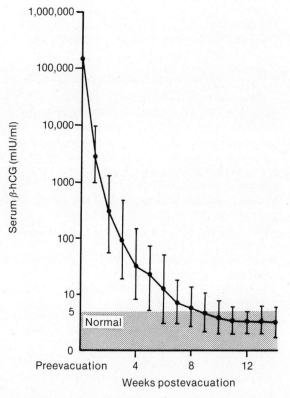

FIG. 10-2. Normal postmolar regression of serum HCG measured by radioimmunoassay. (From Morrow, C.P., and associates: Am. J. Obstet. Gynecol. **128:**428, 1977.)

going to occur, HCG levels should be followed closely and compared to a standard regression curve as outlined by Morrow and associates (1977; Fig. 10-2). This curve indicates that the HCG levels should progressively decline and by 10 to 12 weeks be nondetectable. Second, the nurse must help the patients work through the loss of an expected baby, a defective pregnancy, the fear of the development of proliferative trophoblastic disease, and the fear of recurrence in subsequent pregnancies.

REFERENCES

Curry, S., and others: Hydatidiform mole, Obstet. Gynecol. **45**:1, 1975.

Czernobilsky, B., Barash, A., and Lancet, M.: Partial moles: a clinicopathologic study of 25 cases, Obstet. Gynecol. **59**:75, 1982.

Delfs, E.: Quantitative chorionic gonadotropin: prognostic value in hydatidiform mole and chorioepithelioma, Obstet. Gynecol. **9**:1, 1957.

Delfs, E.: Hydatidiform mole, Obstet. Gynecol. **45**:95, 1975.

DiSaia, P.J., Morrow, C.P., and Townsend, D.E.: Gestational trophoblastic disease. In Synopsis of gynecologic oncology, New York, 1975, John Wiley & Sons, Inc.

Fasoli, M., and others: Management of gestational trophoblastic disease: results of a cooperative study, Obstet. Gynecol. **60**:205, 1982.

Garrett, W.J., Crowe, P.H., and Robinson, D.E.: The interpretation of ultrasonic echograms in abdominal pregnancy, Aust. N.Z. J. Obstet. Gynaecol. **9**:26, 1969.

Goldstein, D.P., Berkowitz, R.S., and Cohen, S.M.: The current management of molar pregnancy, Obstet. Gynecol. **3**:5, 1979.

Goldstein, D.P., and others: A rapid solid-phase radioimmunoassay specific for human chorionic gonadotropin in gestational trophoblastic disease, Obstet. Gynecol. **45**:527, 1975.

Hanson, M.B.: Trophoblastic disease. In Nagell, J.R., and Barbar, H.R., editors: Modern concepts of gynecologic, oncology, London, 1982, John Wright & Sons, Ltd.

Hershman, J.M., and Higgins, P.: When mole causes thyroid dysfunction, Contemp. Obstet. Gynecol. **12**:79, 1978.

Horlacher, J.: 100% remission is possible with trophoblastic disease, OB/GYN News **15**(4):13, 1981.

Jones, W.B., and Lauersen, N.H.: Hydatidiform mole with coexistent fetus, Am. J. Obstet. Gynecol. **122**:267, 1975.

Jones, W.B., and Lewis, J.L.: Treatment of gestational trophoblastic disease. Am. J. Obstet. Gynecol. **120**:14, 1974.

Kajii, T., and Ohama, K.: Androgenetic origin of hydatidiform mole, Nature **268**:633, 1977.

LaVecchia, C., and others: Gestational trophoblastic neoplasms in homozygous twins, Obstet. Gynecol. **160**:250, 1982.

Lewis, J.L.: Treatment of metastatic gestational trophoblastic neoplasms, Am. J. Obstet. Gynecol. **136**:163, 1980.

Martin, P.: High frequency of hydatidiform mole in native Alaskans, Int. J. Gynecol. Obstet. **15**:395, 1978.

McDonald, T., and Ruffolo, E.: Modern management of gestational trophoblastic disease, Obstet. Gynecol. Surv. **38**(2):67, 1983.

Menczer, J., Modan, M., and Serr, D.M.: Prospective followup of patients with hydatidiform mole, Obstet. Gynecol. **55**:346, 1980.

Morrow, C.P., and others: Clinical and laboratory correlates of molar pregnancy and trophoblastic disease, Am. J. Obstet. Gynecol. **128**:424, 1977.

Novak, E.R., and Woodruff, J.D.: Novak's gynecologic and obstetric pathology, ed. 7, Philadelphia, 1974, W.B. Saunders Co.

Pardue, S.F.: Hydatidiform mole: a pathological pregnancy, AJN **77**:836, 1977.

Pastorfide, G.B., and Goldstein, D.P.: Pregnancy after hydatidiform mole, Obstet. Gynecol. **42**:67, 1973.

Pritchard, J., and MacDonald, P.: Williams obstetrics, ed. 16, New York, 1980, Appleton-Century-Crofts, Inc.

Richart, R.: New ways to manage trophoblastic disease, Contemp. Obstet. Gynecol. **20**:159, 1982.

Surwit, E.A., and Hammond, C.B.: Gestational trophoblastic neoplasia. In Pitkin, R.M., and Zlatnik, F.J., editors: 1980 Yearbook of obstetrics and gynecology, Chicago, 1980, Yearbook Medical Publishers, Inc.

Suzuki, M., and others: Hydatidiform mole with a surviving coexisting fetus, Obstet. Gynecol. **56**:384, 1980.

Szulman, A.E., and Surti, U.: The syndromes of hydatidiform mole, I. cytogenetic and morphological correlations, Am. J. Obstet. Gynecol. **131**:665, 1978.

Szulman, A.E., and Surti, U.: The clinicopathologic profile of the partial hydatidiform mole., Obstet. Gynecol. **59**:597, 1982.

Szulman, A.E., Surti, U., and Berman, M.: Patient with partial mole requiring chemotherapy, Lancet **2**:1099, 1978.

Twiggs, L.B., Morrow, C.P., and Schlaerth, J.B.: Acute pulmonary complications of molar pregnancy, Am. J. Obstet. Gynecol. **135**:189, 1979.

Vassilakos, P., Riotton, G., and Kajii, T.: Hydatidiform mole: two entities, Am. J. Obstet. Gynecol. **127**:167, 1977.

Walden, P., and Bagshawe, K.D.: Reproductive performance of women successfully treated for gestational trophoblastic tumors, Am. J. Obstet. Gynecol. **125**:1108, 1976.

CHAPTER 11

Third trimester bleeding: abruptio placentae and placenta previa

About 5% of all pregnant women experience some type of vaginal bleeding during the third trimester of pregnancy (Huff, 1982). The major causes of this bleeding are abruptio placentae and placenta previa. This chapter will focus on these two main causes and will contrast the treatments of both. Other causes of third trimester bleeding are heavy bloody show, cervical carcinoma, polyps, infection of the cervix or vagina, placenta accreta, and vasa previa.

ABRUPTIO PLACENTAE

An abruptio placentae is the premature separation, either partial or total, of a normally implanted placenta from the decidual lining of the uterus after 20 weeks of gestation. It is normally classified into one of three categories: mild, moderate, or severe (Table 11-1). Maternal bleeding in any class can be marginal, concealed, or both (Fig. 11-1), depending on whether or not it is trapped in the uterus, and is classified as one of the following.
1. Marginal or apparent; the separation is near the edge of the placenta and the blood is able to escape
2. Central or concealed; the separation is somewhere in the center of the placenta, and the blood is trapped
3. Mixed or combined; part of the separation is near the edge and part is concealed in the center area

INCIDENCE

The incidence of abruptio placentae is 1 in 120 pregnancies (Knab, 1978) or 0.5% to 2.5% risk (Huff, 1982). The risk increases with increased age and parity. The incidence of recurrence in subsequent pregnancies is 5.6% (Paterson, 1979).

ETIOLOGY

The actual cause of abruptio placentae is unknown. Conditions frequently associated with an abruption are listed below.

223

1. Pregnancy-induced or chronic hypertension present in 47% of patients (Pritchard et al., 1971)
2. Maternal age over 35 years
3. Multiparity greater than five children
4. Previous abruption; 10% increased risk after one abruption and a 25% risk of recurrence after two abruptions (Knab, 1978)
5. Trauma from a direct blow to the uterus or needle puncture during amniocentesis
6. Short umbilical cord
7. Folic acid deficiency; this has not been supported by research but is frequently discussed
8. Cigarette smoking causing vasoconstriction of the spiral arteriola; Naeye, Harkness, and Utts (1977) found that decidual necrosis corresponds closely to the number of cigarettes smoked; findings in their study indicate that cigarette smoking is a major contributory factor in abruptio placentae when compared to abruption caused by a short umbilical cord and abdominal trauma

TABLE 11-1. *Comparison of three classifications of abruptio placentae*

Mild	Moderate	Severe
DEFINITION		
Less than one sixth of the placenta separates prematurely	From one sixth to two thirds of the placenta separates prematurely	More than two thirds of the placenta separates prematurely
SIGNS AND SYMPTOMS		
Vague lower abdominal or back discomfort or uterine tenderness	Gradual or abrupt onset of abdominal pain with uterine tenderness	Usually abrupt onset of uterine pain described as tearing, knifelike, and continuous
Dark vaginal bleeding (absent or slight)	Dark vaginal bleeding (absent to moderate)	Dark vaginal bleeding (moderate to excessive)
Total blood loss less than 500 ml	Total blood loss between 500 and 1,000 ml	Total blood loss more than 1,000 ml
Uterine irritability (absent or slight)	Uterine tone increased; fails to relax completely at any time.	Uterus boardlike and highly reactive to stimuli
Shock and DIC rare	Mild shock and DIC common	Moderate to profound shock common; DIC usual unless the condition is treated immediately
FETAL EFFECTS		
Fetal distress rare	Fetal distress present or not	Fetal distress frequent and death can occur

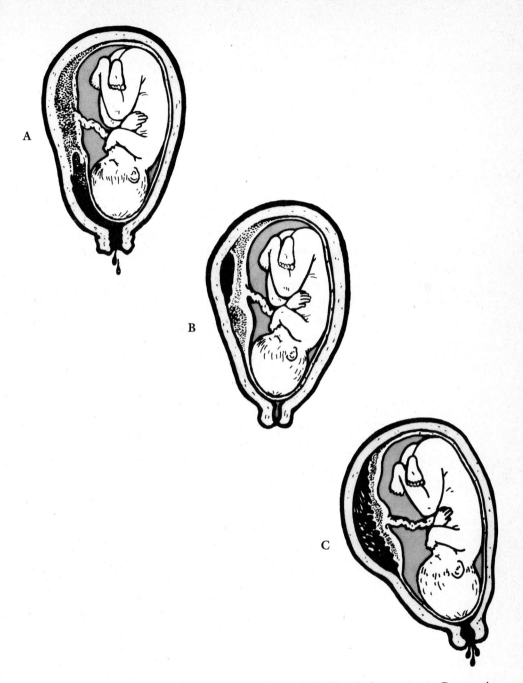

FIG. 11-1. Classification of abruptio placentae. **A,** Marginal or apparent; **B,** central or concealed; **C,** mixed or combined. (Illustrated by Vincenza Genovese, Phoenix, Ariz. Modified from Netter, F.: In Oppenheim, E., editor: Ciba collection of medical illustrations, vol. 2, reproductive system, Summit, N.J., 1965, Ciba Pharmaceutical Co.)

PHYSIOLOGY
Normal

The blastocyst normally implants into the endometrium, now called the *decidua*, by sending out threadlike projections called chorionic villi from the trophoblast cells. These villi open up intervillous spaces, which fill with maternal blood. These spaces are supplied by the spiral arteries. At the same time, the trophoblast cells send out anchoring cords to attach themselves to the uterus.

Pathophysiology

An abruptio placentae is theoretically thought to be caused by degeneration of the spiral arterioles that nourish the decidua (endometrium) and supply blood to the placenta causing decidual necrosis. When this process takes place, rupture of that blood vessel occurs and bleeding quickly results because the uterus is still distended and cannot contract sufficiently to close off the opened bleed vessels. Separation of the placenta takes place in the area of the hemorrhage. If the tear is at the margin of the placenta or if it separates the membranes from the decidua, then vaginal bleeding is evident. Otherwise, the blood is concealed between the placenta and the decidua. If it is concealed, pressure can build up enough for blood to be forced through the fetal membranes into the amniotic sac or into the myometrial muscle fibers, which is called *Couvelaire uterus*. This increases uterine tone and irritability. Clotting occurs simultaneously with the hemorrhage because the decidua tissue is rich in thromboplastin. This leads to the formation of a retroplacental or a subchorionic hematoma, causing the release of large quantities of thromboplastin into the maternal circulation. This can lead to disseminated intravascular coagulation (DIC) (see Chapter 12).

Signs and symptoms

The classic manifestations of an abruptio placentae are the following.
1. Uterine rigidity
2. Uterine tenderness or low back pain
3. Dark vaginal bleeding
4. Signs and symptoms of fetal distress
5. Signs of shock

The presence and degree of each sign are related to the amount of concealed blood trapped behind the placenta and the degree of separation. If the separation occurs at the margin of the placenta, the blood usually tears the membranes away from the decidua and escapes externally. If the separation is in the center of the placenta, blood is trapped behind the placenta. Concealed blood causes pressure and myometrial contractions, and this results in uterine rigidity and tenderness. With no way to escape, pressure builds up and can force blood into the myometrial tissue of the uterus causing increased uterine irritability. Increasing uterine size and decreasing serial hematocrits are other signs of concealed bleeding. If some of this trapped blood is forced through the fetal membranes into the amniotic cavity, the amniotic fluid will be bloody. Vaginal bleeding, according to LoBue (1980), is present in 80% of cases in varying amounts. It is not present in 20% of cases because the outer edges of the placenta remain intact. The blood that finds its way out appears dark because it has had some time to begin clotting.

Mild forms of abruptio placentae usually develop gradually and produce slight uterine tenderness, vague lower abdominal discomfort, and mild to moderate dark vaginal bleeding. In a few instances, the bleeding is totally concealed and no vaginal bleeding is evident. Signs of fetal distress are usually absent, and the mother's vital signs remain stable. This type of abruption can be self-limiting or can progress into a more advanced form.

Moderate abruptio placentae can develop gradually or abruptly and produce persistent abdominal pain accompanied by visible dark vaginal bleeding. The uterus may be very tender on palpation and may remain firm between contractions if the mother is in labor. This can make auditory appraisal of the fetal heart rate difficult. Fetal distress may be present depending on the extent of placental separation and the amount of maternal blood loss. Signs of shock may or may not be present.

Severe abruptio placentae usually develops suddenly, causing excruciating, unremitting abdominal pain often referred to as *knifelike* or *tearing*. The uterus is often boardlike and tender and fails to relax. Profuse bleeding results, although it may not be evident vaginally if the blood is trapped behind the placenta. In these cases the uterus will show signs of enlarging. Shock can ensue, though the signs of shock may not be in proportion to the amount of visible blood loss. Signs of fetal distress are usually evident.

In a few instances, when an abruptio placentae occurs in a posteriorly implanted placenta, no signs of uterine tenderness and pain are manifest. Notelovitz and associates (1979) found in these cases that the classical signs are only vaginal bleeding and backache.

In summary, the typical patient with abruptio placentae presents with various amounts of abdominal pain and dark vaginal bleeding. Usually the bleeding from the site of separation continues until delivery of the placenta. Sometimes a clot blocks the bleeding. Normally uterine activity is stimulated and labor is initiated.

Complications that can develop as a result of abruptio placentae are shock and disseminated intravascular coagulation (DIC).

Shock. Shock results as the body attempts to protect the vital organs, especially the brain and heart, from a reduction in effective circulating blood volume. When blood is lost from the vascular system, venous return is diminished, and consequently cardiac output is reduced. Physiologic compensatory mechanisms are then activated. The decrease in arterial pressure initiates powerful sympathetic reflexes that stimulate vasoconstriction of the arterioles and venules in the kidney, liver, lungs, gastrointestinal tract, muscles, skin, and uterus. Blood is then redistributed to the heart and brain from these areas.

The heart and respiratory rates increase in an attempt to compensate by delivering increased volume and better oxygenated blood to the vital organs. A slower compensatory mechanism is activated that stimulates the absorption of fluid from the intestinal tract and stimulates the kidneys to increase reabsorption of sodium and water. Therefore the results are classic signs of hypovolemic shock, which include hypotension, rapid, thready pulse, shallow, irregular respirations, cold and clammy skin, pallor, syncope, and thirst.

Should severe bleeding continue, the compensatory mechanisms cannot keep up with tissue needs, and cardiac deterioration, loss of vasomotor tone, and release of toxins by ischemic tissue result; cellular death ensues.

Because of the normally increased maternal blood volume during pregnancy, the classic signs of shock are not always present until after the fetal circulation is affected. During pregnancy, signs of shock usually do not present until after 30% of maternal blood volume is lost. Shunting of blood away from the placenta occurs prior to this 30% blood loss.

Disseminated intravascular coagulation (DIC). According to Sher (1978), DIC occurs in all cases of abruptio placentae. Of the total number of cases, 30% will develop severe maternal and fetal complications related to DIC while the fetus remains alive (Pritchard and MacDonald, 1980). In these cases the clotting will become intravascular as well as retroplacental. This coagulation defect usually occurs in patients with a severe, concealed abruptio placentae due to one or more of the following.

1. Depletion of the clotting factors, especially platelets, fibrinogen, and prothrombin
2. Release of thromboplastin into the maternal circulation activating the clotting mechanism throughout the body
3. Activation of the anticoagulant effect stimulated by the presence of increased fibrin degradation products; when a coagulation defect occurs, hypofibrinogenemia results and massive bleeding occurs (see Chapter 12)

Maternal effects

In less than 1% of cases, maternal death occurs from hemorrhagic shock. This low maternal mortality is mainly because of the availability of blood-replacement therapy. However, maternal morbidity is significant. Because of the potential for massive bleeding, the patient is at high risk for developing shock and disseminated intravascular coagulation (DIC) at any time prior to delivery. Hurd and associates (1983) found that during the postpartum period 52% developed anemia, 30% developed an infection, 17% developed postpartum hemorrhage, and 14% developed disseminated intravascular coagulation (DIC). Other complications that can develop as a result of ischemia are renal failure and pituitary necrosis (Sheehan's syndrome).

Fetal and neonatal effects

Perinatal mortality ranges from 25% to 60% (Knab, 1978; Notelovitz et al., 1979; Huff, 1982). This depends on the degree of placental separation and the method of treatment. In the United States, 15% to 25% of all perinatal deaths are attributed to abruptio placentae (Knab, 1978).

Whenever the placenta detaches from the decidual lining of the uterus, the surface area for perfusion is decreased in proportion to the degree of separation. Therefore fetal life support is affected and fetal distress develops in proportion to the degree of separation.

As placental separation increases from mild to severe, the uterine muscle begins to retract and hypertonus develops. This further jeopardizes fetal well-being by *(1)* decreasing the intervillous space and thereby decreasing the exchange surface, and *(2)* impeding the transport of oxygen and essential nutrients via maternal blood to the intervillous spaces. Fetal blood supply is compromised even more by the maternal compensatory mechanism that begins to decrease blood flow to "nonessential organs" and thereby decreases the blood supply to the uterus.

If the circulation to the fetus is affected strongly enough to cause fetal distress, intrauterine asphyxia will occur. This can cause brain damage and neurological abnormalities. If the fetus is not delivered (Notelovitz et al., 1979), total anoxia and fetal death will ensue. When the fetus must be delivered before 36 weeks of gestation, the mortality and morbidity associated with prematurity affect neonatal outcome. Therefore early recognition, rapid correction of the maternal blood volume, continuous monitoring of fetal well-being, and delivery at the opportune time can greatly decrease perinatal mortality.

Even if the bleeding and separation stop, the fetus is at risk for developing distress at any time as the pregnancy progresses. This is related to the decreased placental surface area that remains intact to meet the increased needs of the growing fetus. Therefore intrauterine growth retardation can develop.

MEDICAL DIAGNOSIS

Diagnosis usually is made on the basis of presenting symptoms and a physical assessment. Severe and moderate abruptio placentae are easily diagnosed; a patient presents with one or more of the classic symptoms of uterine tenderness or rigidity, dark vaginal bleeding, and varying degrees of shock. Mild abruptio placentae is more difficult to diagnose; it is easily confused with a placenta previa, because vaginal bleeding may be the only presenting symptom. Therefore ultrasound or a double set-up vaginal examination must be done to rule out a placenta previa. Ultrasound can also identify the presence of a retroplacental clot (Spirt et al., 1979). There is no diagnostic method available to determine the degree of placental separation.

USUAL MEDICAL MANAGEMENT

Treatment of an abruptio placentae depends on the following.
1. The severity of blood loss
2. Fetal maturity
3. Fetal well-being

If the abruptio placentae is mild, gestational age of the fetus is determined first. With an immature fetus of less than 36 weeks of gestation, expectant management is usually the treatment. The components of expectant management are listed below.
1. Close observations for signs of concealed or external bleeding
2. Monitoring fetal well-being with nonstress tests and serial estriols to determine when the placenta becomes inadequate in meeting the needs of the fetus (see Chapter 3)

When the fetus is older than 36 weeks of gestation, delivery is usually the treatment of choice. If the fetus is in a cephalic presentation, a vaginal delivery is usually attempted. If the woman is not in labor, it can be initiated by an amniotomy or a labor stimulant such as oxytocin, provided that the patient is in a tertiary care center where rapid emergency measures can be taken if further abruption occurs with contractions. If the fetus is not in a cephalic presentation or if, during the induction of labor, bleeding increases, the uterus fails to relax between contractions, fetal distress occurs, or labor fails to progress actively, a cesarean delivery will be performed.

If the abruptio placentae is moderate to severe, the following are the objectives of treatment.
1. Restore blood loss quickly
2. Monitor the fetus
3. Correct coagulation defect if present
4. Expedite delivery

Replacement of maternal blood loss is the first medical consideration to prevent the life-threatening effects of shock. This is usually accomplished by fluid replacement using a Ringer's lactate solution and whole blood as soon as it is available. Intravenous Ringer's lactate and blood are usually administered at a rate adequate to maintain the hematocrit at 30% and urinary output at 30 ml/

hr or greater (Pritchard and MacDonald, 1980). In rare instances, the patient's blood loss is rapid and massive, leading to severe shock. In such cases, volume expanders or immediate transfusions with type O Rh-negative blood may be given until properly matched blood is available.

The fetus must be monitored closely until delivery takes place. It should be kept in mind that a maternal heart beat may be picked up through the fetal scalp electrode in the event of fetal death. Therefore fetal heart tones should be compared to the maternal pulse.

If a coagulation defect such as DIC develops, replacement of the clotting factors is the usual treatment. This can be accomplished by the administration of cryoprecipitate or fresh frozen plasma to replace fibrinogen and a platelet transfusion if the platelet count is below $50,000/mm^3$. Heparin was once used to treat DIC in the presence of an abruptio placentae, but it is no longer an acceptable treatment. Within 24 hours following delivery, the coagulation defect normally corrects itself. The platelets may take 2 to 4 days before they return to their normal level (Pritchard and MacDonald, 1980).

Vaginal delivery is usually attempted with a moderate abruptio placentae only in tertiary care centers. The labor can be facilitated by an amniotomy if the fetus is mature. If the fetus is immature, the labor usually progresses faster with an intact sac. If fetal distress occurs, labor does not progress steadily, the uterus fails to relax adequately between contractions, or bleeding cannot be controlled with intravenous therapy and blood replacement, then a cesarean birth will be performed.

In the presence of a severe abruptio placentae, if the fetus is alive, a cesarean birth should be performed as soon as possible. If the fetus is dead, a vaginal delivery may be attempted.

PLACENTA PREVIA

Placenta previa occurs when the placenta attaches to the lower segment of the uterus, near or over the internal os, instead of in the body or fundal segment of the uterus. It is normally classified into one of three categories depending on the degree of coverage of the cervix (Fig. 11-2).

1. Marginal, when the placenta is near but does not cover any part of the internal os
2. Partial, when the placenta implants near and partially covers the interal os
3. Total, when the placenta completely covers the internal os

INCIDENCE

The incidence of placenta previa is approximately 1 in 200 pregnancies or a 0.5% risk (Pritchard and MacDonald, 1980; Cotton et al., 1980). The highest

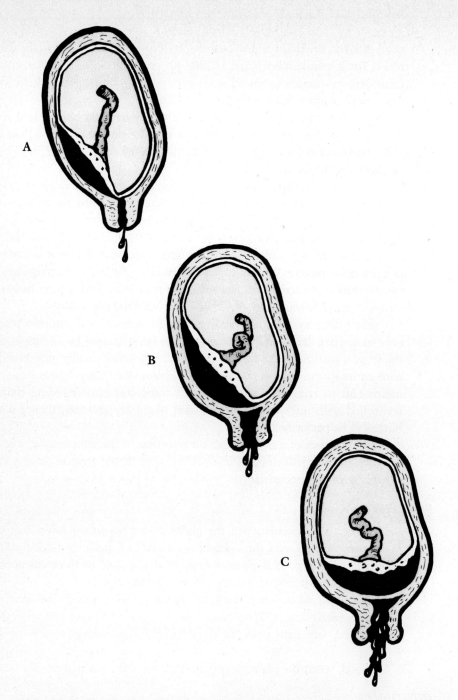

FIG. 11-2. Classifications of placenta previa. **A,** Marginal placenta previa; **B,** partial placenta previa; **C,** total placenta previa. (Illustrated by Vincenza Genovese, Phoenix, Ariz. Modified from Netter, F.: In Oppenheim, E., editor: Ciba collection of medical illustrations, vol. 2, reproductive system, Summit, N.J., 1965, Ciba Pharmaceutical Co.)

incidence has been found in multigravidas, and this is associated with age rather than parity (Abdul-Karim and Chevli, 1976). It has been found that, once placenta previa occurs, the risk of its recurrence in a subsequent pregnancy increases fivefold (Cotton et al., 1980). The incidence of placenta previa doubles following one or more previous abortions and increases sixfold following a cesarean delivery; it occurs twice as often in the pregnant addict (Butnarescu et al., 1980; Cotton et al., 1980; Brenner et al., 1978).

ETIOLOGY

The actual cause of placenta previa is unknown. However, it is frequently associated with factors that cause uterine scarring or interfere with blood supply to the endometrium (Pritchard and MacDonald, 1980). Predisposing factors that can scar the uterine lining are abortion, cesarean delivery, increased parity, a prior placenta previa, uterine infection, or closely spaced pregnancies (Brenner et al., 1978). Predisposing factors that interfere with adequate blood supply to the endometrium are uterine tumors, multiple pregnancy, or maternal age over 35.

PHYSIOLOGY
Normal

The blastocyst normally implants into the upper anterior portion of the uterus, where the vascular blood supply is rich. After implantation of the blastocyst, the trophoblastic tissue sends out threadlike projections, the chorionic villi, that grow into the decidua (endometrium). At first these chorionic villi surround the blastocyst, but, soon after, the portion of the chorionic villi in contact with the decidua basalis proliferates to form the placenta, and the villi, in contact with the decidua capsularis, atrophy. Therefore, according to Young (1978), the cells that make up the placenta have the ability to grow in one area and to remain dormant or to atrophy in another.

The chorionic villi are of two types. One type opens up intervillous spaces, which fill with maternal blood to form an area of exchange between the embryonic and fetal and maternal circulatory systems. Another type of villi forms anchoring cords to stabilize the placenta and embryo or fetus in the uterus. According to Young (1978), these villi can be uprooted and will then reroot themselves.

Pathophysiology

With placenta previa, the blastocyst implants itself in the lower uterine segment, over or very near the internal os. Why it fails to implant in the upper third of the uterus is unknown. However, this appears to be related to a defect in the vascularization of the decidua. Because the vascularization is less favorable in the lower uterine segment than in the fundus, the placenta will often be larger and thinner. This is a compensatory mechanism to increase its efficiency by increasing the placenta's surface area for perfusion. Although placenta previa is related to problems associated with implantation, abruption is related to problems of adherence to the uterine wall.

Signs and symptoms

Normally, during the latter half of pregnancy, the lower uterine segment elongates as the fundal segment of the uterus hypertrophies. Toward the end of the pregnancy, the cervix begins to efface and dilate. When the placenta is implanted in the lower uterine segment over or around the internal cervical os, separation or tearing of portions of the placenta can occur with subsequent bleeding. Usually, the greater the percent of placenta covering the os, the earlier the first episode of bleeding occurs. Because the normal uterine changes occur very gradually until labor begins, the initial bleeding episode is usually slight and ceases spontaneously as clot formation occurs. This is not always the case, however. The bleeding is usually painless and bright red in color without associated uterine tenderness because the blood is not trapped behind the placenta. Recurrence is unpredictable and can take place at any time.

Vital signs may be misleadingly normal even in the presence of severe blood loss. This is related to the normal increase of 40% to 50% in the circulatory blood volume during pregnancy. In fact, after week 32 of gestation, the pregnant patient can lose 30% of her blood volume without exhibiting signs of shock. However, the blood supply to the placenta is affected prior to this 30% decrease in the maternal blood volume. Decreased urinary output is probably the most reliable sign indicating excessive blood loss; the rate of urine formation reflects the amount of renal perfusion, which in turn reflects the blood volume in the circulatory system (Pritchard and MacDonald, 1980).

Fetal heart rate is usually normal unless the placental exchange is compromised by excessive blood loss, maternal shock, or major placental detachment. The presenting part of the fetus usually remains high even in late pregnancy because the placenta occupies the lower uterine segment. For this same reason, there is an increased risk of malpresentations such as transverse, oblique, or breech lie.

Maternal effects

The maternal mortality rate associated with placenta previa is less than 1%. The risk of maternal morbidity is much higher. The mother is at risk for many of the same complications experienced by the abruptio placentae patient. She is at a lesser risk for disseminated intravascular coagulation (DIC), renal damage, and cerebral ischemia than the woman with abruptio placentae. This is probably because the visual blood loss is a more accurate manifestation of the true blood loss. The risks of postpartum hemorrhage, anemia, and infection, however, are as high or higher than in abruptio placentae.

Fetal and neonatal effects

Perinatal mortality currently ranges from 12% to 20% (Goplerud, 1982; Cotton et al., 1980). The steady decline in mortality is related to adequate blood replacement prior to delivery, the utilization of expectant management, use of ultrasound to locate the placenta, cesarean deliveries, and improved neonatal care. The major cause of perinatal mortality today is prematurity and intrauterine hypoxia (Huff, 1982; Brenner et al., 1978) related to inadequate placental oxygenation and the chance of cord prolapse.

MEDICAL DIAGNOSIS

When any pregnant woman complains of vaginal bleeding after 20 weeks of gestation, placenta previa should be considered. To diagnose a placenta previa, the location of the placenta must be determined. If the patient is not bleeding profusely, ultrasound is the preferred method. If ultrasound is not available, radiographic studies can be used. Because vaginal or rectal examinations can cause further separation of a placenta previa, resulting in profuse bleeding, they should *never* be done in the presence of vaginal bleeding unless delivery is imminent. If the fetus has reached a gestational age of 36 weeks or more, a double set-up may be used. A double set-up vaginal exam is done by taking the patient to an operating room prepared for immediate cesarean delivery and doing the vaginal examination with blood available for transfusion. However, double set-up vaginal examination is practiced less often because ultrasound is so highly accurate and easily done.

A speculum examination is usually done to rule out other causes of bright red vaginal bleeding such as cervicitis, cervical polyps, heavy show, or cervical carcinoma.

An amniocentesis may be included in the diagnosis workup to determine fetal lung maturity. If the lecithin/sphingomyelin (L/S) ratio is 2:1 or phosphatidylglycerol (PG) is present, delivery is probably the choice of treatment.

If a placenta previa is found by ultrasound during the second or early third trimester, especially if the patient is asymptomatic, it may cure itself by placental migration toward the fundus (King, 1973). The two mechanisms by which placental migration takes place have been hypothesized by Young (1978). First, the placenta is able to grow in one area and remain dormant or atrophy in another area. Therefore it may multiply in the direction of the fundus and atrophy near or over the cervical os as the pregnancy progresses. This is probably related to the increased vascularity of the fundus as compared to the lower uterine segment. Second, as the uterus grows in size, the various lobules of the placenta appear to be torn up at different times, normally, during pregnancy and then rerooted in the decidua in a different area to allow for this uterine growth. The placenta can thereby gradually change its location.

USUAL MEDICAL MANAGEMENT

Treatment depends on the gestational age and the extent of bleeding. If the gestational age is less than 36 weeks, and the bleeding is mild, less than 250 ml (Rabello, 1981), and the patient is not in labor, then the treatment of choice is expectant management. The sole purpose is to allow the fetus time to mature to improve perinatal mortality from prematurity (Huff, 1982). When expectant management is chosen, it usually includes the following.

1. Hospitalization
2. Bed rest for 72 hours in an attempt to use the fetus as a tamponade
3. Close observation for bleeding
4. Continuous fetal monitoring to facilitate early detection of fetal distress during bleeding episodes; otherwise, assess every 4 hours with a Doppler or fetoscope
5. Intravenous infusions, unless bleeding is minimal; then a heparin lock left in place and changed as needed
6. Type and cross match for at least 2 units of blood
7. No vaginal or rectal examination
8. Daily determination of hemoglobin or hematocrit to detect hidden bleeding
9. If the patient is allowed to return home after stabilization, she should be instructed to limit her activity and to avoid douching, enemas, or coitus

Close supervision by family or significant others in the home is necessary. Discharge is not the most desirable choice of care but may be necessary for social or financial reasons. Fetal activity charts should be kept daily, and a nonstress test (NST) should be done biweekly. Expectant management is terminated as soon as the fetus is mature, excessive bleeding occurs, active labor begins, or any other obstetrical reason to terminate the pregnancy develops, such as pregnancy-induced hypertension or intraamniotic infection.

If the bleeding is profuse, the gestational age is 36 or more weeks, or the L/S ratio is 2:1 or PG is present, immediate delivery is usually the treatment of choice.

If the patient has partial or total placenta previa, a cesarean delivery is indicated to prevent the following.

1. Profuse hemorrhage that can occur from separation of that portion of the placenta lying over the cervical os as the cervix dilates and effaces
2. Cervical lacerations, a frequent complication of a vaginal delivery with a placenta previa

3. Fetal hypoxia due to a large maternal blood loss or premature separation of a large segment of the placenta prior to delivery

When the placenta previa is marginal, many physicians attempt a vaginal delivery if the fetus is in a cephalic presentation in hopes that the presenting part will be able to press the detached part of the placenta against the implantation site and tamponade the blood vessels. An amniotomy is usually performed and intravenous oxytocin given to facilitate the labor. If at any time during the trial labor fetal distress is noted, vaginal bleeding increases, or labor does not progress, then a cesarean delivery will be performed.

An asymptomatic placenta previa, which is identified prior to the latter half of the third trimester, has a 90% chance of changing to a normal placenta (Rizos et al., 1979). Therefore the patient should be followed with serial ultrasound every 6 to 8 weeks to determine if the placenta previa will persist.

NURSING PROCESS FOR ABRUPTIO PLACENTAE AND PLACENTA PREVIA
Prevention

Because inadequate blood supply to the decidua (endometrium) prior to implantation may be the underlying cause of a placenta previa and inadequate blood supply to the decidua (endometrium) during pregnancy may be the underlying cause of an abruptio placentae, any condition that would decrease the blood supply to the uterus should be avoided if possible. Because cigarette smoking decreases uterine blood supply, it should be avoided by the childbearing mother. Adequate contraceptive instructions should be given so that couples can plan the time and number of their children, preventing therapeutic abortions and closely spaced pregnancies. Hypertensive disorders of pregnancy should be monitored closely for an abruptio placentae; this condition increases the risk of an abruptio placentae. All pregnant women should be instructed to avoid the vena cava syndrome during late pregnancy; this decreases uterine blood flow and can trigger abruptio placentae as well. Use of the street drug cocaine is known to cause transient acute hypertensive episodes, which could initiate abruption of the placenta.

Assessment

When any patient experiences bleeding during the last half of pregnancy, the first nursing responsibility is to gather an in-depth data base to assess the cause of the bleeding and the severity of the condition. There is one exception to the rule. If the bleeding is life threatening, immediate care must be implemented without a complete data base. If possible, the following data should be obtained.

1. The patient's perception of what is happening
2. When the bleeding started and its frequency
3. The amount, color, and consistency of the blood present (The bleeding is usually bright red with placenta previa and dark with an abruption.)
4. The patient's activity just prior to and at the time the bleeding started
5. What self-treatment, if any, was used by the patient (If tampons are being used to collect the bleeding, then there is concealed bleeding.)
6. Whether or not any pain or uterine contractions accompanied this bleeding and whether or not the uterus feels firm or tender to touch
7. Whether or not the uterus is contracting, to determine if the patient is in labor
8. Whether or not any previous bleeding episodes occurred during this pregnancy
9. The EDC, to determine appropriate management
10. Vital signs and fetal heart rate
11. Fundal height, to recognize continued concealed bleeding
12. A clot-observation test for DIC if the bleeding is moderate to severe
13. Fetal presentation and state of engagement if near term by abdominal palpation (Transverse or oblique lie is common with a placenta previa, because the placenta usually interferes with engagement.)

In determining the amount of blood lost, the nurse should assist the patient in using measurable terms in describing the amount instead of vague terms. For example, how many pads were saturated in a certain period of time or how many cupfuls were lost. It has been estimated that a saturated pad contains 30 ml of blood. If the nurse changes the pad, it can be weighed to obtain a more accurate assessment by applying the conversion that 1 ml of blood weighs 1 gm.

No vaginal or rectal examinations should be performed until a placenta previa is ruled out because they can initiate further separation, and profuse bleeding would result. In the presence of an abruptio placentae, when delivery is not to be initiated immediately, no vaginal or rectal examinations should be carried out so as not to disturb the injured placenta any further.

Unless profuse bleeding is present, the nurse should be prepared to assist with ultrasound or a double set-up vaginal examination to determine placenta location and an amniocentesis to determine fetal lung maturity. The obstetrician might also want to do a speculum examination to rule out other causes of bleeding. If the patient presents with signs of severe hemorrhage or shock, much of the data base must be omitted and immediate intervention must be implemented.

When the diagnosis of mild abruptio placentae or placenta previa is confirmed and expectant management is ordered, the nurse must continually assess for hemorrhage, fetal distress, level of maternal anxiety, and for signs of labor. Further bleeding is assessed thus.

1. Visually inspecting the amount of external bleeding present on the pads, Chuxs, or linen
2. Marking the fundal height on the abdomen then observing for a change to detect concealed blood loss
3. Following serial hematocrits or hemoglobins
4. Taking frequent vital signs and observing for other signs and symptoms of shock

The well-being of the fetus should be monitored closely by evaluating fetal heart rate with a fetal monitor or a Doppler and carrying out nonstress tests. The uterus should be palpated with each set of vital signs to assess for uterine contractions, tenderness, and rigidity. The patient should also be instructed to notify the nurse if bleeding recurs or if she experiences any uterine contractions, abdominal pain, tenderness, or hardness. Uterine irritability increases the likelihood of bleeding.

Parents are usually very concerned about the health and well-being of the baby and the mother's safety. They may also be experiencing some unusual fears or worries such as "what they did to cause this to happen." Therefore the nurse should encourage the expectant parents to express their feelings and concerns. In this way, the nurse will know better how to individualize emotional support.

Antepartum intervention

When expectant management is ordered, the nurse's role, in addition to an ongoing, thorough assessment, is one of facilitating adaptation to the stresses associated with the diagnosis, implementing care that will facilitate an optimal outcome, and being prepared at all times for emergency intervention should the need arise.

The expectant parents need a clear explanation of the condition, the plan of care, including the various procedures that are to be done, and the prognosis. They are usually very concerned about the well-being of the mother and baby. The nurse should encourage them to talk about their fears, clarifying any misconceptions. There should be an attempt to allay anxiety by focusing the attention of the expectant parents on the positive signs of fetal well-being such as a normal fetal heart rate, fetal activity, and reactive nonstress tests. The mother should be complimented for her cooperation in adhering to medical therapy. The nurse should facilitate problem solving with the mother regarding work- and family-related responsibilities that must be relinquished during this time. A social service referral may be appropriate if long-term hospitalization is required. Some diversional activities should be provided that are of interest to the patient to facilitate her ability to cope with the time of limited activity. Such activities may include reading, crafts, and education on childbirth, since the expectant couple will probably be unable to attend a regular series. The diversional therapy department may be helpful in this area also. Discuss with the expectant parents the possibility of a cesarean delivery. The parents will then be more prepared if the event arises.

To optimize the outcome, the patient is placed on bed rest in a quiet environment. Activity and sensory stimulation can increase the bleeding and elevate the basal metabolic rate, which increases oxygen consumption. To facilitate tamponade with the fetal head, the head of the bed should be elevated 20° to 30°. The mother should be encouraged to lie on either side to prevent pressure on the vena cava and further compromise of fetal circulation. No vaginal or rectal examinations are performed and no enemas or douches given. Intravenous fluid administration is to be started with an 18-gauge intravenous catheter to allow for blood administration if necessary. Oxygen equipment should be available in the patient's room if signs of shock or fetal distress occur. Because the loss of blood increases the risk of anemia, the patient should be encouraged to eat foods high in iron and to take her supplemental iron or prenatal vitamins consistently as ordered. The patient's hemoglobin level is followed daily and, if the level drops to 10 gm or less, the obstetrician should be notified; blood transfusions are then usually started (Buchhiet and Price, 1981).

If the bleeding stops and the patient is discharged home, she is instructed in the following.

1. To notify her obstetrician at the first signs of bleeding, uterine tenderness, or uterine contractions
2. To limit her activity
3. Not to douche or have sexual intercourse, since these can stimulate further separation
4. To recognize the importance of keeping all appointments with her obstetrician and with the testing center

Fetal maturity and well-being tests such as biweekly nonstress, ultrasound, and amniocentesis are usually ordered on a frequent basis in an attempt to determine the optimal time for delivery.

When the placenta is partially detached from the uterine wall, even without further bleeding, the placenta may not be able to keep up with the growing needs as the fetus matures because of the decreased surface area available for perfusion.

In the presence of a mild abruptio placentae or a placenta previa with slight vaginal bleeding and a gestational age of 36 weeks or greater, the nurse should prepare for delivery. In the presence of mild abruptio placentae or a marginal placenta previa, a vaginal delivery is usually attempted. Otherwise, the patient should be prepared for a cesarean delivery.

If the nursing and medical assessment reveals a moderate or severe abruptio placentae or a placenta previa with profuse bleeding, immediate intervention by replacing the blood lost and expediting delivery is indicated. An intravenous line is started immediately with an 18-gauge intravenous catheter to allow for blood administration, and blood should be drawn for type and cross matching of 2 to 5 units of blood. A lactated Ringer's solution can be administered until blood is available; it is a better volume expander than dextrose in water (Pritchard and MacDonald, 1980). Volume expanders can also be ordered while waiting for properly matched blood. The nurse should give the patient nothing by mouth unless it is ordered. The pulse, blood pressure, respiration, and fetal heart tones are monitored at appropriate intervals, usually every 15 minutes. Continuous fetal monitoring is preferred. Hourly intake and output should be noted. In the presence of an abruption, assessment for changes in uterine size should be made. Laboratory studies such as hematocrit, hemoglobin, fibrinogen determination, and clotting time should be carried out as ordered. If for any reason the patient must be kept on her back, the uterus should be tilted to the left to keep the gravid uterus off the vena cava. This can be done by placing a folded sheet under the patient's right hip.

Hypovolemia is a grave problem that can develop whenever there is bleeding. Hypovolemic shock can ensue, causing inadequate organ blood flow and tissue oxygenation. If shock is allowed to develop, it can cause fetal death, maternal DIC, renal failure, or pituitary necrosis. Therefore the nurse should be observant, endeavoring to detect the early signs of hypovolemic shock to implement emergency care immediately and prevent these complications. During pregnancy, due to the increased blood volume, the classic early signs of shock such as hypotension, tachycardia, and hyperpnea are less pronounced. Therefore shock is more difficult to detect. In patients with an abruption, the signs of shock can ensue without notice, even more often than with a placenta previa. This is because the signs of bleeding may be masked if the bleeding is concealed behind the placenta.

On the other hand, if a patient is treated too vigorously with intravenous intervention or blood replacement, fluid overload can result. The most accurate way to determine the patient's fluid needs and prevent fluid overload is by pulmonary wedge or central venous pressure. If these lines cannot be placed, then fluid management must be regulated by other means.

Urinary output is the best noninvasive indicator of circulatory volume. Because the kidneys are very sensitive to lack of perfusion from hypovolemic shock, a urinary output of 60 ml/hr to 100 ml/hr suggests normal kidney function and therefore adequate circulatory volume. Less than 30 ml/hr indicates decreased circulatory volume. However, this indicator is not effective in assessing fluid overload. Another indicator of fluid volume is hematocrit. A hematocrit of 30% or greater indicates an appropriate circulatory volume. Therefore, the nurse should use pulmonary wedge pressure or central venous pressure if available, urinary output, and hematocrit to determine accurately the patient's fluid needs and to prevent fluid overload. The nurse should also watch for signs of pulmonary edema, such as dyspnea, cough, and rales, which, if present, can indicate fluid overload.

If signs of shock develop, oxygen should be administered by mask at 7 liters to increase the oxygen concentration of the blood. The patient should be placed in a modified Trendelenburg position in which only the legs are elevated to increase blood return without contributing to respiratory impairment.

About 10% of all patients with a severe abruption develop DIC (Sher, 1977). Therefore these patients should be followed closely using such laboratory studies as the following.

1. Fibrinogen determination
2. Platelet count
3. Prothrombin or partial thromboplastic times
4. Clotting time

A simple clot-observation test may be done every 30 to 60 minutes at the bedside by the nurse to assess for DIC. To carry this out, the nurse places 5 ml of venous blood in a test tube, hangs it in the room, and observes the time it takes to clot. If it does not form a clot within 8 to 12 minutes, a coagulation defect is usually present (see Chapter 12).

Intrapartum intervention

With adequate intravenous fluids and blood available, delivery should be facilitated as the condition demands. If the abruption is severe and the fetus is alive, or if the placenta previa is marginal with other than a cephalic presentation, or if the placenta previa is partial or total, a cesarean delivery is usually indicated. A trial labor is usually attempted in all other cases provided that there is no other obstetric reason for a cesarean delivery. During this trial labor, the patient's physiologic parameters should be monitored. In addition, the progress of labor is monitored closely. In the presence of a placenta previa, the monitoring must be done without vaginal examination. In evaluating the progress of labor for a patient with severe abruptio placentae, vaginal examination can be done, and the cervical change is usually one of effacement followed by rapid dilatation (Pritchard and MacDonald, 1980). The uterine contractions and fetal heart rate should be monitored with an internal or external monitor. The patient's temperature should be monitored every hour, since these patients are at a higher risk for developing an infection owing to partial separation of the placenta.

The nurse should be prepared to assist with an amniotomy and administer a labor stimulant as ordered. The side-lying position is encouraged to decrease the risk of compressing the vena cava and intensifying the problem of uterine profusion.

All patients having any degree of abruption or placenta previa should be prepared by the nurse for a possible cesarean delivery.

1. Obtain a signed consent.
2. Insert a Foley catheter.
3. Perform an abdominoperineal prep.
4. Administer an antacid every hour as ordered to decrease the risk of aspiration pneumonia if cesarean delivery is necessary.

The pediatrician and nursery are notified of a possible high-risk delivery so that they can be prepared for the arrival. The physician should be notified so that the trial labor can be terminated and a cesarean delivery performed if any of the following conditions develop.

1. Signs of fetal distress, because there is minimal or no placental reserve in a placenta that has separated to some degree
2. Hypertonic uterus
3. Increased signs of bleeding
4. Poor progress in labor

(See Table 11-2 for a comparison of placenta previa and abruptio placentae.)

Even though abruptio placentae generally takes place prior to labor, in a few cases it develops during the first or second stage of labor. Therefore all labor patients should be evaluated by assessing the amount and kind of vaginal discharge present, by listening to the patient's description of the kind of pain she is experiencing, and by palpating the uterus between contractions for relaxation or noting the resting tone on the internal fetal monitor strip. A patient experiencing an abruption may complain of coliclike abdominal pain and the uterus may not relax and return to a normal resting tone between contractions.

Postpartum intervention

Following an abruptio placentae or placenta previa, the patient is at risk for developing the following complications.

1. Hemorrhage
2. Anemia
3. Renal failure
4. Pituitary necrosis
5. Uterine infection

The most common cause of postpartum hemorrhage following an abruption is a poorly contracted uterus; the myometrium that has been infiltrated with blood may not contract effectively. However, following a placenta previa, hemorrhage can occur even if the uterus is firmly contracted. This is because

TABLE 11-2. *Comparison of placenta previa and abruptio placenta*

	Placenta previa	Abruptio placenta
Definition	Implantation of the placenta in the lower segment of the uterus, near or over the internal os	Premature separation of a normally implanted placenta after 20 weeks of gestation
Classification	1. Marginal: the placenta is implanted near but does not cover any part of the internal os	1. Mild: less than one sixth of the placenta is separated, there is minimal bleeding, and no or mild abdominal pain; maternal vital signs and FHR normal
	2. Partial: the placenta implants near and partially covers the internal os	2. Moderate: one sixth to two thirds of the placenta is separated; there is increased bleeding, abdominal pain, and uterine tone; maternal vital signs may show mild hypovolemia and FHR may indicate distress
	3. Total: the placenta completely covers the internal os	3. Severe: over two thirds of the placenta is separated; there is profuse bleeding, persistent and severe abdominal pain, and increased uterine tenderness; signs of shock or coagulopathy are frequently present with fetal distress or death resulting
Etiology	Unknown—theoretic considerations include a defective vascularization of the decidua resulting from uterine scarring or an interference with adequate blood supply to the endometrium	Unknown—theoretic considerations include degeneration of the spiral arteriola, which causes rupture of the involved blood vessels and bleeding; the bleeding under the placenta separates the placenta from the decidua
	Associated conditions include: 1. Maternal age greater than 35 2. Multiparity over five children 3. Prior uterine scar due to a previous abortion or cesarean delivery 4. Prior uterine infection 5. Uterine tumor 6. Multiple pregnancy	Associated conditions include: 1. Maternal age greater than 35 2. Multiparity over five children 3. Trauma or short umbilical cord 4. Pregnancy-induced or chronic hypertension 5. Previous abruption 6. Cigarette smoking
Signs and symptoms	Painless bright red bleeding; onset of bleeding usually slight to moderate and ceases spontaneously	Painful dark red bleeding unless only marginal; onset of bleeding is slight to profuse and usually continues
	Presenting part high or displaced	Presenting part engaged
	Uterus soft and nontender	Uterus tender or rigid (moderate to severe abruption)
	During labor, uterus relaxes between contractions	During labor, uterus usually has increased tone between contractions
	Blood usually clots normally	Clotting defects may be present
Diagnosis	Ultrasound No vaginal examination except under double set-up	According to signs and symptoms

TABLE 11-2. *Comparison of placenta previa and abruptio placenta—cont'd*

	Placenta previa	*Abruptio placenta*

Treatment	If the initial bleeding episode is slight and gestational age less than 37 weeks, then expectant management is the usual choice of treatment and includes:
	1. Close observations of fetal well-being and amount of bleeding
	2. Limited physical activity
	3. No douches, enemas, or sexual intercourse
	4. Delivery when fetus is mature or hemorrhage dictates
	When the bleeding is profuse, gestational age is greater than 36 weeks, or the L/S ratio is 2:1 or greater, delivery is the choice of treatment; if the placenta previa is:
	1. Marginal, a vaginal delivery is attempted
	2. Partial or complete, a cesarean delivery is performed
		In the presence of a mild abruptio placentae and a gestational age less than 36 weeks, expectant management is the usual choice of treatment and includes:
		1. Close observation of fetal well-being and amount of bleeding
		2. Limited physical activity
		3. Serial hematocrits to assess concealed bleeding
		4. Delivery when fetus is mature or hemorrhage dictates
		
		In the presence of a mild abruptio placentae, with a gestational age of 36 weeks or greater, delivery is the usual choice of treatment.
		In the presence of a moderate to severe abruptio placentae:
		1. Restore blood loss
		2. Correct coagulation defect if present
		3. Facilitate delivery
		  a. Vaginal delivery is attempted if there is no evidence of fetal or maternal distress with fluid and blood replacement, the fetus is in a cephalic presentation, labor progresses actively, or fetus is dead
		  b. Cesarean delivery is indicated for severe abruptio if fetus is alive, fetal or maternal distress develops with fluid and blood replacement, labor fails to progress actively, or fetal presentation other than cephalic

Maternal outcome	Less than 1% maternal mortality	Less than 1% maternal mortality
Fetal outcome	Perinatal mortality 12% to 24% Prematurity Intrauterine hypoxia	Perinatal mortality 25% to 60% Prematurity Intrauterine hypoxia
Maternal postpartum complications	Hemorrhage and hypovolemic shock Puerperal infection Anemia DIC Renal failure Pituitary necrosis	Hemorrhage and hypovolemic shock Puerperal infection Anemia DIC Renal failure Pituitary necrosis Couvelaire uterus

Third trimester bleeding: abruptio placentae and placenta previa

Potential patient problem	Outcome criteria
Antepartum care	
A. Potential hypovolemia related to: Premature separation of placenta	Vital signs stable for patient Urinary output 30 ml/hr or greater No signs of shock Hematocrit 30% to 45% Blood loss 250 ml or less

Assessment and intervention

Dx. Assess blood loss:

Obtain history of onset, duration, amount, color, and consistency of bleeding

Obtain history regarding associated symptoms, prior bleeding episodes,
and activity at onset of bleeding

Record visual blood loss by pad count (1 pad = 30 ml) or weigh saturated pads, Chuxs, or linen (1 gm = 1 ml)

Record blood pressure, pulse, and respirations as indicated (depending on
severity)

Observe for signs of shock

Check for abdominal pain, uterine tenderness, or rigidity

Keep an accurate I&O record

Evaluate urinary output as indicated (depends on severity)

Refer to such lab data as hemoglobin and hematocrit

Mark fundal height and observe for change

Th. Expectant management for mild bleeding:

No vaginal or rectal examinations, enemas, or douches until placenta previa
is ruled out

Bed rest for 72 hrs in a quiet environment unless otherwise ordered

Prevent vena cava syndrome by having patient lie on either side; if patient
must be on her back, place a folded sheet under her right hip to tilt the
uterus off the vena cava

Start IV with 18-gauge intravenous catheter

Order blood for type and cross match for 2 to 5 units as ordered

Have blood available for infusion

Prepare for double set-up vaginal examination if ordered

Management for moderate to severe bleeding:

NPO unless otherwise ordered

Bed rest in quiet environment unless otherwise ordered

Start IV with 18-gauge intravenous catheter

Administer Ringer's lactate until blood is available

Order blood for type and cross-match for 5 units as ordered

Prepare for blood transfusion as ordered by having 250 ml normal saline
available

Administer blood replacements or volume expanders as ordered

Notify nursery of possible high-risk infant

If signs of shock develop:

Place patient in modified Trendelenburg position (only elevated legs)

Administer oxygen with mask at 7 liters

Dx., diagnostic; Th., therapeutic; Ed., education; Ref., referral.   *Continued.*

Third trimester bleeding: abruptio placentae and placenta previa—cont'd

Potential patient problem	Outcome criteria
Antepartum care—cont'd	
B. Potential fetal distress related to: Blood loss Decrease placental perfusion	Fetal heart rate baseline between 120 and 160 Reactive NST Negative CST At least four fetal movements in 1 hr
C. Potential anxiety related to: Fear of unknown outcome Possible fetal loss Fear for her own safety Finances	Verbalizes fears and concerns Participates in decisions affecting care Share realistic hopes for maternal and fetal outcome

Assessment and intervention

Ed. If patient is sent home, instruct
  Regarding importance of limiting activity
  Not to douche or have sexual intercourse
  If bleeding recurs or if she experiences any abdominal pain, tenderness, or hardness to contact her physician immediately
  To eat foods high in iron and consistently to take the supplemental iron and prenatal vitamins as ordered to prevent anemia

Dx. Determine EDC
  Check FHR as indicated (depending on severity)
  Evaluate FHR for tachycardia, bradycardia, late or variable decelerations, and loss of long- or short-term variability
  Check fetal positions
  During labor:
    Check uterine contractions for duration, frequency and uterine resting tone
    Observe amniotic fluid for meconium staining
Th. Keep patient positioned on left or right side; if must be on back tilt uterus to the left by placing folded sheet under the right hip
  During labor apply external monitor or assist with internal monitor placement
  Administer oxygen as indicated with mask at 7 liters
Ed. Prepare patient for ordered procedures such as ultrasound, NST, CST, and amniocentesis
Ref. Notify physician if a baseline or periodic fetal heart rate change is noted or if there is a nonreactive NST or a positive CST

Dx. Assess family's coping strategies and resources
  Assess expectant parents' fears and concerns
Th. Encourage verbalization
  Explain procedures and reasons for each
  Keep patient and significant others informed as to plan of treatment
  Facilitate problem solving with the mother and family regarding mother's work and family responsibilities
  Provide diversional activities
Ed. Prepare patient for possibility of cesarean delivery
  Explain that cause of condition is unknown but not related to patient's activity at time of occurrence
Ref. Refer to social service if note ineffective coping, family difficulties in problem solving, or financial difficulties
  Refer to pastor, priest, or chaplain per patient's request

Continued.

Third trimester bleeding: abruptio placentae and placenta previa—cont'd

Potential patient problem	Outcome criteria

D. Potential DIC related to:
    Depletion of clotting factors
    Release of thromboplastin and
      fibrinogen
	Clotting factors within normal limits for
	    pregnancy
	Clotting time 8 to 12 min
	Fibrinogen levels 400 mg/100 ml
	Platelets 150,000 to 350,000 mm^3
	Partial prothrombin time (PTT) 18 to 38
	    sec

E. Potential fluid overload related
    to:
      Replacement therapy
	Urinary output between 30 and 60 ml/hr
	No signs of pulmonary congestion
	CVP 5 to 12 cm H$_2$O
	PWP 10 to 12 mm Hg

Intrapartum Care
A. Potential cesarean delivery related
    to:
      Degree of separation
	Delivery of a healthy neonate for their
	    level of development

Postpartum Care
A. Potential infection related to:
    Opened blood vessels near cer-
      vical os
    Premature separation of the
      placenta
	Temperature less than 38° C (100.4° F)
	No foul-smelling lochia

Assessment and intervention

Dx. Observe for signs of DIC such as oozing of blood from IV site, easy bruising, or petechia

Refer to such lab data as fibrinogen, platelets, PTT, and clotting time

Th. Be prepared to carry out a quick bedside test for DIC by placing 5 ml of blood in test tube

If DIC develops, see DIC suggested plan of nursing care

Ref. Report to physician at first sign of DIC

Dx. Assess for signs of pulmonary congestion such as dyspnea, cough, or rales

Keep an accurate I&O record

Check CVP or PWP if a CVP line or Swan-Ganz catheter is in place

Th. Auscultate lung field every shift for rales

Ref. Notify physician immediately of any signs of fluid overload or changes in the CVP or PWP

Dx. Monitor progress of labor:

Without vaginal exams if placenta previa

Check uterine contractions for frequency, duration, intensity, and uterine resting tone

Assess blood loss

Th. Prepare patient for possible cesarean delivery by

Obtaining signed consent

Placing a Foley catheter

Completing an abdominal placental prep

Notifying the pediatrician and nursery of possible high-risk delivery

Ed. Explain the possibility of a cesarean delivery

Ref. Notify physician if the following develop

Signs of fetal distress

Hypertonic uterus

Increased signs of bleeding

Labor progresses abnormally slow according to the Friedman curve

Dx. Check temperature qid until 48 hr postdelivery; if greater than 100.4° F check every 2 hr

Check vaginal discharge, lochia for odor every shift

Th. Use aseptic technique in care of patient

Ed. Explain perineal care and adequate hand washing

Ref. Notify physician if temperature elevated over 100.4° F (39° C) or if any other signs of infection develop

Continued.

Third trimester bleeding: abruptio placentae and placenta previa—cont'd

Potential patient problem	*Outcome criteria*
B. Potential postpartum hemorrhage related to: Opened blood vessels near os Couvelaire uterus Poor contractility of the uterus DIC	Vital signs stable for patient Adequately contracted uterus
C. Potential pituitary necrosis (Sheehan's syndrome) related to: Shock Vascular spasms DIC	Onset of lactation by the fourth or fifth postpartum day
D. Potential renal failure related to: Shock Vascular spasm DIC	Urinary output greater than 30 ml/hr or 120 ml/4 hr
E. Anxiety related to: Effect on neonate Effect on self	Verbalize fears and concerns Participates in infant care

Assessment and intervention

Dx. Record blood pressure, pulse, and respiration every 15 min eight times, every 30 min two times, every 1 hr two times, every 4 hr two times, then qid
Check firmness of uterus and vaginal flow with each vital sign check
Keep pad count
Refer to such lab data such as hematocrit and hemoglobin
Th. Keep bladder empty
Manually massage relaxed, boggy fundus very gently until firm
Maintain oxytocics and IV fluids as ordered
Administer blood replacements as ordered
Ref. Notify physician if excessive bleeding occurs in the presence of a contracted uterus or if uterus fails to contract or stay contracted with massage

Dx. Assess for onset of lactation by fourth or fifth postpartum day
Th. Administer no lactation suppressant if patient experienced shock during pregnancy or labor and delivery
Ed. If patient is bottle feeding explain the reason for the delay in lactation-suppressant therapy
Instruct patient to notify physician if onset of lactation does not occur by the fifth postpartum day

Dx. Keep an accurate I&O record
Ref. Notify physician if urinary output is less than 30 ml/hr or 120 ml/4 hr

Dx. Assess family's anxiety over neonatal and maternal well-being
Assess level of attachment
Th. Encourage verbalization of feelings and labor experiences
Ed. Instruct if infant survives delivery, rarely any long-term negative effect
Ref. Refer to social worker if inadequate coping or attachment is noted

the lower uterine segment does not have the contractility of the upper uterine segment and, as a consequence, there is less compression of the open vessels resulting from the removal of the placenta. The risk of hemorrhage is further increased by the larger than normal surface area denuded by the removal of the placenta. If DIC developed in connection with either an abruption or a placenta previa, the patient is at a greater risk for developing hemorrhage due to the inability of the uterus to contract. Following an abruption, uterine massage and a high concentration of intravenous oxytocin are usually effective in stimulating uterine contractions, but, when these are ineffective, prostaglandin F_{2a} has been successful (Hayaski et al., 1981). Following a placenta previa, uterine packing may be needed to control the hemorrhage. In rare cases, the bleeding cannot be controlled and a hysterectomy must be performed.

Renal failure can develop if shock, vascular spasms, or DIC have occurred. Therefore urinary output must be monitored closely. Pituitary necrosis (Sheehan's syndrome) occasionally results from the same conditions that cause renal failure. Since pituitary hormones regulate lactation, the nurse can assess for this condition by watching for the onset of lactation, which should occur by the fourth or fifth postpartum day. Therefore lactation should not be suppressed with medication in patients who experienced hypovolemic shock, vascular spasms, or DIC until after the onset of lactation has occurred.

There is an increased risk of infection following a placenta previa; the opened blood vessels are near the cervical os and can become infected easily. Following an abruption, the patient has an increased risk of uterine infection due to prolonged separation of the placenta. Thus strict asepsis should be used in administering perineal care. The nurse should assess the vaginal discharge for odor every shift and check the patient's temperature four times per day for 48 hours.

The parents will be apprehensive about the long-term effects of the placental separation on their newborn. According to Niswander (1981), if the fetus lives through the separation, the neonate rarely has any long-term negative effects except for the normal risks of prematurity if he or she is born early. These parents will need more time with their infant and should be encouraged to examine their baby closely. The nurse should point out reassuring characteristics.

Evaluation

The ultimate goal in the treatment of both an abruptio placentae and a placenta previa is early recognition and appropriate intervention to prevent hemorrhage and its resulting complications of shock, DIC, pituitary necrosis, renal failure, and ultimately death to mother or fetus. At the same time, premature delivery should be avoided as long as intrauterine hypoxia is not present.

REFERENCES

Abdul-Karim, R., and Chevli, R.: Antepartum hemorrhage and shock, Clin. Obstet. Gynecol. **19**:533, 1976.

Basu, H.: Some observations on the aetiology and management of coagulation failure complicating abruptio placenta, Obstet. Gynecol. Surv. **28**:551, 1972.

Brenner, W., Edelman, D., and Hendricks, C.: Characteristics of patients with placenta previa and results of "expectant management," Am. J. Obstet. Gynecol. **132**:180, 1978.

Brome, R.G., and others: Maternal risk in abruption, Obstet. Gynecol. **31**:224, 1968.

Buchhiet, K., and Price, J.: Obstetrical hemorrhage emergency care. In Perez, R., editor: Protocols for perinatal nursing practice, St. Louis, 1981, The C.V. Mosby Co.

Burke, L.: Abruptio placenta. In Friedman, E., editor: Obstetrical decision making, St. Louis, 1982, The C.V. Mosby Co.

Butnarescu, G.F., Tillotson, D.M., and Villarrael, P.P.: Perinatal nursing: reproductive risk, vol. 2, New York, 1980, John Wiley & Sons, Inc.

Cotton, C., and others: The conservative aggressive management of placenta previa, Am. J. Obstet. Gynecol. **137**:687, 1980.

Crosby, W.: Trauma during pregnancy: maternal and fetal injury, Obstet. Gynecol. Surv. **29**:687, 1974.

Gillieson, M., Winer-Muram, H., and Muram, D.: Low-lying placenta, Radiology **144**:577, 1982.

Goldberg, B.: The identification of placenta previa, Radiology **128**:255, 1978.

Golditch, I., and Boyce, N.E.: Management of abruptio placenta, JAMA **212**:288, 1970.

Goplerud, C.: Bleeding in late pregnancy. In Danforth, D., editor: Obstetrics and gynecology, ed. 4, Hagerstown, Md., 1982, Harper & Row Inc.

Hayaski, R.H., Castillo, M.S., and Noah, M.L.: Management of severe postpartum hemorrhage due to uterine atony using an analogue of prostaglandin F_{2a}, Obstet. Gynecol. **58**:426, 1981.

Huff, R.W.: How to handle third-trimester bleeding, Contemp. Obstet. Gynecol. **20**:39, 1982.

Hurd, W.W., and others: Selective management of abruptio placenta: a prospective study, Obstet. Gynecol. **61**:467, 1983.

Jensen, M.D., and Bobak, I.M.: Maternity and gynecologic care: the nurse and the family, ed. 4, St. Louis, 1985, The C.V. Mosby Co.

Kilker, R., and Wilkerson, B.: Nursing care in placenta previa and abruptio placenta, Nursing Clin. North Am. **8**:479, 1973.

King, D.L.: Placental migration demonstrated by ultronsonography, Radiology **109**:163, 1973.

Knab, D.: Abruptio placentae, Obstet. Gynecol. **52**:625, 1978.

LoBue, C.: Third trimester bleeding. In Niswander, K., editor: Manual of obstetrics, Boston, 1980, Little, Brown & Co.

Naeye, R.L., Harkness, W.L., and Utts, J.: Abruptio placentae and perinatal death: a prospective study, Am. J. Obstet. Gynecol. **128**:740, 1977.

Netter, F.: The Ciba collection of medical illustrations: vol. 2, reproductive system, Summit, N.J., 1965, Ciba Pharmaceutical Co.

Niswander, K.: Obstetrics, ed. 2, Boston, 1981, Little, Brown & Co.

Notelovitz, M., and others: Painless abruptio placentae, Obstet. Gynecol. **53**:270, 1979.

Paterson, M.E.L.: The aetiology and outcome of abruptio placentae, Acta Obstet. Gynecol. Scand. **58:**31, 1979.

Pillitteri, A.: Maternal-newborn nursing: case of the growing family, ed. 2, Boston, 1981, Little, Brown & Co.

Pritchard, J.A., and Brekken, A.: Clinical and laboratory studies on severe abruptio placentae, Am. J. Obstet. Gynecol. **97:**681, 1967.

Pritchard, J., and MacDonald, P.: Williams' obstetrics, ed. 16, New York, 1980, Appleton Century Crofts, Inc.

Pritchard, J., and others: Genesis of severe placental abruption, Obstet. Gynecol. Surv. **26:**236, 1971.

Puls, K.: Abruptio placentae, Nursing '82 **12**(9):69, 1982.

Rabello, Y.: Nursing assessment and management of hemorrhage in the obstetric patient, Paper presented at the Western Symposium on Maternal-Infant Health, Anaheim, Calif., March 6-8, 1981.

Rizos, N., and others: Natural history of placenta previa ascertained by diagnostic ultrasound, Am. J. Obstet. Gynecol. **133:**287, 1979.

Sher, G.: Pathogenesis and management of uterine intertia complicating abruptio placentae with consumption coagulaopathy, Am. J. Obstet. Gynecol. **129:**164, 1977.

Sher, G.: A rational basis for the management of abruptio placentae, J. Reprod. Med. **21:**123, 1978.

Spirt, B.A., Kagan, E.H., and Rozanski, R.M.: Abruptio placentae: sonographic and pathologic correlation, Am. J. Roentgenol. **133:**877, 1979.

Young, G.: The peripatetic placenta, Radiology **128:**183, 1978.

CHAPTER 12

Disseminated intravascular coagulopathy

Disseminated intravascular coagulopathy (DIC) is not a primary disease but rather a secondary event activated by a number of severe illnesses. It is also called *consumptive coagulopathy* or *intravascular coagulation and fibrinolysis*. It occurs when a severe illness causes a generalized activation of the coagulation process. If coagulation factors are consumed faster than the liver can replace them, depletion occurs. At that point the process of fibrinolysis is activated in response to coagulation. The result is rampant coagulation and massive fibrinolysis at the same time.

INCIDENCE

The incidence of disseminated intravascular coagulopathy is unknown.

ETIOLOGY

Certain stimuli, known to activate the coagulation process, are listed below.
1. Infusion of tissue extract from injured tissue
2. Severe injury to endothelial cells
3. Red cell or platelet injury seen in hemolytic processes
4. Bacterial debris or endotoxins
5. Immune reactions
6. Thrombocytopenia
7. Chemical and physical agents

PHYSIOLOGY
Normal

The processes of clot formation and clot breakdown (fibrinolysis) must be understood to understand DIC. Clot formation and fibrinolysis are intertwined with the activation of factors maintaining a homeostasis under normal circumstances.

Whenever blood vessels or tissue become damaged and bleeding occurs, several factors attempt hemostasis. First, central nervous system reflexes cause vascular spasms, reducing blood flow to the area. Second, platelets attempt to plug the break. Finally, clot formation occurs. Clot formation can be activated by intrinsic and extrinsic factors. The intrinsic factors exist within the vascular system and are activated upon blood vessel damage. The extrinsic factors are within the tissue and are activated in response to tissue trauma. When either process is activated, prothrombin activator is formed. Prothrombin activator, along with calcium and phospholipids, acts as a catalyst to convert inactive plasma prothrombin into thrombin. The enzyme thrombin converts inactive plasma fibrinogen into fibrin. Fibrin, along with platelets, causes the red blood cells and plasma to mesh, and a clot is then formed (Fig. 12-1).

Fibrinolysis normally occurs simultaneously with clot formation as long as activators are present. Plasminogen, a plasma euglobulin, is activated into plasmin. Plasmin then breaks fibrin down into fibrin-split products and fibrinogen into fibrinogen-split products. This process consumes factors V, VIII, and XII, (intrinsic factors) and prothrombin. Anticoagulants, antithrombin III, and heparin also facilitate fibrinolysis. Antithrombin III neutralizes thrombin, plasmin, and factors VII, IX, XI, and XII, which are intrinsic and extrinsic factors. Heparin greatly enhances the action of antithrombin III (Fig. 12-2).

In pregnancy, fibrinogen, platelet adhesiveness, and factor VIII are increased. Antithrombin III and the activators for plasminogen are decreased. Plasminogen itself is increased. Therefore the equilibrium of coagulation and fibrinolysis is skewed toward procoagulation. Factors in pregnancy that can promote this include the following.

1. Entry of placental thrombin into maternal circulation through the vascular interfaces
2. Fetoplacental hormones
3. Pregnancy-specific hormones
4. Immunologic complexes

Pathophysiology

DIC occurs when factor consumption of the coagulation-fibrinolysis processes exceeds the liver's capacity to produce factors. When factors are depleted, equilibrium is disrupted and bleeding occurs because of deficient coagulation factors. The body continues to attempt clot formation in the presence of bleeding, which further depletes coagulation factors.

This disruption of the equilibrium of clot formation and breakdown can be triggered by severe illnesses as such those listed below.

1. Abruption of the placenta
2. Intrauterine fetal death, especially if longer than 5 weeks' duration
3. Preeclampsia/eclampsia
4. Postpartum hemorrhagic sepsis
5. Rapid, traumatic labor and delivery
6. Amniotic fluid embolism

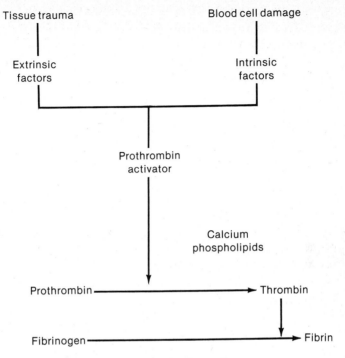

FIG. 12-1. Clot formation.

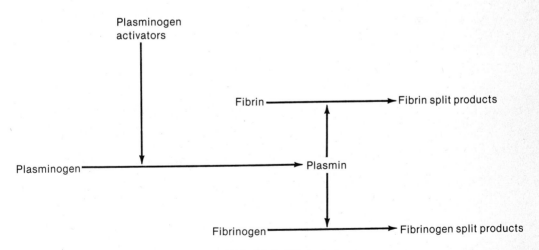

FIG. 12-2. Fibrinolysis.

When the placenta separates from the wall of the uterus, a retroplacental clot forms. Part of the products of clot formation, and placental thrombin, can be pushed into the maternal circulation, and massive consumption of clotting factors results.

Amniotic fluid embolism causes an extravasation of amniotic fluid with vernix, squamous cells, and mucus into the maternal circulation. Maternal immunologic defenses attempt to wall off the huge quantities of these foreign substances. This attempt initiates a cascade of activation of both the coagulation and the fibrinolysis processes.

When the products of conception are retained after intrauterine fetal demise, thromboplastic material can seep into the maternal circulation. This infusion of tissue extract activates the overwhelming depletion of coagulation factors.

In preeclampsia and eclampsia, damage to vessel walls occurs secondary to vasospasm and hypoxia. The vessel wall damage causes products of cellular breakdown to come in contact with the surface of the platelets and the coagulation-fibrinolysis occurs simultaneously. Massive amounts of coagulation-fibrinolysis factors are then consumed by the process, and the liver is unable to replace factors as rapidly as is necessary.

Hemorrhage and shock can also precipitate disequilibrium of coagulation-fibrinolysis. Hypovolemia causes decreased cardiac output, decreased arterial pressure, and decreased systemic blood flow. This leads to decreased nutrition to the brain and vascular system. The hypoxic vascular endothelium triggers intravascular coagulation. Intravascular coagulation releases toxins that increase capillary permeability, further diminishing circulating volume. Brain anoxia results in cardiac depression and further compromises cardiac output.

Signs and symptoms

Early symptoms of DIC include ecchymoses and bleeding into the urine or at the site of an intravenous line. As DIC develops, these early signs may rapidly progress to severe signs of shock.

1. Respirations progress from rapid and deep to rapid, shallow, and irregular and finally to barely perceptible.
2. Pulse rate becomes rapid, weaker, irregular, and thready.
3. Blood pressure may initially be normal, but then begins falling until the systolic is below 60 mm Hg or is not palpable.
4. Skin color may then begin to pale and cool, progressing rapidly to being cold, clammy, and cyanotic.
5. Urinary output initially remains stable, then quickly begins to decrease to less than 30 ml/hr.
6. Level of consciousness changes from apprehension to increasing restlessness, lethargy, and finally coma.
7. CVP and PAWP drop.

Laboratory signs of DIC include hypofibrinogenemia, decreased platelet count, abnormal prothrombin and partial thromboplastic times, and an increase in fibrin and fibrinogen split products. Normal coagulation factor values are given below.

1. Fibrinogen—400 mg/dl
2. Platelets—150,000 to 350,000 mm^3
3. Prothrombin time—10 to 14 seconds
4. Partial thromboplastic time—18 to 38 seconds
5. Fibrin-split products—less than 10 μg/ml.

Maternal effects

DIC can result in maternal death.

Fetal and neonatal effects

DIC can result in fetal death or severe hypoxia. Possible neonatal sequelae to severe hypoxia are intracranial bleeding and brain death.

MEDICAL DIAGNOSIS

The medical diagnosis is made from a history of predisposing conditions and the early signs of ecchymosis formation and bleeding from the intravenous site or urinary tract. Definitive diagnosis is made by the laboratory data previously listed.

USUAL MEDICAL MANAGEMENT

When DIC occurs in the antepartum period, the initial treatment is to empty the uterus by the most expeditious means. Blood replacement with packed cells, fresh frozen plasma, cryoprecipitate, and platelets is necessary to replace volume and depleted coagulation factors. Simultaneously, the primary disease must also be stabilized and corrected.

Supportive measures for monitoring fluid replacement and cardiac output must also be instituted. These include cardiac monitoring, hemodynamic monitoring, and blood pressure recordings every 5 to 15 minutes. Because clinical signs of DIC may be rapid in onset, the emergency initially threatens the mother's life and fetal considerations are excluded. Once factor replacement is instituted for the mother, the fetus is often delivered before continuous monitoring of the fetal heart rate can be initiated.

NURSING PROCESS
Prevention

When the mother has a condition that might predispose her to development of DIC, the nurse must be alert for early signs of ecchymosis and bleeding. A simple test to confirm possible early signs of DIC is the clot-retraction test; 5

Disseminated intravascular coagulopathy

Potential nursing diagnosis	Outcome criteria
A. Potential depletion of clotting factors related to: Factor consumption exceeding liver capacity to produce	Normal clotting factors clotting time 8 to 12 min Fibrinogen levels 400 mg/dl Platelets 150,000 to 350,000 mm^3 Partial thromboplastin time 12 to 14 sec
B. Potential hypovolemia related to: Depletion of clotting factors Shock	Blood pressure within normal range (90/50 to 120/80) Pulse 70 to 100/min Respiration 12 to 18 per min Urinary output greater than 30 ml/hr CVP, PAP, and PAWP within normal limits
C. Potential for fetal distress related to: Maternal shock Decreased utero-placental profusion	FHR baseline between 120 and 160 with adequate variability and no ominous periodic pattern changes

O F   N U R S I N G   C A R E

Assessment and intervention

Dx. Observe for signs of DIC such as oozing of blood from IV site, easy bruising, and petechia
Refer to appropriate laboratory data
Observe those patients who are preeclamptic, have third trimester bleeding, or have hemorrhage for early signs of DIC

Th. Be prepared to carry out bedside clot-retraction test by placing 5 ml of blood in test tube
Prepare to administer a blood transfusion, cryoprecipitate, or fresh frozen plasma as ordered
Prepare for hemodynamic monitoring

Ref. Notify physician if signs of DIC develop

Dx. Assess BP, pulse, and respiration as condition indicates
Observe for mental changes and skin temperature and color changes consistent with impending shock
Check urinary output each hr
Check CVP, PAP, or PAWP as ordered

Th. Have 16 or 18-gauge IV started with a solution such as Ringer's lactate or normal saline
Be prepared to transfuse cryoprecipitate or fresh frozen plasma

Ref. Report changes in vital signs, renal function, and hemodynamics immediately to the physician

Dx. Observe for signs of fetal distress while stabilizing mother

Th. Apply fetal monitor for continuous observation
Turn mother to left side, increase IV fluids, administer oxygen by tight face mask at 6 to 10 liters/min
Prepare for emergency cesarean delivery if mother is stable and fetus is viable

Dx., diagnostic; Th., therapeutic; Ed., education; Ref., referral.

Continued.

Disseminated intravascular coagulopathy—cont'd

Potential nursing diagnosis	*Outcome criteria*

D. Potential renal failure or pituitary necrosis related to:
    Hypovolemia
    Depletion of clotting factors
	Urinary output greater than 30 ml/hr
	Onset of lactation by 4 to 5 days postpartum

E. Potential postpartum infection related to: Depletion of immunologic factors	No evidence of infection during recovery phase (2 to 7 days postpartum)
F. Potential anxiety or grief	Verbalizes fears and discusses events for reality testing Seeks acquaintance time with infant whether alive, ill, or dead

ml of blood are drawn into a test tube, capped, and taped to the bedside wall. If a clot has not formed and separated the serum from the cells within 8 to 10 minutes, DIC is possible and the physician should be notified.

Assessment

Early signs of disequilibrium of the coagulation-fibrinolysis process should be assessed in any of the diseases or conditions known to predispose the pregnant woman to DIC. These signs include unusual ecchymosis formation; bleeding from the gums, intravenous insertion site, or other venous punctures; and bleeding into the urine.

Failing to recognize early signs, the nurse should be alert for the progressive changes in respiration, pulse, blood pressure, skin color, and urinary output that indicate mild to moderate shock.

In the recovery phase (2 to 7 days), the woman should also be observed for signs of infection and potential transfusion hepatitis. These problems are usually readily remediable with medical management.

Assessment and intervention

Dx. Keep accurate I&O record
Observe for onset of lactation by the fourth or fifth postpartum day
Th. Administer no lactation suppressant if shock was experienced
Ed. Explain reason for no lactation suppression to mother
Ref. Report decreased urinary output to physician
Report failure of lactation

Dx. Observe for signs of an infection such as increased fever greater than 100.4°
F, foul lochia, urinary tract infection
Th. Be prepared to administer IV antibiotics as ordered
Ref. Report early signs of infection to physician

Dx. Assess parent's level of anxiety or grief
Assess for signs of withdrawal, depression, anxiety, and grief
Th. Encourage discussion of feelings and events
Provide time for woman and significant other to discuss events and be with
infant
Ref. Grief counselor or clergy as appropriate
Utilize institutional support person, that is, clergy, social worker, nurse spe-
cialist
Refer to community support group especially if fetal/neonatal death has oc-
cured

Intervention

Interventions are the same for antepartum, intrapartum, and postpartum periods. An IV should be started with a 16-gauge angiocatheter and a solution
such as lactated Ringer's or normal saline. Preparations should be made for
hemodynamic monitoring (see Chapter 6) and cardiac monitoring. A Foley
catheter should be inserted for hourly determinations of urinary output.

In the recovery phase, replacement of blood and specific coagulation factors
may be reinstituted. Antibiotic therapy might be necessary if signs of infection
occur as a result of depleted immunologic factors. Hepatitis may occur as a
result of contaminated blood products.

The emergent nature of obvious DIC can cause a persistent need to talk
through the events. The nurse should provide opportunities for the woman to
discuss the experience. If the events resulted in fetal or neonatal death, grief
counseling will be valuable. Various institutions may delegate this to a social
service worker, a nurse specialist, or to the clergy. Follow-up referrals should
be made to community support groups.

EVALUATION

The goal of care of the woman with DIC is, first, to prevent shock and its sequelae. Early recognition of conditions that can precipitate this event will assist in prevention of maternal death or other sequelae such as infection or hepatitis.

REFERENCES

Brandt, P., and Jespersen, J.: Renal diseases, disseminated intravascular coagulation, and antithrombin III (letter), Nephron **34**(3):203, 1983.

Clark, A., and Alfonso, D.: Childbearing: a nursing perspective, Philadelphia, 1979, F.A. Davis Co.

Danforth, D.: Obstetrics and gynecology, Hagerstown, Md., 1982, Harper & Row, Inc.

Davison, J.: Physiological adjustments in pregnancy. In Hytten, E., editor: Clinics in obstetrics and gynecology, Philadelphia, 1975, W.B. Saunders Co.

Giles, C.: Intravascular coagulation in gestational hypertension and pre-eclampsia: the value of haematological screening tests, Clin. Lab. Hematol. **4**:351, 1982.

Hurd, W.W., Miodovnik, M., and Stys, S.J.: Pregnancy associated with paroxysmal nocturnal hemoglobinuria, Obstet. Gynecol. **60**:742, 1982

Hytlen, F., and Leitch, I.: The physiology of human pregnancy, Oxford, 1971, Blackwell Scientific Publications, Ltd.

Jensen, M., and Bobak, I.: Maternity and gynecologic care: the nurse and the family, ed. 4, St. Louis, 1985, The C.V. Mosby Co.

Liebman, H.A., and others: Severe depression of antithrombin III associated with disseminated intravascular coagulation in women with fatty liver of pregnancy, Ann. Intern. Med. **98**:330, 1983.

Lox, C.D., Dorsett, M.M., and Hampton, R.M.: Observations on clotting activity during pre-eclampsia, Clin. Exp. Hypertens. Series B **2**:179, 1983.

Niswander, K.: Manual of obstetrics, Boston, 1980, Little, Brown & Co.

Olds, S. and others: Obstetric nursing, Menlo Park, Calif., 1980, Addison Wesley Publishing Co.

Perez, R.: Protocols for perinatal nursing practice, St. Louis, 1981, The C.V. Mosby Co.

Pritchard, J., and MacDonald, P.: Williams' obstetrics, New York, 1980, Appleton Century Crofts, Inc.

Purdie, F.R., and others: Rupture of the uterus with DIC, Ann. Emergency Med. **12**:174, 1983.

Reeder, S., Mastroianni, L., and Martin, L.: Maternity nursing, ed. 15, Philadelphia, 1983, J.B. Lippincott Co.

Skelly, H., and others: Consumptive coagulopathy following fetal death in a triplet pregnancy, Am. J. Obstet. Gynecol. **142**:595, 1982.

Suzuki, S., Murakoshi, T., and Sakamoto, W.: Studies on the various causal factors related to hypercoagulability in the field of obstetrics—with special reference to the onset of DIC as viewed from the changing of kinin-kallikrein system and fibrinopeptide A, Adv. Exp. Med. Biol. **156**(B):1055, 1983.

Taenaka, N., and others: Survival from DIC following amniotic fluid embolism: successful treatment with a serine proteinase inhibitor, FOY, Anaesthesia **36**:389, 1981.

CHAPTER 13

Hypertensive Disorders
of Pregnancy

Hypertensive disorders of pregnancy commonly have been referred to as *toxemia*, but the term is inappropriate; research has revealed that there is no known toxin involved. Therefore the Committee on Terminology of the American College of Obstetricians and Gynecologists has recently developed a new classification of the various hypertensive states of pregnancy. In this classification, pregnancy-induced hypertension (PIH) is differentiated from concurrent hypertension and pregnancy (CHP). Pregnancy-induced hypertension includes hypertensive disorders peculiar to pregnancy that have their onset during pregnancy and subside completely following delivery. Concurrent hypertension and pregnancy includes hypertensive disorders that are etiologically unrelated to pregnancy. Table 13-1 defines the various pregnancy-induced hypertensive and concurrent hypertensive disorders. This chapter will focus on pregnancy-induced hypertension (PIH), and particularly on preeclampsia and eclampsia.

INCIDENCE

Approximately 6% to 30% of all pregnant women have been shown to have a hypertensive disorder (Welt and Crenshaw, 1978). Of this 80% is pregnancy-induced hypertension (PIH). A primigravida woman is six times more likely to have PIH than a multigravida woman, especially if the primigravida is under 17 or over 35. PIH is five times greater in the lower socioeconomic groups. Other factors associated with a higher than normal incidence of PIH include the following.

1. Familial history
2. Diabetes
3. Multiple gestation
4. Polyhydramnios
5. Persistent hypertension
6. Hydatidiform mole
7. Rh incompatibility

TABLE 13-1. *Classification of the hypertensive states of pregnancy*

Type	Description
PREGNANCY-INDUCED HYPERTENSION (PIH)	
Gestational hypertension	The development of hypertension after 20 weeks of gestation in a previously normotensive woman without proteinuria; the blood pressure returns to normal within 10 postpartum days
Preeclampsia	The development of hypertension and proteinuria with or without edema in a previously normotensive woman after 20 weeks of gestation or early postpartum; in the presence of trophoblastic disease it can develop prior to 20 weeks of gestation
Eclampsia	The development of convulsions or coma in a preeclamptic patient
Superimposed preeclampsia or eclampsia	The development of preeclampsia or eclampsia in a patient with concurrent hypertension
CONCURRENT HYPERTENSION AND PREGNANCY (CHP)	
Chronic hypertension	Hypertension that develops before pregnancy or week 20 of gestation that is not pregnancy associated

ETIOLOGY

The cause of PIH remains unknown. However, there are many current theories as to its possible cause. A few of the more common theories are:

1. Nutritional deficiency. According to Brewer (1966), nutritional deficiency, especially in protein and calories, causes hepatic insufficiency, which leads to significant impairment in hepatic conjugation of the placental steroid hormones estrogen and progesterone. Therefore the steroid hormones accumulate within the body and may trigger PIH. According to Belizan and Villar (1980), a deficient calcium, iron, and vitamin intake during pregnancy may trigger PIH. DeAlvarez (1978) indicates that PIH may be related to an inadequate utilization of nutrients, particularly lipids. This would interfere with prostaglandin synthesis and lead to an increased sensitivity to angiotensin. This might partially explain why teenagers and lower socioeconomic group patients are at a greater risk for PIH.

2. Immunologic deficiency. Another current theory being studied is immunologically based. According to Beer (1978), PIH might be the result of an overwhelming immune response, similar to organ rejection, activated by the woman's body against the placenta and fetus. This reaction is being proposed as the result of insufficient "blocking" or enhancing antibodies or insufficient B and T lymphocyte production to immunoprotect the expanding invasive trophoblast. These antibodies, if present, prevent the development of effector lymphocytes and humoral antibodies against the cytotrophoblast tissue. If effector lymphocytes and humoral

antibodies are produced against the trophoblastic tissue, lipid is accumulated, fibrin is deposited, and ultimately occlusion of some placental blood vessels can result. This resulting damage might cause the release of thromboplastin and fibrin/fibrinogen products, which are deposited in the liver and renal glomerulus and cause generalized vasospasms. This might partially explain why primigravidas and multigravidas who are having their first baby with a new father are at greater risk for preeclampsia. These women have had shorter exposure to the father's sperm.

According to Alanen and Lassila (1982), PIH may be the result of a deficiency in maternal natural killer cell activity; during pregnancy these cells are responsible for identifying and engulfing fetal cells that reach the maternal circulatory system before antibodies can be formed against them. This deficiency in natural killer cell activity might be related to a deficiency in prostaglandins or prostaglandinlike substances.

3. Genetics. Cooper and Liston (1979) studied the possibility of PIH being related to a single recessive gene and found a high correlation between daughters and their mothers who experienced PIH. This seems to indicate that there is a hereditary tendency involved in the development of PIH. No specific chromosome abnormality has been identified.

4. Uterine ischemia. According to this theory, decreased blood flow through the uterus initiates the release of vasoconstricting substance into the circulatory system, triggering vasospasms (Dennis et al., 1982).

PHYSIOLOGY
Normal

Even though the triggering factor of this disease remains unknown, much of the pathophysiology of the disease is understood. In order to understand the pathophysiology of PIH, the nurse should be familiar with the normal physiologic changes of pregnancy. The normal physiologic changes of pregnancy that are affected by PIH are summarized as follows.

1. Total blood volume is increased 30% to 50% and cardiac output is maximized.

2. The normal glomerular filtration rate is increased by approximately 50% and tubular reabsorption is enhanced.

3. Renin, angiotensin II, and aldosterone levels are increased related to increased estrogen. These substrates facilitate the normal expansion of the blood volume by 30% to 50% above nonpregnant levels.

4. Aldosterone stimulates the kidney tubules to reabsorb sodium and water. Progesterone exerts a sodium-losing influence on the kidney tubules by blocking the effect of aldosterone. The net effect is sodium depletion (Ehrlich, 1978).

5. Angiotensin II is a potent pressor substance that stimulates a rise in blood pressure. In normal pregnancy, even though the levels of angiotensin II are elevated, blood pressure does not rise. This is because normal pregnant women have an increased resistance to the pressor effects of angiotensin II (Abdul-Karim and Assali, 1961). This increased resistance, normally found in pregnancy, is postulated by Valenzuela, Harper, and Hayashi (1983) to be related to increased levels of vasodilator prostaglandins, such as prostaglandin E_2 and prostacyclin.

6. Peripheral vascular resistance decreases during pregnancy to accommodate the increased blood volume, and the blood pressure normally drops slightly during the second trimester followed by a return to nonpregnant levels during the third trimester (Henry, 1963).

7. Fluid moves from the intravascular space to the extracellular space in the dependent limbs. This is related to decreased plasma colloid osmotic pressure secondary to the normal hemodilution of the blood. This is also related to the increased venous capillary hydrostatic pressure in the dependent limbs secondary to the gravid uterus pressing on the inferior vena cava interfering with the blood returning to the heart. The net result is physiologic edema in the dependent limbs during the last trimester of pregnancy. Physiologic edema should disappear after 8 to 12 hours of bed rest.

Pathophysiology

In PIH disorders, there is an increased vascular sensitivity to angiotensin II, which means that it takes very little angiotensin II to raise the blood pressure (Chesley, 1966; Gant et al., 1973). According to Gant and associates (1973), this increased vascular sensitivity occurs before the onset of hypertension. When the normal resistance to angiotensin II is lost, blood vessel spasms occur. This causes constriction of the blood vessels, decreasing their diameter, impeding blood flow, and leading to a rise in blood pressure to propel the blood through the constricted cardiovascular system.

Because blood flow to all body organs is decreased, especially to the placenta, kidneys, liver, and brain, impairing their function by 40% to 60%, the following pathophysiologic changes result.

1. Blood supply to the placenta and the uterus is decreased. This leads to a premature, exaggerated, progressive degenerative aging of the placenta, and intrauterine growth retardation of the fetus can result. Uterine activity is increased and the use of oxytocin for induction may result in an increased susceptibility to the effects of the drug.

2. Blood supply to the kidneys is decreased, which reduces glomerular filtration rate and leads to degenerative changes in the glomeruli. Protein,

mainly in the form of albumin, is lost into the urine and uric acid clearance is decreased. Therefore proteinuria and increased plasma uric acid levels are signs of preeclampsia.

3. Sodium and water retention result from impaired renal function.
4. Serum albumin is decreased, which results from impaired renal function causing a decrease in the plasma colloid osmotic pressure.
5. Fluid shifts from the intravascular to the intracellular space because of the decrease in colloid osmotic pressure. As a result, the blood becomes more viscous and edema increases. The increase in the viscosity of the blood is referred to as an increase in the *hemoconcentration* or concentration of red blood cell mass. This is seen as a rise in hematocrit. Therefore hematocrit readings can be an indicator as to whether the condition is improving or deteriorating. In severe preeclampsia the blood volume may fall to nonpregnant levels as fluid leaves the intravascular space resulting in severe edema.
6. Blood supply to the liver is decreased, which leads to impairment of liver function and can result in hemorrhagic necrosis, indicated by epigastric pain (a sign of impending eclampsia). Liver enzymes are elevated when liver tissue is necrosed.
7. Blood supply to the eyes is decreased, which causes retinal arteriolar spasms leading to visual changes such as blurring.
8. Loss of fluid from the blood vessels in the brain leads to cerebral edema and hemorrhages, causing CNS irritability. Signs of CNS irritability are headaches, hyperreflexia, and ankle clonus.
9. As the disease progresses, damage to the lining of the blood vessel wall occurs and platelets, fibrinogen, immunoglobulin, and components of complement are deposited at the damaged sites. Therefore disseminated intravascular coagulation (DIC) can develop in the microcirculation.

See Fig. 13-1 for a summary of the pathophysiologic changes of PIH.

Signs and symptoms

There are three cardinal signs of PIH: (1) hypertension, (2) proteinuria, and (3) sudden and excessive edema. An elevated blood pressure is usually the first sign to develop in the early stages of this disease; therefore the disease may be diagnosed without the presence of proteinuria or edema. Hypertension is diagnosed if one of the following is present.

1. The blood pressure is 140/90 mm Hg or more on two occasions 6 hours apart.
2. There is an increase of 30 mm Hg or more in the systolic pressure or 15 mm Hg or more in the diastolic pressure from the baseline reading obtained on the initial prenatal visit.

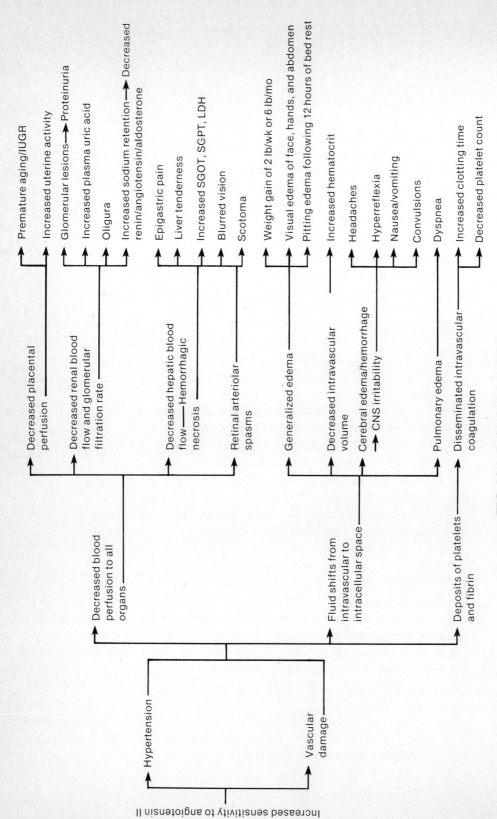

FIG. 13-1. Pathophysiology of PIH.

Some facts should be kept in mind when evaluating the blood pressure reading.

1. The diastolic pressure is the most prognostic of the disease.
2. Blood pressure normally drops slightly during the second trimester of pregnancy.

It is very difficult to differentiate between normal physiologic edema and pathologic edema caused by PIH. It is best determined by a sudden weight gain that exceeds 2 pounds in 1 week or 6 pounds in 1 month. This usually occurs before visual signs of edema of the face, hands, and abdomen appear. It is also considered pathologic edema if pitting edema is still present in the feet or legs after 12 hours of bed rest.

Proteinuria is usually the last of the three signs to appear and is diagnosed if one of the following is present.

1. More than 0.3 gm of protein per liter of urine is found in a 24 hour urine collection
2. More than 1 gm of protein per liter is found in at least two random urine specimens collected on two or more occasions at least 6 hours apart (This is indicated as +2 or greater on a urodipstix.)

The following guidelines should be kept in mind when evaluating the urine for protein.

1. Vaginal discharge, blood, amniotic fluid, and bacteria can contaminate the specimen and give a false positive reading.
2. The specimen should be collected by either a voided midstream or catheterization to avoid contamination with vaginal discharge.

Subjective signs of preeclampsia are listed below.

1. Headaches
2. Visual changes such as blurred vision
3. Increased edema of the face and pitting edema of the extremities
4. Oliguria
5. Hyperreflexia
6. Nausea or vomiting
7. Epigastric pain

Preeclampsia is usually categorized in grades of either mild or severe for the purpose of treatment (see Table 13-2 for comparison).

Mild preeclampsia is diagnosed thus.

1. Blood pressure 140/90 or greater but less than 160/110, or systolic blood pressure increased 30 mm Hg or more but less than 60 mm Hg, or diastolic blood pressure increased 15 mm Hg or more but less than 30 mm Hg from the nonpregnant baseline
2. Proteinuria greater than 0.3 gm but less than 5 gm/24 hr or persistent proteinuria in a clean-catch urine specimen on two or more successive days

3. Urinary output greater than 500 ml/24 hr
4. Generalized edema, without pulmonary edema
5. No subjective signs or symptoms such as headache, visual disturbances, epigastric pain, or hyperreflexia

Severe preeclampsia is diagnosed thus.

1. Blood pressure 160/110 or greater, systolic blood pressure increased 60 mm Hg or more, or diastolic blood pressure increased 30 mm Hg or more
2. Proteinuria 5 gm or more/24 hr
3. Urinary output less than 400 ml/24 hr
4. Subjective signs such as headache, visual disturbances, epigastric pain, dyspnea, or hyperreflexia

If coma or convulsions occur, it is then classified as eclampsia. Epigastric pain, hyperreflexia, or clonus are usually signs of an approaching convulsion. However, in the presence of only edema, some normal women have hyperreflexia.

Maternal effects

PIH is a very serious disease and is the third leading cause of maternal mortality. If treated early and effectively, maternal mortality is very low. If the disease is allowed to progress to eclampsia, the maternal mortality increases to as high as 13%. The most common causes of death are related to congestive heart failure, renal failure, and cerebral hemorrhage (Zuspan, 1978).

Fetal and neonatal effects

Perinatal morality related to preeclampsia ranges from 1% to 8% and, if the disease is allowed to progress to eclampsia, perinatal mortality is as high as

TABLE 13-2. *Comparison of mild and severe preeclampsia*

	Mild	*Severe*
Blood pressure	140/90 to 160/110 mm Hg	160/110 mm Hg or greater
Systolic	30 to 60 mm Hg increase	60 mm Hg or greater increase
Diastolic	15 to 30 mm Hg increase	30 mm Hg or greater increase
Proteinuria	0.3 gm to 4 gm	5 gm/24 hr or greater
Dipstick	+2/+3	+4
Urinary output	Greater than 30 ml/hr	Less than 20 ml/hr
	Greater than 650 ml/24 hr	Less than 400 ml/24 hr
Edema	+1/+2	+3/+4
Headaches/visual disturbance	Not present	Can be persistent
Other subjective signs, such as epigastric pain, hyperreflexia, clonus, and dyspnea	Not present	Can be present

37% (Zuspan, 1978). The majority of perinatal losses are related either to placental insufficiency causing intrauterine growth retardation or to prematurity associated with preterm delivery.

MEDICAL DIAGNOSIS

There are no diagnostic tests available to detect PIH. One must depend on the recognition of signs and symptoms in order to detect its development. Since edema is common in normal pregnancy and proteinuria can occur in the presence of other conditions, the most diagnostic symptom is a rise in blood pressure. To detect blood pressure diagnostic of early PIH, one must consider two things. First, the blood pressure normally drops slightly during the second trimester of pregnancy and then gradually returns to its original baseline level during the third trimester. Second, a significant increase in blood pressure can be small. Therefore it is important to obtain an accurate baseline blood pressure early in pregnancy and at every prenatal visit.

To obtain an accurate blood pressure reading, the blood pressure cuff must cover approximately two thirds of the upper arm. Because position can lead to variability in the blood pressure reading, blood pressure should be measured in the same arm and with the patient in the same position each time. It is also preferable to record the muffled diastolic sound instead of the disappearance of diastolic sound (Hill, 1980).

Because the hypertensive disease process begins long before signs and symptoms appear, the health team should determine those patients at risk for PIH and conduct screening tests on them. Two tests currently being used to screen patients at risk for PIH are the rollover test and the angiotensin II test.

The rollover test was first described in 1974 when Gant and associates observed that a pregnant woman between 28 and 32 weeks of gestation whose blood pressure increased 20 mm Hg or more when turned from side to back had a higher risk of developing hypertension. Karbhari, Harrigan, and LaMagra (1977) found the rollover test 93% accurate in predicting PIH. About the same time, Marshall and Newman (1977) conducted a similar study and found the test approximately 90% accurate in predicting PIH. Spinapolice, Feld, and Harrigan (1983) found it very reliable in the study they conducted. However, not all research studies confirm that the rollover test is accurate in predicting PIH. Kasser, Aldridge, and Quirk (1980) found the rollover test to have a 29.6% false negative rate and to be only 25.5% accurate.

The test is performed by taking the woman's blood pressure every 5 minutes at least three times or until stable while she is resting on her left side. She is then asked to turn onto her back and her blood pressure is recorded immediately and at 5-minute intervals until stable. A 20 mm Hg or more increase is a positive result and indicates a high probability of her developing preeclampsia.

The angiotensin II test is based on the observation that most women who develop hypertension during their pregnancy have an increased sensitivity to the pressor effects of angiotensin II. Everett and associates (1978) found that women who had an increased blood pressure response of 20 mm Hg or more after receiving 8 ng/kg/min of angiotensin II had a 90% chance of developing PIH. Gant and associates (1974) found very similar results.

USUAL MEDICAL MANAGEMENT

The only cure for PIH is termination of the pregnancy. Because many fetuses are immature when the disease develops, the severity of the disease and the maturity of the fetus must be considered in determining when delivery should take place. If the pregnancy has progressed 36 weeks or more or fetal maturity is confirmed by a lecithin/sphingomyelin (L/S) ratio of 2:1, delivery is the choice of treatment after the condition is stabilized. If the pregnancy is of less than 36 weeks' gestation or the fetus is immature, interventions will be instituted to alleviate the symptoms and allow time for the fetus to mature.

The medical treatment for PIH depends on the degree of severity of the disease. In mild preeclampsia bed rest in the lateral recumbent position or limited activity is usually instituted. Resting in bed in the lateral recumbent position takes the pressure of the gravid uterus off the inferior vena cava. This facilitates venous return, thereby increasing the circulatory volume, which increases renal blood flow and promotes diuresis. The release of angiotensin II is also decreased (Gant et al., 1974). Blood pressure normally drops as a result, enhancing blood flow to the placenta and fetus.

A high-protein diet of 80 to 100 gm is therapeutic in replacing the protein being lost in the urine. Protein also increases the plasma colloid osmotic pressure. As the plasma colloid osmotic pressure increases, it pulls fluid from the intracellular spaces back into the circulatory system.

Sodium intake should not exceed 6 gm (3 teaspoons) daily. An excessive salt intake can increase antiotensin II sensitivity and cause increased vasoconstriction. According to Jaspers, DeJong, and Mulder (1983), a large intake of sodium can increase the production of vasoconstrictor prostaglandins. On the other hand, an inappropriate dietary sodium restriction below 2.5 gm can further reduce the blood volume and decrease placental perfusion (Nolten and Ehrlich, 1980). It can also activate the renin-angiotensin-aldosterone cycle excessively and cause increased vasoconstriction.

In the past, a sedative such as phenobarbital was administered to allay anxiety and promote rest. It is used less today for several reasons.

1. Its benefit is unproved.
2. Patients build up a tolerance to its sedative effect in a couple of days and require ever increasing amounts to achieve desired effects.
3. It may cause a nonreactive nonstress test if the test is done within 8 hours of the medication administration.

Although diuretics were part of the treatment of preeclampsia not many years ago, they are not used today. It has been shown that diuretics further decrease blood flow to the placenta by decreasing blood volume, disrupt the normal electrolyte balance, which can impair certain aspects of placental function such as estrogen production, and create further stress on already compromised kidneys. Therefore diuretics should be used for the treatment of PIH only in the presence of heart failure.

There is a controversy among clinicians as to the best place for this treatment to be implemented. Some hospitalize all women with mild preeclampsia; others allow selected women to stay at home. The second biggest controversy is the amount of bed rest required to promote effective results. Most clinicians advocate complete bed rest with bathroom privileges only (Haesslein, 1980; Dennis et al., 1982). There are others, however, who advocate only limiting activity. This is based on research done at Parkland Memorial Hospital in Dallas where several doctors conducted a study in which their mild preeclamptic nulliparous patients were admitted to a special 28 bed unit. While hospitalized, they were allowed to ambulate as desired and to eat a regular diet while being monitored closely. Within 5 days, 94% of the women demonstrated a drop in blood pressure and 81% were normotensive. Therefore continuation of gestation was possible until fetal maturity was reached in all of these patients (Gilstrap et al., 1978). In light of this study, the question remains whether or not complete bed rest is necessary for therapeutic effects. However, a need for close monitoring of the patient, even when an initial drop in blood pressure occurs, is emphasized by this study, because many of the patients experienced recurrent hypertension.

If selected patients are treated as outpatients, a protocol for routine screening should be developed. Criteria used in selecting a patient who can be treated as an outpatient are listed below.

1. The diastolic pressure dropping below 90 mm Hg after 10 to 15 minutes in a lateral recumbent position
2. Proteinuria as measured by dipstick trace or less
3. The patient being responsible and dependable
4. No subjective symptoms such as headache, blurred vision, hyperreflexion or epigastric pain

If the disease is severe, the patient is always hospitalized for treatment and absolute bed rest is usually instituted. Magnesium sulfate ($MgSO_4$) and hydralazine hydrochloride (Apresoline) are two common drugs used to stabilize the severely preeclamptic patient. Plasma volume expanders such as dextran, plasmanate, or albumin are used by some clinicians to pull fluid back into the intravascular space. Sehgal and Hitt (1980) found them to improve substantially the hemoconcentration and the urine output and to lower the blood pressure. Cunningham and Pritchard (1978) and Assali and Vaughn (1977) question this practice because the intravascular space is constricted, but adequately filled, even though the volume is decreased. They feel this practice could lead to circulatory overload or pulmonary edema.

To prevent the development of permanent maternal vascular damage and eclampsia, and intrauterine fetal hypoxia, the well-being and maturity of the fetus and the mother's response to treatment must be monitored closely. Nonstress tests, estriol determinations, contraction stress tests, and ultrasound measurements of fetal growth are frequently used to detect signs of intrauterine fetal distress. Amniocentesis is usually done to determine fetal pulmonary lung maturity. If the patient's condition stabilizes and improves with hospitalization as indicated by lower blood pressure and diuresis, and if the fetus appears to be growing appropriately, delivery is delayed until labor begins or the fetus is mature. If the patient's condition does not improve with hospitalization, she must be delivered after stabilization of her condition to prevent serious complications such as fetal death, maternal convulsion, intracranial hemorrhage, or death. Laboratory studies used to monitor the condition are plasma uric acid levels, hematocrit, platelet count, and liver enzyme studies such as SGOT, SGPT, and LDH.

NURSING PROCESS
Prevention

Because the etiology of the disease is unknown, it is difficult to outline a protocol for prevention. Based on scientific studies, there are some general prenatal principles, however, that appear to decrease the incidence of this disease.

1. Adequate nutrition. Dr. Tom Brewer (1974) and others have noted a correlation between a low-protein diet and the development of PIH. On a high-protein diet with all the essential elements of good nutrition, Dr. Brewer's low socioeconomic patients do not develop PIH. On the average, in the United States, the incidence of PIH is five times greater in the lower socioeconomic groups. Prinrose and Higgins (1971) suggest based on their studies that higher levels of plasma protein might prevent preeclampsia. This might occur because protein increases the colloid osmotic pressure, which helps maintain the normal fluid volume in the circulatory system. Therefore all pregnant patients should receive instructions regarding the benefits of eating a nutritious, balanced diet containing at least 80 to 100 gm of protein per day.
2. Adequate fluid intake. Atkinson (1972) maintains that a larger fluid intake may aid in the prevention of preeclampsia by combating intravascular hemoconcentration. Whether this is true or not, 8 to 10 glasses of water or fluid per day is therapeutic for the pregnant patient.

3. Adequate rest. Bed rest facilitates venous return, increasing the circulatory volume, enhancing renal and placental perfusion, and lowering blood pressure. Therefore high-risk patients may benefit from 8 to 12 hours of sleep each night with a rest period in the middle of the day. Bed rest also mobilizes edematous fluid back into the intravascular space. Spinapolice, Feld, and Harrigan (1983) found this regime 94% effective in preventing the development of PIH if diagnosed early by a positive rollover test.

4. No smoking. Smoking causes vasoconstriction, which leads to decreased uterine blood flow. Since uterine ischemia is either a triggering or resulting factor of preeclampsia, all prenatal patients should be provided information regarding the effects of smoking on the health of the mother and fetus. That smoking has any influence on the development of preeclampsia has not been proven, but it can accentuate the uterine ischemia associated with the disease.

5. Early, appropriate treatment. Early, appropriate treatment is effective in preventing the severe form of preeclampsia or eclampsia. Therefore early detection of its development is effective in lowering the high maternal and fetal mortality associated with the disease. This should begin on the first prenatal visit. The nurse should then obtain an in depth patient history that includes age and parity and a medical history of such things as diabetes, persistent hypertensive disorders, and familial history of preeclampsia/eclampsia. Because subjective symptoms that the patient might experience are late signs, early detection of the disease is dependent on: (1) changes in blood pressure from the baseline established on the first prenatal visit, (2) abnormal patterns of weight gain and increased signs of edema after 12 hours of bed rest, and (3) the presence of protein in the urine. Therefore on each prenatal visit, the patient should be weighed, an accurate blood pressure reading obtained, and an early morning urine specimen checked for protein. If protein is noted in the urine, it should be checked for bacteria and another specimen obtained by clean catch midstream or minicatheterization, because bacteria, vaginal discharge, blood, and amniotic fluid can give a false positive result.

Assessment

When any patient is diagnosed with PIH, the nurse must continually gather in-depth data to detect early indicators that the condition is deteriorating.

Vital signs should be checked every 4 hours while awake or more often if indicated. The blood pressure should be taken on the same arm with the patient in the same position each time. An increase in blood pressure indicates that the condition is deteriorating. The urine should be evaluated for protein, specific gravity, pH, and glucose every 8 hours or more often if indicated. The gram equivalent of protein as indicated on the dipstick is outlined in Table 13-3. A 24-hour urine collection for protein may be ordered. The loss of 5 gm or more of protein per 24 hours indicates severe preeclampsia. A daily weight should be obtained before breakfast and an intake and output kept. If the urinary output is less than 30 ml/hr or 120 ml/4 hr and oliguria is present, this indicates that the condition is deteriorating. The degree of edema should be evaluated every 8 hours and scored as shown in Table 13-4. Deep tendon reflexes (DTR) should be checked every 8 hours or more often if indicated. The easiest DTR to check is the patella reflex (knee jerk). The response elicited should be graded as shown in Table 13-5. At the same time, it should be determined whether or not clonus is present. If present, dorsiflexion of the foot causes spasms of the muscle. This is seen as convulsive movements of the foot and indicates neuromuscular irritability. Each clonus beat is counted. The nurse should also assess the patient for subjective signs and symptoms that indicate that the condition is deteriorating. Such signs are headache, blurred vision or scotoma (blind spots before the eyes), epigastric pain, nausea or vomiting, and dyspnea. Because decreased uteroplacental blood flow can contribute to a hyperirritable uterus, the nurse should also assess for the presence of uterine contractions.

Because of the reduced blood supply to the fetus, constant surveillance is critical. Therefore fetal heart rate should be checked every 4 hours with a Doppler or a continuous electronic fetal monitor should be used if the condition so indicates. Fetal activity should also be monitored; this has been shown to correlate with fetal well-being. Fetal movements reduced from the patient's previous pattern might indicate fetal hypoxia. Rayburn (1983) has developed a protocol for interpreting fetal activity. According to his protocol, inactivity is indicated when there are less than four fetal movements per hour for 2 consecutive days. Other fetal assessment tests will be used to assess uteroplacental sufficiency, such as a nonstress or contraction stress test. One or the other of these tests is usually performed weekly.

Laboratory tests that can be helpful in evaluating the disease are listed below.

1. Hematocrit, to determine the amount of intravascular fluid loss
2. Liver enzymes, such as SGOT, SGPT, and LDH, to evaluate liver function
3. Uric acid and blood urea nitrogen, to evaluate kidney function
4. Coagulation studies, such as platelet count, prothrombin time, and partial thromboplastin time, to evaluate for disseminated intravascular coagulation (DIC)

On admission, a diet profile should be obtained to determine what types of

TABLE 13-3. *Proteinuria*

Dipstick reading	Protein
Trace	—
+1	300 mg/liter
+2	1 gm/liter
+3	3 gm/liter
+4	10 to 20 gm/liter

Combistic package insert, Miles Laboratory, Ames Division, Elkhart, Ind. 1982.

TABLE 13-4. *Degree of edema*

Physical finding	Score
Minimal edema of lower extremities	+1
Marked edema of lower extremities	+2
Edema of lower extremities, face, hands	+3
Generalized massive edema including the abdomen and sacrum	+4

Data from Dennis, E., McFarland, K., and Hester, L.: The preeclampsia/eclampsia syndrome. In Danforth, D., editor: Obstetrics and gynecology, ed. 4, Hagerstown, Md., 1982, Harper & Row Publishers.

TABLE 13-5. *Deep tendon reflex (DTR) grading*

Physical result	Grade
None elicited	0
Sluggish or dull	+1
Active, normal	+2
Brisk	+3
Brisk with transient clonus	+4
Brisk with sustained clonus	+5

Data from Dennis, E., McFarland, K., and Hester, L.: The preeclampsia/eclampsia syndrome. In Danforth, D., editor: Obstetrics and gynecology, ed. 4, Hagerstown, Md., 1982, Harper & Row Publishers.

foods the patient has been eating. The diet should then be evaluated for protein, salt, caloric, and vitamin content. Based on the findings, instructions regarding needed changes can be given, keeping in mind the patient's likes and dislikes. Thus a palatable therapeutic dietary plan for the patient can be developed.

The mother's responsibilities should be identified so that the changes in lifestyle that must be made to implement bed rest can be determined. The resources available to the family should also be evaluated so that problems in this area can be identified. At the same time, the interests of the mother should be determined to discover which diversional activities within the limitations of her condition can be provided.

Complications that can develop as a result of severe preeclampsia are abruptio placentae, disseminated intravascular coagulation (DIC), pulmonary edema, necrosis of the liver, glomerular endotheliosis, and cerebral hemorrhage. To assess for abruptio placentae, the nurse should check for uterine tenderness or rigidity, low back pain, or the presence of vaginal bleeding. Signs of DIC are blood oozing from the intravenous site, easy bruising, bleeding gums, or petechiae. Signs of pulmonary edema are dyspnea or rales; however, these are late signs. If the patient is at high risk for developing pulmonary edema, such as a patient placed on volume expanders, a Swan-Ganz pulmonary artery catheter or a central venous pressure line is the best way to assess for volume overload, which can lead to pulmonary edema. Signs of cerebral hemorrhage are mental confusion, intense headaches, or hyperreflexia.

Antepartum intervention

If the patient is a candidate for home care, education becomes an important role of the nurse.

1. The patient must be instructed regarding the importance of bed rest in the lateral recumbent position even though she feels reasonably well. She should be instructed not to lie on her back because the weight of the gravid uterus can further occlude blood flow to the placenta.
2. The patient's home environment and responsibilities should be assessed to determine difficulties she will face in implementing the prescribed bed rest. Discussion of her resources regarding available help for household responsibilities and available diversional activities should be included. The patient should be encouraged to pursue interests such as crafts, reading, and puzzles that can be done in bed.
3. Her diet should be evaluated for protein, caloric, and essential nutrient content, and she should be counseled in areas of deficiency. The patient should be instructed to avoid foods high in sodium, such as processed foods or ready-prepared foods, potato chips, and salted nuts. She should

also avoid adding salt at the table. The nurse should determine the patient's resources for buying food and cooking it. If a problem is identified in this area, a referral to a social worker should be made.

4. Because of the possible effect of the disease on uterine blood flow, the well-being of the fetus must be evaluated. One or more fetal well-being tests, such as ultrasound for amount of amniotic fluid, the nonstress test, the contraction stress test, and serum and/or urine estriols should be carried out weekly. The patient should be instructed regarding the importance of keeping her appointments for these tests, what the tests are for, and what she can expect to experience during the tests. The mother should also be instructed to evaluate fetal well-being daily by counting the number of fetal movements felt in 1 hour while she is resting. If there are three or fewer movements felt in that hour, she should notify her physician right away; fetal activity decreases if hypoxia develops (Rayburn, 1983).

5. Accurate assessment of patient progress is very important to determine if the treatment is effective and to provide identification of a deteriorating condition. The most critical parameter in the evaluation of the progress is blood pressure. For the medical staff to assess the patient adequately, medical visits twice weekly are advised. A family member should be instructed to take a blood pressure twice daily. If elevated, the blood pressure should be reported to the doctor. The patient should be taught to check her urine for protein twice each day and weigh herself each morning before breakfast.

6. If the patient smokes, she should be instructed that smoking further decreases the blood flow to the uterus. Then the nurse should support the patient in her decision to quit or continue to smoke.

7. The patient should be made aware of the subjective symptoms indicating that the condition is deteriorating and be instructed to call her physician immediately if she experiences any symptoms such as headaches, blurred vision, dizziness, or epigastric pain.

8. Time should be provided so that the patient and her family can ask questions. A brief explanation of PIH and the complications the disease can present for mother and baby should be given. Time spent in teaching the patient about her condition and her responsibility in the management will be very beneficial. Patient understanding usually correlates directly to compliance to the prescribed treatment program.

9. Provide time for the patient and her family to express their concerns regarding the possible outcome for the baby and inconvenience to the mother and family during the treatment. Encourage the patient to vent any feelings, fears, and anger she may be experiencing.

The same time should be spent in instructing the patient and her family if she is treated in the hospital, and the same information should be shared. She should also be encouraged to participate in her care. A quiet, pleasant environment with limited lighting should be provided so as not to activate further the already overstimulated central nervous system. Visitors should also be limited, but the patient's significant others should be encouraged to visit. Seizure precautions should be instituted. An eclamptic tray should be at the patient's bedside. Oxygen, suction, a padded tongue blade, and supplies to pad the side rails should be at the bedside.

The nurse should report to the attending physician an increase of 10 mm Hg or more in blood pressure, +3 or greater deep tendon reflex (DTR), +2 or greater proteinuria, any change in fetal heart rate, or any subjective signs that develop such as headache, epigastric pain, blurred vision, or urinary output of less than 30 ml/hour or 120 ml/4 hours.

Boredom is also a real problem in the hospital and increases the patient's fear and anxiety regarding herself, her family, and the outcome for the baby. Thus the nurse should use her creativity in helping these patients combat boredom. A diversional therapist or volunteer can be called on to provide reading material, hand crafts, or other interesting things. A class in preparation for childbirth regarding relaxation and breathing could be given, because the hospitalization usually occurs prior to her attendance of a prepared childbirth class.

Exercises are important in keeping the muscles in tone and in increasing blood flow. The patient should be instructed to do leg exercises such as foot circles at least twice each day. She should also be instructed to do the Kegel and abdominal tightening exercises to keep the perineal and abdominal muscles in tone. If the patient complains of back pain, the pelvic rock can be effective in relieving this discomfort (see Table 1-1).

Intervention for magnesium sulfate therapy

Magnesium sulfate is the most effective drug in the prevention and treatment of convulsions related to PIH. Magnesium sulfate acts by

1. Decreasing neuromuscular irritability and blocking the release of acetylcholine at neuromuscular junctions. Acetylcholine is the excitatory substance that transmits nerve messages across the synapse.
2. Depressing the vasomotor center by acting on the peripheral vascular system. This causes slight vasodilatation, which increases blood flow to the uterus and can cause a transient episode of lowered blood pressure for 30 to 45 minutes after administration.
3. Depressing the central nervous system, thereby decreasing central nervous system irritability.

Therapeutic administration of magnesium sulfate usually consists of an initial loading dose of 3 to 4 gm intravenous push administered over 10 minutes, followed by a maintenance dose of 1 to 2 gm/hr diluted in 5% dextrose and lactated Ringer's solution administered by an infusion pump to maintain hyporeflexia. The maintenance dose can also be administered intramuscularly. The normal dosage is usually 5 gm per buttock or a total of 10 gm administered after the intravenous loading dose. This is followed by 5 gm every 4 hours. Intramuscular injections of magnesium sulfate are seldom used because the rate of absorption cannot be controlled, tissue necrosis can develop, and the injections are painful. If administered intramuscularly, Z track technique should be utilized with a 3 inch long 20-gauge dry needle, to ensure that the medication is injected deep into the gluteal muscle, and the site gently massaged to facilitate absorption. A local anesthetic agent can be added to the magnesium sulfate solution to minimize the discomfort.

Because magnesium blocks neuromuscular transmission of nerve impulses and depresses the central nervous system, respiratory paralysis and cardiac arrest can result if serum magnesium levels rise too high. Plasma levels of 4 to 7.5 mEq/liter are very effective in preventing convulsions, demonstrated by depressed deep tendon reflexes (DTR). Plasma levels between 10 and 12 mEq/liter cause a loss of DTR, which is a sign of toxicity. Plasma levels above 15 mEq/liter can cause respiratory paralysis, and levels greater than 25 mEq/liter can cause cardiac arrest (Table 13-6). Therefore serum magnesium levels should be assessed daily.

Based on the action of the drug, the nurse should assess any patient on magnesium sulfate for early signs of magnesium toxicity. The DTR should be checked every hour if the patient is on continuous IV drip and before administering each dose if the patient is on intermittent therapy (Table 13-6). Respiratory rate, pulse, and blood pressure should be checked every 15 to 30 minutes if the patient is on continuous IV drip or before administering each dose if the patient is on intermittent therapy.

TABLE 13-6. *Serum magnesium levels*

Magnesium level	Interpretation
1.5 to 2.5 mEq/liter	Normal
4 to 7.5 mEq/liter	Therapeutic
10 to 12 mEq/liter	Loss of DTR
15 mEq/liter	Respiratory paralysis
25 mEq/liter	Cardiac arrest

Data from information in Thomas, R.: Calcium: The desirable electrolyte. In Jackson, E., editor: Nursing skillbook: monitoring fluid and electrolytes precisely, Horsham, Pa., 1978, Intermedical Communications, Inc.

Magnesium is excreted largely in the urine so the patient with kidney involvement can develop toxicity very quickly. Therefore, the patient's intake and output should be monitored closely. If the patient is on continuous IV drip, the urinary output should be at least 30 ml/hr. If the patient is on intermittent doses of magnesium, the urinary output should be obtained every 4 hours and should be at least 120 ml.

Magnesium sulfate should be discontinued or withheld and the physician notified if any of the following signs are present.

1. No DTR or a sudden change in the DTR
2. Respirations less than 12/min
3. Urinary output less than 30 ml/hr or 120 ml/4 hr
4. A significant drop in pulse or blood pressure
5. Signs of fetal distress

Serum magnesium levels are also a useful guide in assessing for magnesium toxicity. Therapeutic levels are between 4 and 7.5 mEq/liter.

Calcium gluconate is the antidote for magnesium toxicity because calcium stimulates the release of acetylecholine at the nerve synapse. Ten milliliters of a 10% solution (1 gm) is the normal dose given by intravenous push. This should be administered by the physician over 3 minutes to avoid undesirable reactions such as bradycardia, arrhythmias, and ventricular fibrillation. It can also be administered intravenously at a rate of 1 gm/hr if needed.

Intervention for antihypertensive therapy

If the diastolic blood pressure is greater than 110 mm Hg or if evidence of impending cerebrovascular accident (CVA) is present, hydralazine (Apresoline) is the antihypertensive drug normally used. Hydralazine acts on the following systems.

1. On the arterioles, causing them to relax, thereby decreasing arteriolar spasms
2. On the vasomotor center, thereby decreasing blood pressure
3. On the heart, stimulating cardiac output

Because of these three actions, peripheral blood flow is increased, which increases renal, cerebral, liver, and placenta blood flow (Woods, 1975).

The normal method of administration is 2 to 5 mg intravenous push administered over 10 minutes. The nurse is responsible for checking the blood pressure every minute for the first 5 minutes following administration and then every 5 minutes for the next 30 minutes. This is best accomplished with an automatic blood pressure cuff, if available. The dose can be repeated every 5 minutes until the diastolic blood pressure is between 90 and 100 mm Hg or an intravenous infusion is started and continuous infusion is administered by an infusion pump. The diastolic blood pressure should not be allowed to fall below 90 mm Hg to prevent further reduction in blood flow to the placenta. Hydralazine is administered whenever the diastolic blood pressure again reaches 110 mm Hg. Side effects the patient can experience are tachycardia, dizziness, faintness, headache, palpitation, numbness and tingling of the extremities, and disorientation.

Intervention for eclampsia

Preeclampsia progresses into eclampsia whenever a convulsion or seizure occurs. Therefore all patients with any degree of PIH should be monitored closely for signs of impending eclampsia.

1. Epigastric pain
2. Headache
3. Visual disturbances
4. Restlessness
5. Blood pressure of 160/110 mm Hg or greater
6. Hyperreflexia
7. Oliguria related to preeclampsia

Although early, proper treatment of preeclampsia should adequately control the disease, eclampsia is always a possible complication of preeclampsia and the nurse should be prepared to care for the woman who does convulse. An eclamptic tray should be available on the unit and should contain the following.

1. Intravenous and intramuscular magnesium sulfate
2. Intravenous diazepam (Valium)
3. Calcium gluconate
4. Hydralazine (Apresoline)
5. Amobarbital sodium (Amytal Sodium)
6. Syringes and needles
7. A padded tongue blade
8. An airway
9. Oxygen tubing with a nasal cannula
10. A tourniquet

Oxygen and suction should be available at the bedside.

The convulsive activity begins with facial twitching followed by generalized muscle rigidity (Pritchard, 1978). During the convulsion, respiration ceases because of muscular spasms. Coma usually follows the seizurelike activity.

The first nursing action should be to assess and establish the airway patency by lowering and turning the head to one side to keep the airway open and minimize aspiration. If possible, a padded tongue blade should be inserted with care between the teeth to prevent tongue injury and to facilitate the insertion of an airway if needed. Suction should be available and used as needed.

The patient should be protected from injury by making sure the side rails are up and padded if possible. After these initial actions the nurse should call for help by turning on the patient's call light. Oxygen should be administered to increase the maternal oxygen concentration and improve the oxygen supply to the fetus, which is lessened during a convulsion.

Diazepam (Valium) and amobarbital sodium (Amytal Sodium) should be available and are used to inhibit seizure activity. Magnesium sulfate therapy is usually initiated as soon as the seizure has stopped. An intravenous line should be started if it has not already been. Delivery of intravenous fluid should be monitored closely with an infusion pump to prevent fluid overload of the constricted intravascular space.

The seizure activity should be observed for time of occurrence, length of seizure, and type of activity. The blood pressure should be checked as soon as possible to determine whether or not a hypertensive agent such as hydralazine will be needed. A Foley catheter should be inserted once the convulsive state has passed, and urine should be checked for protein. Because DIC is a possible complication resulting from eclampsia, especially if abruptio placentae develops, clotting studies may be requested (Pritchard and MacDonald, 1981). The nurse can run a clot retraction test at the bedside by placing 5 ml of blood in a glass test tube and taping the tube to the wall. If the clotting mechanism is normal, a firm clot should form within 8 to 10 minutes. Other signs that indicate the development of DIC are easy bruising, the oozing of blood from puncture sites such as the IV site, or petechia.

During the coma phase, the nurse should assess frequently for uterine contractions; a seizure frequently stimulates labor. This may be indicated by restlessness. The fetal heart rate should be assessed frequently. Normally the hypoxic and acidotic state of a seizure causes bradycardia in the fetus. Delivery should not take place until stabilization of mother and fetus has been achieved. The environment should be kept as quiet as possible, and bright lights should be avoided to decrease central nervous system stimulation.

Labor, if not already underway, is usually initiated once the patient is oriented. If there is no obstetric contraindication precluding a vaginal delivery, induction by a labor stimulant is usually attempted and delivery should take place within 12 hours. The eclamptic patient will be continued on magnesium sulfate during labor and for at least 24 to 48 hours postpartum.

Intrapartum intervention

Delivery is indicated in the PIH patient in any of the following cases.
1. Fetal distress is noted
2. Treatment is ineffective in improving the disease
3. Eclampsia is present

Vaginal delivery is usually attempted and achieved after induction with oxytocin, unless the following conditions are present; then cesarean birth is the method of delivery.

1. Labor does not begin promptly after attempted induction
2. Vaginal delivery is contraindicated for other obstetric reasons
3. The fetus weighs less than 1,500 gm

The same precise care that was outlined for the antepartum period should be continued throughout the intrapartum period.

If oxytocin is used, the contractions must be assessed frequently for hypertonus because the uterus may be more sensitive to oxytocin than usual (Pritchard, 1978). This may not be true in patients who are receiving magnesium sulfate. Some clinicians have found that patients on magnesium sulfate are difficult to induce with oxytocin because of the suppressant effect of magnesium sulfate on the uterus (Keegan, 1981). The progress of labor should be monitored closely because the patient may not be aware of the strength and frequency of her contractions.

Analgesia during labor is limited to small doses and withheld during the 2 hours prior to delivery. If the fetus is premature, analgesics should be avoided; they further depress an already compromised fetus. Regional anesthesia such as spinal, caudal, and epidural is rarely used in the preeclamptic or eclamptic patient because of the risk of hypotension.

The fetus should be monitored very closely because the uteroplacental blood flow is already compromised and the added stress of labor may be too much. Magnesium sulfate crosses the placenta readily. It can cause decreased beat to beat variability as seen on the fetal monitor strip. However, there is no indication that it adversely affects the fetus as long as the mother's serum magnesium does not reach toxic levels.

The patient is usually very anxious about the well-being of the fetus and her own condition. Most women with preeclampsia or eclampsia are transferred to a high-risk center. This can mean that they are a long way from home with or without any significant others. This adds to the anxiety and stress of the condition. Therefore, it is important for nurses who are providing skilled care to attempt to allay the anxiety level.

Postpartum intervention

If the patient has been on magnesium sulfate, it is continued for 24 to 48 hours following delivery. During this time, the patient's condition should be monitored as closely as before; her condition can still deteriorate. This risk may be enhanced by normal postpartum diuresis. As diuresis takes place, there is an increased loss of magnesium leading to a drop in serum magnesium below therapeutic levels, and a convulsion could result.

Blood loss is not tolerated as well as in the normal postpartum patient because of the reduced blood volume caused by the disease process. Therefore the nurse should monitor the blood loss very closely by noting the estimated blood loss during delivery, frequently assessing the status of the uterus, evaluating the amount and type of lochia, closely monitoring the vital signs, keeping an accurate intake and output, and evaluating the hematocrit daily. Nursing measures to decrease blood loss should include massaging the fundus as needed and keeping the bladder empty to facilitate uterine contractions.

A drop in blood pressure accompanied by an increase in urinary output are positive signs that preeclampsia is subsiding. However, an abrupt fall in blood pressure should be considered a sign of hypovolemia until proven otherwise. Oliguria is another sign of hypovolemia and is treated by increasing fluids and administering blood replacements. As the condition improves and the blood volume expands, anemia is a common problem. This occurs because of blood volume expansion without red blood cell increase.

Vasomotor collapse is a very rare but a possible postpartum complication resulting from low serum sodium levels. Serum sodium can be as low as 115 mEq/liter as opposed to the normal 150 mEq/liter level. If this condition ensues, the mother will develop symptoms of shock and fall into a coma. Intravenous sodium chloride and 100 mg of hydrocortisone is usually effective treatment. Therefore the nurse should be alert for signs and notify the attending physician immediately.

Psychologic needs are great during the postpartum period. If the mother was not fully alert for all or part of the labor and delivery, it is important to fill in the gaps in the event for her. Most parents are also very concerned about their neonate's well-being. If the neonate was born prematurely or has intrauterine growth retardation and is in the neonatal intensive care unit (NICU), the mother should be shown pictures of the infant and kept informed regarding the infant's condition. The father should be encouraged to visit the NICU. Then, when the mother's condition becomes stable, arrangements should be made and she should be encouraged to visit the NICU. Even if the neonate is healthy, the mother will need extra support, because she will be separated from her infant for a large portion of the first day or two following delivery. This is because the mother needs limited neuromuscular stimulation and therefore will be kept in a dark, quiet environment with limited visitors.

The parents might be concerned about the effects of magnesium on their neonate. They should be reassured that it has no long-term negative side effects. The neonate may appear hypotonic at first. The parents should be informed that this is a temporary condition, and it does not indicate neurologic damage. Green and associates (1983) found no neuromuscular differences in comparing full-term neonates to the term neonates whose mothers had received magnesium. The mother may also be concerned about breast feeding and the effects of magnesium. Cruikshank, Varner, and Pitkin (1982) found no negative effects if the mother breastfed while taking high levels of magnesium.

After her condition stabilizes, the mother may be concerned about the residual effects of the disease. Zuspan (1978) found in his long-term follow-up study that the disease is reversible unless hypertensive vascular disease either existed before the pregnancy or the patient would have developed it anyway. Chronic hypertension does not result from PIH. The mother should also be reassured that she does not have a significantly increased risk of developing PIH in a future pregnancy (Chesley, 1978) unless one of the major predisposing factors is present.

1. Diabetes
2. Multiple gestation
3. Chronic hypertension
4. Hydatidiform mole
5. Rh incompatibility

Evaluation

The ultimate goal of the nurse is to prevent PIH. PIH is a much studied disease of pregnancy, but the triggering factor still remains unknown. This makes prevention difficult; however, because research indicates that several factors such as adequate fluid and nutrients (especially protein) play an important role, the nurse should include these in the prenatal instructions. When a patient develops preeclampsia during pregnancy, the goal becomes the prevention of eclampsia and uteroplacental insufficiency while attempting to facilitate fetal maturity. Therefore PIH is treated in hopes of stabilizing the condition until fetal maturity is reached. If treatment is effective, diuresis should occur within 18 to 36 hours. Positive signs of stabilization are increased output and a decrease in weight, blood pressure, edema, and proteinuria. If PIH does not respond to treatment, then delivery is the choice of treatment to prevent eclampsia and uteroplacental insufficiency.

Hypertensive disorders of pregnancy

Potential patient problem	Outcome criteria

Antepartum and intrapartum care for preeclampsia

A. Potential deterioration of condition from mild to severe related to:

    Eclampsia

Blood pressure stable for patient
Less than +2 proteinuria
Stable weight
No signs of headache, visual changes, epigastric pain, and nausea or vomiting
Reflexes +2

Assessment and intervention

Dx. Take pulse, respiration, and blood pressure every 4 hr or as ordered
Take temperature qid or as ordered
Assess fluid retention by:
  monitoring I&O
  daily weight before breakfast each day
  observing for signs of edema
Check urine for pH, specific gravity, protein, and glucose every shift
Collect a diet profile for protein, essential nutrients, and calories
Assess for hemoconcentration by checking urine daily or as ordered
Observe for signs that indicate condition is deteriorating such as:
  headaches
  blurred vision or scotoma (blind spots)
  epigastric pain
  oliguria
  blood pressure 160/110 or greater
  dyspnea
Check DTR every shift

Th. Bed rest or limited ambulation (encourage left lateral position)
Provide diet high in protein with no sodium restriction unless ordered
Leg exercises qid
Have eclamptic tray on unit or at bedside; it should include:
  IV and IM MgSO$_4$
  IV diazepam
  calcium gluconate
  hydralazine
  amobarbital sodium
  syringes and needles
  padded tongue blade
  airway
  oxygen tubing with nasal cannula
  tourniquet
Implement seizure precautions by having oxygen, suction, a padded tongue
  blade, and supplies to pad side rails at bedside

Ed. Explain disease, routine management, and possible complications for mother
  and baby in broad terms
Teach self-care such as:
  the therapeutic effects of bed rest or limited activity
  significance of an adequate diet high in protein and ways to combine foods
    to make a complete protein
  how to check urine for protein
  danger signs
  if patient smokes, the effects of smoking on the already decreased uterine
    blood flow

Dx., diagnostic; Th., therapeutic; Ed., education; Ref., referral.   *Continued.*

Potential patient problem	*Outcome criteria*
Antepartum and intrapartum care for preeclampsia—cont'd	
B. Potential fetal distress related to: Uteroplacental insufficiency	Fetal heart rate between 120 and 160 Negative CST Reactive NST At least four fetal movements in 1 hr
C. Potential anxiety, stress, and boredom related to: Possible outcome Bed rest or limited activity	Express inconvenience regarding life-style and fear of possible outcome Participate in decisions affecting self-care
D. Potential complication of abruptio placentae, DIC, pulmonary edema related to: Preeclampsia	No signs of complications

Ref. Notify physician if:
      blood pressure increases 10 mm Hg or more
      DTR is +3 or greater
      proteinuria is +3 or greater
      subjective signs develop that indicate condition is deteriorating

---

Dx. Assess fetal well-being by:
      checking FHT with Doppler every 4 hr or use a continuous fetal monitor
        (depends on severity)
      having mother count the number of fetal movements felt in 1 hr
Th. Carry out NST or CST as ordered
Ed. Explain any ordered test such as NST/CST, amniocentesis for L/S ratio and/
      or PG, and ultrasound for amniotic fluid volume
Ref. Notify physician if fetal heart rate drops from baseline

---

Dx. Evaluate family resources and mother's responsibilities
    Assess for problems related to hospitalization such as:
      work
      child care
      household duties
      finances
    Identify diversional activity of interest to patient
Th. Provide diversional activity to decrease restlessness and boredom
    Guide in making changes in life style to implement bed rest
    Provide opportunity for mother to express feelings of anxiety related to diag-
      nosis
    If hospitalized, provide some uninterrupted time for family to be together,
      alone
Ref. Diversional therapist
    Social worker if problems are identified
    Chaplain on parent(s) request

Dx. Assess for signs of abruptio placentae such as:
      uterine tenderness or low back pain
      uterine rigidity
      vaginal bleeding
    Assess for signs of DIC such as:
      oozing blood from IV site
      easy bruising
      bleeding gums
      petechia
    Assess for signs of pulmonary edema such as:
      dyspnea
      rales
    If on volume expanders, evaluate for pulmonary edema
Ref. Notify physician if any of the above signs develop

Continued.

Hypertensive disorders of pregnancy—cont'd

Potential patient problem	Outcome criteria
E. Potential hyperirritable uterus related to: Decreased uteroplacental blood flow	No more than five uterine contractions every 10 min No fetal periodic deceleration patterns Uterine contractions that do not last longer than 70 to 90 sec
(If on MgSO$_4$ therapy) **F.** Potential CNS suppression related to: MgSO$_4$ toxicity	Respiratory rate greater than 12 DTR $+1$ or $+2$ and no clonus present Urinary output greater than 30 ml/hr or 120 ml/4 hr Serum Mg levels between 4 and 7.5 mEq/liter

Assessment and intervention

Dx. Assess uterine contractions
Th. Utilize fetal monitor during labor
Ref. Notify physician if
    a periodic deceleration pattern develops
    contractions occur more frequent than five every 10 min
    contractions last longer than 70 to 90 sec

Dx. Assess for $MgSO_4$ toxicity every 30 min/1 hr if on IV therapy and before
    each dose if on intermittent therapy by:
        checking DTR and clonus
        checking respiratory rate
        monitoring urinary output
    Assess for medication side effects such as hot feeling, flushing, or sweating
    Refer to such lab data as serum magnesium levels
    Assess pulse and blood pressure every 30 min/1 hr (depends on severity)
    Assess fetal heart rate every 30 min/1 hr or continuously with a fetal monitor
        (depends on severity)
    Check urine for specific gravity, pH, protein, and glucose every 1 hr
Th. Administer IM medication by Z track with dry needle
    Administer IV loading dose by IV push over 10 min for every 3 to 4 gm
    Administer IV maintenance dose by infusion pump (Imed, IVAC)
    Discontinue or withhold magnesium if
        DTR is absent
        respirations are less than 12/min
        urinary output is less than 30 ml/hr or 120 ml/4 hr
        a significant drop in pulse or blood pressure occurs
        signs of fetal distress develop
    Have antidote calcium gluconate on unit
    If ordered, administer calcium gluconate IV push over 3 min for every 10
        ml/10% solution (1 gm) to prevent bradycardia and arrhythmias
Ed. Instruct parents that if infant is hypotonic at birth it is not related to neuro-
    logic problems but is medication related
Ref. Notify physician if
        DTR is absent
        Respirations are less than 12/min
        Urinary output is less than 30 ml/hr or 120 ml/4 hr
        A significant drop in pulse or blood pressure occurs
        Signs of fetal distress develop

Continued.

Hypertensive disorders of pregnancy—cont'd

Potential patient problem	Outcome criteria
G. Potential cerebral hemorrhage related to: Hypertension greater than 110 diastolic	Diastolic blood pressure maintained between 90 and 100 mm Hg

Antepartum care for eclampsia

A. Convulsions or seizures related to: CNS irritability	No seizure activity No injuries due to seizure activity

Assessment and intervention

Dx. Following administration of IV push Apresoline check blood pressure every
      1 min five times, then every 5 min six times, then every 30 min two times,
      or as ordered

      Assess for side effects of Apresoline such as tachycardia, headaches, dizziness,
      faintness, palpitations, numbness, and tingling of the extremities

Th. Assist physician with administration of IV push Apresoline

      Administer IV hydralazine (Apresoline) maintenance dose via infusion pump

Ref. Keep physician informed of blood pressure changes

Dx. Assess patency of airway

      Observe seizure activity for

      time of occurrence

      length of seizure

      type of seizure activity

      Following seizure

      check blood pressure to assess for hypertension

      check fetal heart rate (bradycardia may result from the hypoxic and acidotic
          state)

      assess urine for protein

Th. Lower and turn head to one side to keep airway open and decrease risk of
      aspiration

      Insert tongue pad, if possible, to prevent tongue injury and facilitate inser-
      tion of airway if needed

      Call for help by turning on the patient's call light

      Protect patient from injury by having side rails up and pad if possible

      Administer oxygen by face mask to increase fetal oxygenation

      Be prepared to administer diazepam (Valium) or Amytal Sodium as ordered
      IV to stop seizure activity (The usual dose of diazepam [Valium] is 5 to
      10 mg IV push. Do not inject more than 5 mg per min. The usual dose of
      amobarbital sodium [Amytal Sodium] is 250 mg diluted in 2.5 ml of ster-
      ile water. It should be administered IV push 1 ml/min.)

      Start an IV as soon as possible

      Monitor IV fluid closely with infusion pump

      Initial intake of fluid should be based on the need to combat dehydration
      (Usual amount for first 24 hr is 3,000 ml of fluid. Thereafter, if not dehy-
      drated, fluid intake equals amount of urinary output of the previous 24 hr
      plus 1,000 ml except in acute renal failure; then intake should not exceed
      500 ml.)

      Insert Foley catheter once convulsive state has passed if ordered

Ref. Notify physician at the first sign of convulsive activity

Continued.

Hypertensive disorders of pregnancy—cont'd

Potential patient problem	Outcome criteria
B. Potential initiation of labor related to: Convulsion or seizure	

C. Potential DIC related to:
    Damage of the lining of the
    blood vessel wall
	Clotting factors within normal limits for
	  pregnancy
	Clotting time 8 to 12 min
	Fibrinogen levels 400 mg/dl
	Platelets 150,000 to 350,000 mm^3

Postpartum care
A. Potential convulsions or seizures
    related to:
    Diuresis
    Decreased serum magnesium
	Blood pressure stable for patient
	Less than +2 proteinuria
	Stable weight
	+2 reflexes
	No signs of headache, visual changes, epigastric pain, or nausea or vomiting

B. Potential hypovolemia related to: A decreased blood volume	Blood pressure stable for patient Urinary output 300 ml or more per voiding

C. Potential anemia related to:
    Expansion of blood volume
    without expansion of the
    hemoglobin
	Hemoglobin between 12 and 14

Assessment and intervention

Dx. Assess for signs of restlessness after convulsion
Th. Assess for fundal tightening
      Place patient on external monitor if signs of labor are present
Ref. Notify physician of signs of labor

Dx. Assess for signs of DIC such as
        easy bruising
        oozing of blood from IV site
        petechia
Th. Be prepared to carry out a clot retraction test for DIC by placing 5 ml of
        blood in a test tube

Dx. Continue plan A as outlined in the antepartum and intrapartum suggested
        plan of nursing care
Th. If on $MgSO_4$, continue for 24 to 48 hr as ordered
      Continue close monitoring as outlined in plan A antepartum and intrapartum
        suggested plan of nursing care

Dx. Check blood pressure, pulse, and respiration every 15 min eight times, every
        30 min two times, every 1 hr two times, then every 4 hr
      Check firmness of uterus and vaginal flow with each vital sign check
      Keep an accurate I&O record
Th. Decrease blood loss by
        keeping fundus firm
        keeping bladder empty
Ed. Instruct patient in the need to drink six to eight glasses of fluid per day
Ref. Notify physician
        if urinary output is less than 120 ml/4 hr
        if blood pressure falls abruptly

Dx. Refer to such lab data as hemoglobin/hematocrit
Ed. Instruct patient to eat foods high in iron
Ref. Notify physician if hemoglobin is below 11 gm

Continued.

Hypertensive disorders of pregnancy—cont'd

Potential patient problem	Outcome criteria
D. Potential anxiety related to: Fear of residual hypertension Fear of recurrence of condition in future pregnancies Fear for neonate's well-being	Parent(s) will express fears and anxieties
E. Potential vasomotor collapse related to: Decreased serum sodium	Serum sodium 150 mEq/liter No signs of shock

REFERENCES

Abdul-Karim, R., and Assali, N.: Pressor response to angiotonin in pregnant and non-pregnant women, Am. J. Obstet. Gynecol. **82**:246, 1961.

Alanen, A., and Lassila, O.: Deficient natural killer cell function in preeclampsia, Obstet. Gynecol. **60**:631, 1982.

Assali, N., and Vaughn, D.: Blood volume in preeclampsia: fantasy and reality, Am. J. Obstet. Gynecol. **129**:355, 1977.

Atkinson, S.: Salt, water, and rest as a prevention for toxemia of pregnancy, J. Reprod. Med. **9**(5):223, 1972.

Bates, B.A.: Guide to physical examination, ed. 2, Philadelphia, 1979, J.B. Lippincott Co.

Beer, A.: Possible immunologic bases of preeclampsia/eclampsia, Sem. Perinatol. **2**(1):39, 1978.

Belizan, J.M., and Villar, J.: The relationship between calcium intake and edema, proteinuria and hypertension gestosis: a hypothesis, Am. J. Clin. Nutr. **33**:2202, 1980.

Brewer, T.: Metabolic toxemia of late pregnancy, Springfield, Ill., 1966, Charles C Thomas, Publishers.

Brewer, T.: Metabolic toxemia of late pregnancy in a county prenatal nutrition education project: a preliminary report, J. Reprod. Med. **13**(5):175, 1974.

Brunner, H., and others: Antiotensin II vascular receptors: their avidity in relationship to sodium balance the autonomic nervous system, and hypertension, J. Clin. Invest. **51**:58, 1972.

Assessment and intervention

Dx. Assess parent(s) level of concern and fears
Th. Encourage parent(s) to express fears and concerns
   If neonate is in the NICU, encourage parent(s) to visit nursery as soon as possible
Ed. Instruct patient that preeclampsia does not lead to chronic hypertension
   Instruct patient that preeclampsia usually does not recur in a subsequent pregnancy unless one of the major predisposing factors is present:
   diabetes
   multiple gestation
   chronic hypertension
   Instruct parent(s) that magnesium does not negatively affect the neonate
   Instruct patient that it is okay to breastfeed

Dx. Assess for beginning signs of shock
   Refer to such lab data as serum sodium
Ref. Notify physician if
   serum sodium levels are below 140 mEq/liter
   signs of shock develop

Bryans, C., Jr., Southerland, W., and Zuspan, F.: Eclampsia: a long-term follow-up study, Obstet. Gynecol. **21:**701, 1963.

Butts, P.: Magnesium sulfate in the treatment of toxemia, AJN **77:**1294, 1977.

Chesley, L.: Vascular reactivity in normal and toxemic pregnancy, Clinical Obstet. Gynecol. **9:**871, 1966.

Chesley, L.: Eclampsia: the remote prognosis, Sem. Perinatol. **2**(1):99, 1978.

Cooper, D., and Liston, W.: Genetic control of severe preeclampsia, J. Med. Genet. **16:**409, 1979.

Cruikshank, D.P., Varner, M.W., and Pitkin, R.W.: Breast milk magnesium and calcium concentrations following magnesium sulfate treatment, Am. J. Obstet. Gynecol. **143:**685, 1982.

Cunningham, F., and Pritchard, J.: Hematologic considerations of pregnancy-induced hypertension, Sem. Perinatol. **2**(1):29, 1978.

DeAlvarez, R.: Preeclampsia-eclampsia and renal disease in pregnancy, Clin. Obstet. Gynecol. **21:**881, 1978.

Dennis, E., McFarland, K., and Hester, L.: The preeclampsia-eclampsia syndrome. In Danforth, D., editor: Obstetrics and gynecology, 4th ed., Hagerstown, Md., 1982, Harper & Row, Inc.

Ehrlich, E.N.: Mineralocorticoids in normal and hypertensive pregnancies, Sem. Perinatol. **2**(1):61, 1978.

Everett, R., and others: Vascular reactivity to angiotensin II in human pregnancy, Sem. Perinatol. **2**(1):3, 1978.

Ferris, T., Stein, J., and Kauffman, J.: Uterine blood flow and uterine renin secretion, J. Clin. Invest. **51**:2827, 1972.

Foster, S.: Magnesium sulfate: eclampsia management effects on neonates, MCN **6**(5):355, 1981.

Gant, N., and others: A study of angiotensin II pressor response throughout premigravid pregnancy, J. Clin. Invest. **52**:2682, 1973.

Gant, N., and others: The nature of pressor responsiveness to angiotensin II in human pregnancy, Obstet. Gynecol. **43**:854, 1974.

Gant, N., and others: A prospective study of angiotensin II pressor responsiveness in pregnancies complicated by chronic essential hypertension, Am. J. Obstet. Gynecol. **127**:369, 1977.

Gilstrap, L., Cunningham, F., and Whalley, P.: Management of pregnancy-induced hypertension in the nulliparous patient remote from term, Sem. Perinatol. **2**(1):73, 1978.

Goodlin, R.: Severe pre-eclampsia: another great imitator, Am. J. Obstet. Gynecol. **125**:747, 1976.

Green, K., and others: The effects of maternally administered magnesium sulfate on the neonate, Am. J. Obstet. Gynecol. **146**:29, 1983.

Haesslein, H.: Hypertensive disease. In Niswander, K., editor: Manual of obstetrics, Boston, 1980, Little, Brown & Co.

Hauth, J., Cunningham, F., and Whalley, P.: Management of pregnancy-induced hypertension in the nullipara, Obstet. Gynecol. **48**:253, 1976.

Henry, J.: The effect of pregnancy upon the blood pressure, J. Obstet. Gynecol. Br. Empire **43**:908, 1963.

Hill, M.H.: Hypertension: what can go wrong when you measure blood pressure, AJN **80**:942, 1980.

Jaspers, W., DeJong, P., and Mulder, A.: Decrease of angiotensin sensitivity after bedrest and strongly sodium-restricted diet in pregnancy, Am. J. Obstet. Gynecol. **145**:792, 1983.

Jones, M.: Hypertensive disorders of pregnancy, JOGN Nursing **8**:92, 1979.

Karbhari, D., Harrigan, J., and LaMagra, R.: The supine hypertensive test as a predictor of incipient preeclampsia, Am. J. Obstet. Gynecol. **127**:620, 1977.

Kasser, N.S., Aldridge, J., and Quirk, B.: Rollover test, Obstet. Gynecol. **55**:411, 1980.

Keegan, K.: Hypertension in pregnancy. Paper presented at the Western Symposium of Maternal-Infant Health. Anaheim, Calif., March 7, 1981.

Lindheimer, M., and Katz, A.: Sodium and diuretics in pregnancy, N. Engl. J. Med. **288**:891, 1973.

Marshall, G., and Newman, R.: Rollover test, Am. J. Obstet. Gynecol. **127**:623, 1977.

Nolten, W.E., and Ehrlich, E.N.: Sodium and mineralocorticoids in normal pregnancy, Kidney Int. **18**:162, 1980.

Oaks, Q., Chez, R., and Morelli, I.: Diet in pregnancy, AJN **75**:1134, 1975.

Perkins, R.: Management of the hypertensive pregnant patient, Clin. Perinatol. **7**:313, 1980.

Prinrose, T., and Higgins, A.: A study in human antepartum nutrition, J. Reprod. Med. **7**:257, 1971.

Pritchard, J.: Management of severe preeclampsia and eclampsia, Sem. Perinatol. **2**(1):83, 1978.

Pritchard, J.: The use of magnesium sulfate in preeclampsia-eclampsia, J. Reprod. Med. **23:**107, 1979.

Pritchard, J., Cunningham, F., and Mason, R.: Coagulation changes in eclampsia: their frequency and pathogenesis, Am. J. Obstet. Gynecol. **124:**855, 1976.

Pritchard, J., and MacDonald, P.: Williams' obstetrics, ed. 16, New York, 1981, Appleton-Century-Crofts, Inc.

Rayburn, W.: Fetal activity patterns in hypertensive pregnancies, Obstet. Gynecol. Surv. **38**(3):142, 1983.

Scott, J., and Beer, A.: Immunologic aspects of preeclampsia, Am. J. Obstet. Gynecol. **125:**418, 1976.

Sehgal, N., and Hitt, J.: Plasma volume expansion in the treatment of preeclampsia, Am. J. Obstet. Gynecol. **138:**165, 1980.

Sonstegard, L.: Pregnancy induced hypertension: prenatal nursing concerns, MCN **4**(2):90, 1979.

Speroff, L.: Toxemia of pregnancy: mechanism and therapeutic management, Am. J. Cardiol. **32:**583, 1973.

Spinapolice, R., Feld, S., and Harrigan, J.: Effective prevention of gestational hypertension in nulliparous women at high risk as identified by the rollover test, Am. J. Obstet. Gynecol. **146:**166, 1983.

Stone, S., and Pritchard, J.: Effect of maternally administered magnesium sulfate on the neonate, Obstet. Gynecol. **35:**374, 1970.

Taber, B.: Manual of gynecologic and obstetric emergencies, Philadelphia, 1979, W.B. Saunders Co.

Tichy, A., and Chong, D.: Placental function and its role in toxemia, MCN **4**(2):84, 1979.

Thomas, R.: Calcium: the durable electrolyte. In Jackson, E., editor: Nursing skillbook: monitoring fluid and electrolytes precisely, Horsham, Pa., 1978, Intermedical Communications, Inc.

Valenzuela, G., Harper, M., and Hayashi, R.: Uterine venous, peripheral venous, and radial arteriol levels of prostaglandins E and F in women with pregnancy-induced hypertension, Am. J. Obstet. Gynecol. **145:**11, 1983.

Venuto, R., and others: Uterine prostaglandin E secretion and uterine blood flow in the pregnant rabbit, J. Clin. Invest. **55:**193, 1975.

Weir, R., and others: Plasma renin, renin substrate, angiotensin II, and aldosterone in hypertensive disease of pregnancy, Lancet **1:**291, 1973.

Welt, S., and Crenshaw, M.: Concurrent hypertension and pregnancy, Clin. Obstet. Gynecol. **21:**619, 1978.

Wheeler, L., and Jones, M.: Pregnancy-induced hypertension, JOGN Nursing **10**(3):212, 1981.

Willis, S.: Hypertension in pregnancy: pathophysiology, AJN **82:**791, 1982.

Willis, S., and Sharp, E.: Hypertension in pregnancy: prenatal detection and management, AJN **82:**798, 1982.

Woods, J., and Brinkman, C.: The treatment of gestational hypertension, J. Reprod. Med. **15**(5):195, 1975.

Worley, R., and others: Fetal considerations: metabolic clearance rate of maternal plasma dehydroisoandrosterone sulfate, Sem. Perinatol. **2**(1):15, 1978.

Zuspan, F.: Problems encountered in the treatment of pregnancy-induced hypertension, Am. J. Obstet. Gynecol. **131:**591, 1978.

CHAPTER 14

Preterm labor

Preterm labor can be defined as regular uterine contractions that cause progressive dilatation of the cervix after 20 weeks of gestation and prior to 36 completed weeks. The contractions occur a minimum of every 7 to 10 minutes, lasting at least 1 hour.

INCIDENCE

Approximately 8% of all pregnancies end in preterm labor. Of these, only 15% to 20% qualify for a labor suppressant (Garite, 1981). It has also been found that preterm labor is three times more likely to reoccur in subsequent pregnancies (Barden, 1976). Prematurity in the newborn accounts for 75% to 80% of neonatal morbidity and mortality.

ETIOLOGY

The cause cannot be identified in over 50% of patients who experience preterm labor (Oxorn, 1980). Factors frequently related to preterm labor are classified as maternal, uterine, fetal, or placental. Outlined below are these predisposing factors.

Maternal
- Previous preterm labor (single most important factor)
- Low socioeconomic status
- Low maternal weight gain
- Smokes
- Maternal age less than 18 or greater than 40
- Heavy work
- Commute for more than 1 hour to work
- Diethylstilbesterol (DES) exposure in utero
- Abdominal trauma
- Acute diseases
  - Urinary tract infection
  - Vaginal infections
  - Preeclampsia

    Chronic diseases
        Untreated Cushing disease
        Cardiovascular disease
        Renal disease
        Poorly controlled diabetes
Uterine
    Overdistension of the uterus
        Multiple gestation
        Polyhydramnios
    Uterine infection
    Incompetent cervix
    Uterine anomalies
    Retained IUD
    Premature rupture of membranes (PROM)
Fetal
    Death
    Anomalies
    Infection
Placenta
    Abruptio placentae
    Placenta previa

PHYSIOLOGY

Normal

In order to have a physiologic base for the possible causes and current treatments for preterm labor, one must understand the physiology of labor contractions. What actually initiates labor remains unknown. However, several new concepts have developed from research efforts over the past few years.

Currently there is strong scientific evidence that various hormones influence uterine activity. Progesterone has a relaxing effect on the uterine muscle; estrogen, oxytocin, and prostaglandins are all known stimulators of uterine activity. It appears that all of these hormones play a role in labor. Current research suggests that as the fetal adrenal gland matures it secretes increasing amounts of the precursor for estriol, one form of estrogen. The healthy, growing placenta takes this precursor and secretes increasing amounts of estriol as the pregnancy advances. Estriol affects the fetal membranes and decidua vera by stimulating these tissues to deposit glycerophospholipids, prostaglandin precursors (MacDonald et al., 1974). For prostaglandin synthesis to take place, the enzyme phospholipase A_2 must be present to free arachidonic acid from glycerophospholipids converting it to prostaglandins (Schwarz et al., 1977). Phospholipase A_2 is released by the fetal membranes or decidual lysosomes

(Gustavii, 1972; Liggins, 1973). High levels of progesterone appear to prevent the release of phospholipase A_2 by stabilizing the lysosomal membrane and thereby preventing prostaglandin synthesis (Huddleston, 1982; Schwarz et al., 1976b). High levels of estriol appear to stimulate its release. Therefore it would appear that the lysosomes are held stable until progesterone levels drop or estriol levels exceed progesterone levels. Progesterone does not appear to drop prior to labor, but MacDonald and associates (1978) have observed a progesterone binding protein present in the fetal membranes in late pregnancy. Such a protein may account for a decreased effectiveness of progesterone in stabilizing the lysosomes. This might lead to the increase in prostaglandin production and initiate labor (Challis and Mitchell, 1981). Other factors might influence an unstable lysosome state and trigger preterm labor. Petrie (1981) speculates that low magnesium levels might alter the estrogen:progesterone ratio and thereby influence the release of phospholipase A_2 via the lysosomes. Damage to the fetal membranes can also cause unstable lysosomes to occur (Fig. 14-1).

The presence of oxytocin can stimulate uterine contractions in late pregnancy if estrogen levels are high enough. However, increased levels of oxytocin are not ordinarily found until active labor (Huddleston, 1982; Chard, 1973). Therefore oxytocin appears to facilitate uterine contractions once initiated rather than initiate labor.

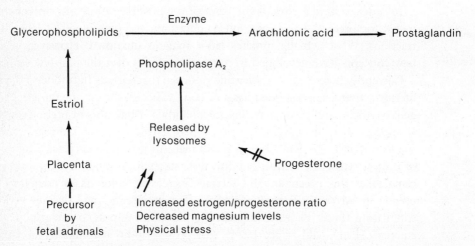

FIG. 14-1. Diagrammatic representation of the interrelationships between the different endocrine factors that contribute to the control of labor (↗↗, stimulate; ✗ , block).

Prostaglandins and oxytocin stimulate the uterus to contract related to their capability of increasing intracellular concentrations of calcium, which activates the muscle to contract. First, prostaglandins and oxytocin block calcium from being bound to the sarcoplasmic reticulum where it is stored. Second, they block the beta-adrenergic receptors from stimulating adenyl cyclase. If stimulated, the plasma enzyme adenyl cyclase accelerates the transport of sodium out of the cell in exchange for potassium. This increases the sodium gradient, and sodium is exchanged for calcium causing an intracellular decrease in calcium (Fig. 14-2). Carsten (1968) noted that there is little difference in the capability of prostaglandins to inhibit storage of calcium in a pregnant or nonpregnant uterus. However, she noted a marked difference in the capability of oxytocin, which is effective only in late pregnancy when estrogen levels are high.

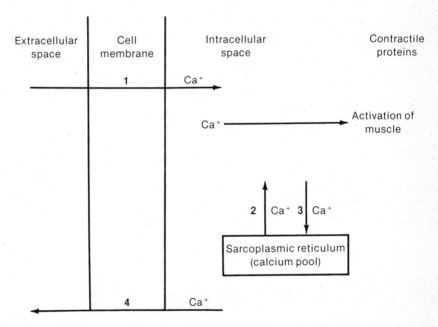

FIG. 14-2. Diagrammatic representation of the final steps that lead to contraction and relaxation of the myometrium. *1,* Calcium flows in from the extracellular space. *2,* Calcium is released from the sarcoplasmic reticulum. Steps 1 and 2 cause an increase calcium level inside the muscle, which activates the muscle to contract. *3,* Calcium returns to the sarcoplasmic reticulum. *4,* Calcium returns to the extracellular space. Steps 3 and 4 cause a decrease calcium level inside the muscle which causes the muscle to relax. (Modified from Forman, A., Andersson, K., and Ulmsten, U.: Sem. Perinatol. **5:**289, 1981.)

Pathophysiology

Each of the aspects of labor may be affected as follows.

Prostaglandin. According to Schwarz and associates (1976a), the fetal membranes and uterine decidua produce or store glycerophospholipids, a prostaglandin precursor. Before prostaglandin synthesis can take place, the enzyme phospholipase A_2 must be present to free arachidonic acid from glycerophospholipid. A decrease in progesterone levels, physical stress such as myometrial stretch, hyperosmolality, and fetal membrane or uterine trauma cause lysosomes to release phospholipase A_2. Thus prostaglandins are produced, and this stimulates the myometrium to contract. Therefore premature rupture of membranes (PROM), abdominal trauma, multiple gestations, and polyhydramnios could stimulate preterm labor. Rush and associates (1976) found that approximately 50% of multiple gestations result in preterm delivery. Bacterial infections can also stimulate preterm labor in this manner, because bacterial organisms release phospholipase A_2 (Bejar et al., 1981).

Oxytocin. In normal labor, the level of oxytocin increases gradually as labor progresses. It appears that oxytocin normally is not the trigger for labor but enhances the progess of labor. However, if high levels of oxytocin are present, they can stimulate labor. According to Seppala and associates (1972), meconium-stained amniotic fluid contains high levels of oxytocin, and therefore a distressed fetus can initiate labor.

Uterine blood flow. Uterine blood flow can influence the onset of labor. Decreased blood flow to the uterus may lead to decidual necrosis, which causes the lysosomes to become unstable and release phospholipase A_2. In this way uterine activity is stimulated. Therefore conditions during pregnancy that interfere with uterine blood flow could trigger preterm labor. Some of these conditions are multiple gestation, polyhydramnios, uterine anomaly causing overdistension of the uterus, preeclampsia, uncontrolled diabetes, heart disease, heavy smoking, abruptio placentae, or placenta previa.

Factors unrelated to physiologic changes. Statistical studies indicate that there are other factors that predispose one to a preterm labor in which the causative mechanism is unknown. One of these is a low socioeconomic status, which appears to play a very dominant role, approximately 60%, in preterm labor (Hemminki and Starfield, 1978). The deterrent factor is unknown, but poor nutrition, bacterial or viral flora of the reproductive tract due to poor habits of hygiene, lack of education, higher incidence of teenage pregnancies, higher frequency of grand multiparity, psychologic and physical stress have all been suggested. Preterm labor also occurs in association with uterine abnormalities. According to Creasy and Herron (1981), approximately 4% of all preterm labors have been associated with uterine anomalies. Kaufman and associates

(1980) studied women who had been exposed to diethylstilbesterol (DES) during fetal life and found they had a 30% chance of a spontaneous abortion, a 35% chance of preterm delivery, and only a 40% chance of a term delivery. According to Garite (1981), 66% of women exposed to DES in utero have uterine abnormalities. As Creasy and Herron (1981) reviewed the literature, they found that the incidence of preterm labor was closely related to previous reproductive performance. For instance, the risk of preterm labor increased after induced or spontaneous abortion and a history of previous preterm labor. In fact Keirse (1979) found the risk of repeat preterm labor to be 25% to 50%. Infections of the urinary tract, vagina, and uterus also increase the risk of preterm labor. The exact relationship has not been identified, but it is hypothesized that bacteria have a stimulating effect similar to oxytocin on the myometrium causing it to contract (Sweet, 1977).

Fetal and neonatal effects

Preterm labor leads to the delivery of an infant whose body processes are immature. Therefore these infants have an increased risk of birth trauma and an increased difficulty adjusting to extrauterine life. Special problems seen in the preterm infant are listed below.

1. Respiratory distress syndrome
2. Intraventricular or pulmonary hemorrhage
3. Hyperbilirubinemia
4. Increased susceptibility to infections
5. Anemia
6. Neurologic disorders
7. Metabolic disturbances
8. Ineffective temperature regulatory mechanism

The severity of each of these problems depends greatly on the gestational age of the infant.

The greatest potential problem of the preterm infant is respiratory distress. If it is severe, hypoxia can ensue and cerebral hemorrhage, seizure disorders, and neonatal death can result. In fact, preterm labor accounts for 75% to 85% of all neonatal mortality and morbidity.

MEDICAL DIAGNOSIS

When a patient comes in experiencing regular, rhythmic uterine contractions, the medical team must first determine whether or not the patient is in true active labor. The diagnosis is usually made in the presence of (1) contractions that occur every 7 to 10 minutes, last at least 30 seconds, and have been present for at least 1 hour; and (2) a cervix that is beginning to dilate or efface.

USUAL MEDICAL MANAGEMENT

When the diagnosis of preterm labor is made, the medical team should attempt to determine the cause and whether further continuation of the pregnancy will be beneficial or harmful to the fetus or harmful to the mother. The choice of treatment depends on the answers to these questions and the age and maturity of the fetus.

Halting labor is contraindicated in the presence of any of the following conditions.

1. Mature fetus as demonstrated by an L/S ratio of 2:1 or greater or the presence of phosphatidylglycerol (PG) in the amniotic fluid
2. Fetal death
3. Fetal anomaly incompatible with life
4. Intrauterine growth retardation related to an unfavorable intrauterine environment
5. Fetal distress
6. Active hemorrhage related to moderate or severe abruptio placentae or placenta previa
7. Chorioamnionitis or intrauterine infection
8. Severe preeclampsia, heart disease, placenta previa, or abruptio placentae

In the presence of premature rupture of membranes (PROM), there are two schools of thought as to whether arrest of labor should be attempted (see Chapter 15). Any patient in advanced active labor as indicated by a cervical dilatation greater than 4 is a poor candidate for suppression of labor.

Suppression of preterm labor is usually attempted if the following factors are present.

1. Fetus is between 20 and 36 weeks of gestation without fetal distress
2. Membranes are intact
3. No obstetric or medical contraindications for prolonging the pregnancy are present

Bed rest in a lateral position combined with adequate hydration is the usual choice of treatment to arrest labor. Labor suppressants may also be used in an attempt to stop contractions; however, only a few patients actually receive the medication. For example, Lipshitz (1981) followed 100 patients in preterm labor. All patients were placed on bed rest and hydrated with intravenous fluids. No labor suppressant drug was administered unless cervical dilatation and effacement could be determined. Of the 100 patients, 40 had spontaneous arrest of uterine activity without any further treatment. Another 42 patients were found to have fetal lung maturity and were not treated with tocolytic agents. Therefore only 18% of the patients who were eligible actually received a labor suppressant.

The next management dilemma arises regarding which labor suppressant should be used. There are many drugs that have been used in an attempt to slow labor, but, because none are without serious undesirable side effects and a statistical history of drug ineffectiveness, the selection is complicated. Currently the drugs of choice are beta-sympathomimetics such as ritodrine (Yutopar) and terbutaline sulfate (Brethine) or magnesium sulfate. Ritodrine is the only drug approved by the Food and Drug Administration for use in suppressing labor.

Whether any of these drugs is effective in arresting labor remains controversial. Hemminki and Starfield (1978) evaluated 13 published research studies that compared a placebo to a labor suppressant drug such as hormones, alcohol, or beta-sympathomimetic agents and found only two of the 13 in which the drug was better than the placebo. However, many research studies indicate that beta-sympathomimetic agents and magnesium sulfate have a 75% to 85% effectiveness in delaying delivery for at least 24 hours. Even if these drugs cannot arrest labor until term in the majority of cases, a delay of delivery for 48 to 72 hours or more can be beneficial to the fetus. During this time glucocorticoids can be administered to accelerate fetal lung maturity. According to Thornfeldt and associates (1978), the incidence of respiratory distress can be reduced to 50% if the patient receives a glucocorticoid 24 hours or more prior to delivery.

NURSING PROCESS
Prevention

Prematurity is the most frequent cause of infant mortality. Preterm labor appears to be the most important cause of prematurity. No treatment is consistently effective for preterm labor. Therefore the best approach to lowering infant mortality is the prevention of preterm labor.

Preventive measures must center around counteracting or improving the conditions that predispose to preterm labor. Adequate diet, prenatal care, and hygiene throughout pregnancy should be helpful in lowering the risk. Prenatally, women at risk for preterm labor should be defined. Because low socioeconomic patients have a 40% to 60% risk for preterm delivery, these patients should be instructed carefully about the importance of proper nutrition and drinking 8 to 10 glasses of water per day to prevent dehydration and to decrease the risk of urinary tract infections. They also need to be educated in the importance of using appropriate perineal hygiene to help decrease the chances of a vaginal or urinary tract infection and in maintaining a balance of exercise and rest and avoiding strenuous physical work. These patients should also be screened frequently for the following.

1. Signs of vaginal or urinary tract infections
2. Anemia
3. Preeclampsia

Every prenatal patient should be screened carefully throughout her pregnancy for diabetes, anemia, infections, and an incompetent cervix. Any identified problem should be cared for early. Treatments for these conditions are usually as follows.

1. Urinary tract infections should be treated with antibiotics.
2. Vaginal infections should be treated early with antibiotics or antifungal agents.
3. Diabetes should be monitored closely to determine the changing insulin needs to control the diabetes.
4. Anemia is treated with iron supplements and diet.
5. Incompetent cervix is treated with cerclage.
6. If an IUD is in place, it should be removed if the string or an end is accessible without dilating the cervix.
7. Any uterine abnormality should be repaired surgically prior to pregnancy.

Patients with (1) a repeated history of abortions or preterm deliveries, (2) multiple gestation, and (3) polyhydramnios have a greater risk of preterm labor. These patients should attempt to protect the uterus as much as possible. Therefore the nurse should instruct these patients thus.

1. To limit their activity as the pregnancy progresses by restricting work, exercise, and increasing their rest periods
2. To limit car riding to no more than 1 hour in length at any one time
3. To limit intercourse, especially in the third trimester of the pregnancy, because orgasm and male seminal fluid increase prostaglandin levels
4. To refrain from preparing the breast for nursing until 2 weeks prior to the due date because nipple rolling stimulates the release of oxytocin

Some obstetricians are treating patients who have a history of preterm labor from an unknown cause prophylactically with progesterone between 18 and 36 weeks of gestation. This is based on the study conducted by Johnson and associates (1975) in which 14 of 36 patients at risk for preterm labor were treated with progesterone and all delivered after 36 weeks. Of the 22 patients who received a placebo, 41% delivered prior to 36 weeks. However, progesterone has been found ineffective in stopping preterm labor once uterine contractions have begun.

During the first prenatal visit, all pregnant women who smoke should be instructed regarding the effects of smoking on the outcome of the pregnancy. There is a well-established relationship between smoking and preterm or small for gestational age (SGA) infants.

Any woman who experiences trauma, especially abdominal trauma, should be observed for signs of preterm labor. An abruption is often the direct result of trauma and leads to preterm labor. The first sign is usually late decelerations on the fetal monitor strip.

Several scoring systems to predict a pregnant woman at risk for preterm labor have been developed so that treatment can be initiated early when it is more effective. Such factors as premature effacement of the cervix, early engagement of the presenting part, and excessive uterine activity have all been identified as possible indicators of preterm labor (Fedrick, 1976). Other subtle signs that can indicate impending preterm labor are low back discomfort different from that which the patient has normally experienced during pregnancy, menstruallike cramps, rhythmic pelvic pressure, a change in vaginal discharge from a thin and clear mucus to a thick mucus, or abdominal cramps with or without diarrhea (Creasy and Herron, 1981; Chez and Creasy, 1982). All high-risk patients should be taught to detect and immediately report any of these subtle signs. When a patient experiences any of these, she should be monitored with an external fetal monitor for 1 to 2 hours to determine uterine activity. If four regular uterine contractions occur within 20 minutes, the patient should be placed on bed rest, encouraged to drink fluids, and unless contraindicated a tocolytic agent should be administered. At the University of California at San Francisco, Herron, Katz, and Creasy (1982) have been able to decrease their preterm delivery rate from 6.75% to 2.4% after introducing such a program.

Assessment

When a patient presents with signs of preterm labor, the nurse should determine whether or not true contractions are occurring by palpating the uterus and placing the patient on an external fetal monitor. If true labor contractions are detected, then the nurse should complete an in-depth assessment to facilitate the decision as to whether or not arrest of labor should be attempted. The following should be included in this assessment.

1. Fetal heart tones, to determine if the fetus is alive
2. Fetal distress with a fetal monitor
3. The presence of bleeding, to rule out an abruptio placentae or placenta previa
4. Urinary tract infection, by obtaining a urinalysis for culture and sensitivity
5. Signs of maternal infection, by temperature and white blood cell count
6. Signs of fetal membrane rupture
7. If membranes are intact, evaluating amount of cervical dilatation
8. Determine EDC

The nurse should be prepared to assist with ultrasound to assess for fetal anomalities and intrauterine growth retardation. The nurse should also assist with an amniocentesis to assess for an intraamniotic infection with amniotic fluid cultures and fetal maturity by amniotic fluid studies for L/S ratio or the presence of phosphatidylglycerol (PG).

As the nurse is assessing the physical status, the patient's psychologic status should also be determined. Parents are highly anxious when preterm labor is suspected because of the threat of long-term hospitalization, potential deformity, or death for their infant. Because of the possibility of death, the parents may pull away from any emotional attachment as a protective mechanism. This can affect later attachment or successful resolution of grief in the event that the infant dies. Therefore the nurse should assess for the level of anxiety. Guilt is often experienced by these parents too. They wonder what they did to cause this to happen. These feelings may be enhanced because the cause of preterm labor can rarely be definitely determined. The nurse should allow the parents an opportunity to express these fears by stating that it is common for parents to feel that they did something to cause the preterm labor and ask them if they have experienced any of these thoughts. This unexpected hospitalization might interfere with many of the woman's everyday responsibilities such as work, child care, and household duties. The nurse should assess for problems in these areas. It is also appropriate to determine the parents' support systems.

Antepartum intervention

If the fetus is immature and is not in distress, and there are no medical or obstetrical contraindications that would be harmful to the fetus or mother if the pregnancy continued, arrest of labor should be attempted. The protocol for suppressing labor usually consists of one or more of the following: (*1*) bed rest, (*2*) sedation, (*3*) hydration, and (*4*) tocolytic agents.

Bed rest is the most beneficial treatment for preterm labor especially in the lateral position. It is intended to keep the pressure of the fetus off the cervix and thereby decrease cervical dilatation and effacement. It is also thought to increase the blood flow to the uterus, stabilizing decidual lysosomes. This decreases myometrial activity by decreasing prostaglandin production. Kneeling or sitting in bed does not keep the pressure of the fetus off the cervix and should not be allowed. To facilitate compliance with bed rest, the nurse should instruct the patient regarding its therapeutic effectiveness. Quiet diversional activities such as TV, radio, and reading material should be provided.

Mental rest should accompany the physical rest. This will be facilitated by peace of mind. Therefore any feelings of guilt, fear, and anxiety identified during the initial assessment should be dealt with appropriately. Allowing time for expression of these feelings is advisable. The possible outcomes of preterm labor should be discussed with the parents. They should understand the benefits and side effects of therapy. Giving false reassurance is not appropriate, but identifying any positive signs can help establish healthy parental attachment. The nurse should encourage the parents to utilize their support systems. If inadequate support is identified, a referral to a social worker may be beneficial. Spiritual assistance can be helpful and should be made available if desired. When the plan of treatment has been determined, the parents should be instructed as to what will happen. When time permits, attention to the couple's need for information adequate to deal with labor and delivery will greatly aid in their coping capabilities as parents of a premature infant.

Boredom is also a real problem in the hospital and increases the patient's fear and anxiety regarding herself, her family needs, and the outcome for the baby. Thus the nurse should use her creativity in helping these patients combat boredom. A diversional therapist or volunteers can be called on to provide reading material, hand crafts, or other interesting things. Instruction in preparation for childbirth regarding relaxation and breathing could be given, because the hospitalization usually occurs prior to her attendance of a prepared childbirth class.

Exercises are important in keeping the muscles in tone and increasing blood flow. The patient should be instructed to do leg exercises such as foot circles at least twice daily. She should also be instructed to do the Kegel and abdominal tightening exercises to keep the perineal and abdominal muscles in tone. If the patient complains of back pain, the pelvic rock can be effective in relieving the discomfort (see Table 1-1).

Sedatives or narcotic analgesics such as meperidine hydrochloride (Demerol) can have an effect similar to oxytocin (Sica-Blanco et al., 1967). Even more serious is the fact that most narcotics depress the respiratory center and enhance respiratory difficulties in the premature infant in the event of delivery. However, hydration is universally thought to aid in the arrest of preterm labor by decreasing the release of antidiuretic hormone (ADH) and oxytocin from the posterior pituitary gland (Niebyl et al., 1978). It also improves the blood flow to the uterus and thereby decreases the release of prostaglandins by stabilizing decidual lysosomes (Huddleston, 1982). A rapid expansion of the maternal vascular volume is contraindicated in patients with a cardiovascular or renal disease because of their potential risk for developing pulmonary edema.

If uterine contractions continue and cervical changes are present, tocolytic agents (which are drugs to inhibit preterm labor) can be used. Because ritodrine (Yutopar) is the only drug approved by the Food and Drug Administration for use in preterm labor, the patient must sign a consent form prior to administration of any of the other beta-sympathomimetic drugs. The benefits and risks of the drug should be discussed with the parent(s) before they are asked to sign the consent.

Intervention—drug therapy for the suppression of labor

Tocolytic agents are currently divided into five classes: *(1)* beta-sympathomimetics, *(2)* magnesium sulfate, *(3)* alcohol, *(4)* calcium antagonists, and *(5)* prostaglandin inhibitors.

Beta-sympathomimetics. Sympathomimetic drugs supplement or mimic the effects of norepinephrine and epinephrine on the body's organs innervated by the adrenergic nerve fibers. There are two types of adrenergic receptors: alpha and beta. Alpha receptors primarily cause contractions of smooth muscle; beta receptors primarily cause relaxation of smooth muscle, except in the heart where they cause cardiac stimulation. There are two types of beta receptors: $beta_1$ and $beta_2$. $Beta_1$ receptors are more predominant in the heart, and their stimulation results in tachycardia and increased myocardial contractility. $Beta_2$ receptors are more predominant in the uterus, blood vessels, bronchioles, and diaphragm. The contractility of the smooth muscle is decreased, which results in uterine and bronchial relaxation and peripheral vasodilation. Contractility of smooth muscle is decreased by binding calcium to the sarcoplasmic reticulum and activating adenyl cyclase, thereby decreasing intracellular concentration of calcium (Fig. 14-3).

Sympathomimetic tocolytic drugs are primarily $beta_2$ stimulators. The most common beta-sympathomimetics that have been used in the United States are ritodrine, terbutaline, and isoxsuprine hydrochloride (Vasodilan). Fenoterol and salbutamol are used in Europe. Isoxsuprine was the first of these types of drugs to be used. It was effective in depressing uterine activity, but severe side effects of hypotension, maternal and fetal tachycardia, nausea, and sweating were frequent. Therefore it is seldom used clinically today. Ritodrine and terbutaline are currently being used. The dose depends on the patient's tolerance. They are effective in relaxing the uterus if a large enough dose is tolerated without side effects. They have a higher therapeutic ratio than isoxsuprine, meaning a larger dose can be administered prior to the development of intolerable $beta_2$ side effects.

When ritodrine and terbutaline are used, it is the nurse's responsibility to administer the drug according to the physician's orders. When intravenous ritodrine is ordered, 150 mg is usually diluted in 500 ml of intravenous fluid such as normal saline or Ringer's lactate yielding a 0.3 mg/ml or 300 μg/ml concentration. It is usually started at 50 to 100 μg/min (0.05 to 0.1 mg/min) and increased 50 μg/min (0.05 mg/min) every 10 minutes until one of the following events occurs.

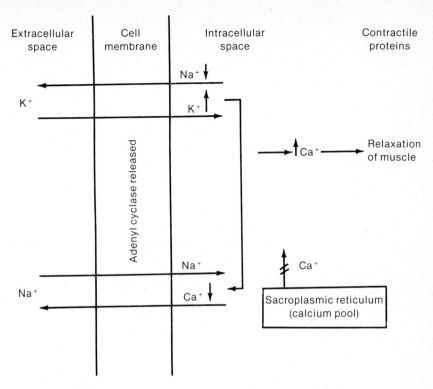

FIG. 14-3. Diagrammatic representation of how beta$_2$-sympathomimetic drugs cause the smooth muscles of the uterus to relax (✗, block). (Modified from Lipshitz, J.: Sem. Perinatol. **5:**252, 1981.)

    1. Uterine contractions stop
    2. Intolerable side effects develop
    3. A maximum dose of 350 μg/minute (0.35 mg/minute) is reached
The patient is usually maintained on the dose that is effective for her for 12 to 24 hours after uterine contractions cease. Then the IV medication is usually tapered off and the patient is placed on oral therapy 30 minutes prior to stopping the IV infusion. The initial oral dosage is 10 mg every 2 to 4 hours for 24 hours and then 10 to 20 mg every 4 to 6 hours.

    When intravenous terbutaline is ordered, 5 mg is usually diluted in 500 ml. It is usually started at 10 μg/min and increased 5 μg/min every 10 minutes until one of the following occurs.

    1. Uterine contractions cease
    2. Intolerable side effects develop
    3. A maximum dose of 80 μg/minute is reached

The patient is usually maintained on a dose that is effective for her for 12 to 24 hours after uterine contractions cease. The medication is then tapered off and the patient is started on subcutaneous injections of 0.25 mg every 4 hours or oral therapy of 2.5 to 5 mg every 4 hours. The frequency of administration may be reduced to three times daily.

Side effects that frequently occur with ritodrine or terbutaline include the following.

1. Slight hypotension, or a widening of maternal pulse pressure related to a slight increase in systolic and a slight decrease in diastolic pressure
2. Light-headedness, tremors, and a flushed feeling related to relaxation of vascular smooth muscle
3. Maternal and fetal tachycardia and heart palpitations related to cardiac stimulation
4. Transient maternal hyperglycemia related to drug stimulation of the liver and muscle causing glycogenolysis, glyconeogenesis, and decreased uptake of glucose by peripheral tissue
5. Elevated lactate and free fatty acids related to hyperglycemia
6. Increased insulin and glucagon secretion related to drug stimulation of the pancreas
7. Decreased serum potassium due to an intracellular shift from the extracellular space
8. Decreased hematocrit by 20% to 25% related to plasma volume expansion
9. Nausea or vomiting related to decreased intestinal motility
10. Bronchial relaxation

Potentially life-threatening complications that have resulted from the administration of ritodrine or terbutaline are listed below.

1. Pulmonary edema, which results from myocardial failure and fluid overload or might not be cardiac-related (Benedetti, 1983)
2. Subendocardial myocardial ischemia (Tye et al., 1980)
3. Cardiac arrhythmias such as premature ventricular contractions, premature nodal contractions, and atrial fibrillation (Benedetti, 1983)
4. Cerebral vasospasm in patients who have a history of migraine headaches (Rosene et al., 1982)

Because of the potential side effects and complications of beta-sympathomimetics, a patient history should be obtained regarding any history of cardiovascular disease, cardiac arrhythmias, uncontrolled maternal hyperthyroidism, or migraine headache. If the mother has a history of any of these disorders, she is not a candidate for this type of labor suppressant therapy. Since beta-sympathomimetics antagonize the body's normal compensatory mechanism for blood loss by its effects on heart rate and systolic and diastolic pressure, these drugs should not be used if there are any indications that bleeding is present. Suppression of labor is always contraindicated in the presence of chorioamnionitis, but especially with beta-sympathomimetics, because of the increased risk of developing pulmonary edema. Therefore an amniocentesis for Gram stain should be done if no signs of chorioamnionitis are present prior to the use of these drugs. Other baseline data should include the following.

1. Fetal heart rate and uterine activity with an external monitor
2. Maternal vital signs
3. Laboratory studies such as complete blood count with differential, blood glucose, urea nitrogen, and serum electrolytes
4. Weight
5. Clean catch midstream or catheterized urine specimen for urinalysis and urine culture to check for urinary tract infection
6. Electrocardiogram

After obtaining the baseline data, an IV infusion of normal saline should be started with an 18-gauge needle to piggyback the intravenous administration of ritodrine and terbutaline. Because incremental titration is essential, an infusion pump should be used.

During intravenous administration, the patient should be encouraged to maintain a left lateral position to minimize the risk of hypotension. An external monitor should be used to record fetal heart tones and uterine activity continuously. Blood pressure, pulse rate and rhythm, fetal heart rate, and uterine activity should be noted and recorded every 15 minutes until 1 hour after the maximum effective infusion rate is reached and then every 30 minutes until intravenous therapy is discontinued. Maternal tachycardia greater than 140, fetal tachycardia greater than 180, a drop in blood pressure below 90/60, or the development of cardiac arrhythmias should be reported to the attending physician. If severe hypotension and tachycardia occur, the drug should be discontinued, mainline IV fluid should be increased, oxygen should be administered via face mask, and the patient should be placed in a modified Trendelenburg position. An appropriate beta-blocking agent such as propranolol (Inderal), 0.25 mg administered intravenously, may be required as an antidote. To avoid fluid overload and pulmonary edema, the total fluid intake for 24 hours should not exceed 2 liters. Strict intake and output measurements and daily weight are obtained during IV therapy. Emergency cardiovascular resuscitation equipment should be available at all times.

The patient on intravenous therapy should be assessed for chest pain regularly. If chest pain develops, the IV therapy is discontinued and oxygen administered by mask. An electrocardiogram is repeated if the heart rate is persistently greater than 130 beats per minute, if the duration of intravenous therapy is greater than 12 hours, or any time the patient complains of chest pain. Laboratory studies such as blood glucose, serum potassium, hemoglobin, hematocrit, and renal function are usually made periodically during the intravenous treatment.

The nurse should assess the patient frequently for signs of hyperglycemia. This can be done by testing a double-voided urine specimen for glucose and ketones four times daily. Testape or Clinistix are used because they are specific for glucose. The blood glucose is checked twice daily with B-G chemstrips or the dextrometer. Diabetic patients can become hyperglycemic if treated with either terbutaline or ritodrine. Therefore they require careful monitoring of plasma glucose and usually require IV insulin administration during treatment with tocolytics.

Hypokalemia can develop as the result of potassium moving from the extracellular space to the intracellular space. However, there is no change in the total body potassium level, and supplemental potassium is usually not necessary. The potassium level will return to normal within 24 hours after the IV therapy is discontinued.

Oral tocolytic therapy is usually continued until 36 weeks of gestation or until medical or obstetric complications necessitate its termination or uterine contractions resume. If uterine contractions resume, IV therapy may be repeated. When the patient is first started on oral therapy, vital signs should be taken every 2 hours for the initial 24 hours and then every 4 hours thereafter. The nurse should evaluate the effectiveness of the therapy in preventing uterine contractions by asking the patient every 2 to 4 hours if she has experienced any contractions, back pain, cramps, or increased vaginal discharge and by palpating the uterus. The patient should also be monitored for drug-related side effects. They are usually mild and can often be reduced by administering the medication with meals or a snack. In the nondiabetic patient, long-term oral therapy does not appear to affect blood glucose. However, long-term oral therapy can cause hyperglycemia in the diabetic.

Every patient discharged and continued on oral therapy at home should be instructed regarding the following.

1. To stay on bed rest as much as possible
2. To refrain from preparing the breasts for nursing until 2 weeks prior to the due date because it can stimulate the release of oxytocin
3. To avoid sexual intercourse and orgasm because they can stimulate uterine activity
4. To check pulse prior to taking the medicine and contact the physician if the pulse is greater than 130 beats/minute
5. To report any side effects to the drug such as heart palpitations, tremors, or nervousness
6. To check temperature daily

7. To report signs of labor such as regular contractions, low back pain, cramping, or increased vaginal discharge
8. To report signs of rupture of membranes, vaginal bleeding, and signs of infection such as elevated temperature
9. To return weekly for antepartum fetal testing

Parents will be interested in the long-term effects of ritodrine or terbutaline on their baby. The only major side effect to the fetus is tachycardia, but no adverse physical or neurologic effects have been noted (Lipshitz, 1981). Freyse and associates (1977) found no developmental effects on children followed for 3 years who had received ritodrine prenatally. In contrast, beneficial effects have been demonstrated by Unbebann (1974) even when delivery was postponed for 24 to 72 hours. The beneficial effects include increased placental blood flow and acceleration of the phospholipid synthesis due to stress on the fetus. Therefore, the incidence of neonatal respiratory distress syndrome was decreased. The only side effect noted in the neonate has been mild, transient hypoglycemia or hyperglycemia during the first 24 hours.

Magnesium sulfate. In the past, magnesium sulfate has been used in obstetrics primarily to treat preeclampsia. Now it is being used more and more in the treatment of preterm labor. Magnesium relaxes the smooth muscle of the uterus by substituting itself in place of calcium (Petrie, 1981). Not only does magnesium act at the cellular level to decrease uterine activity, but it also acts at a nerve transmission level. Magnesium blocks the release of acetylcholine at the nerve synapse by displacing calcium, thus blocking nerve transmission to the muscle (Petrie, 1981). Secondary effects of magnesium such as decreasing arteriole pressure and increasing uterine blood flow can also be therapeutic in suppressing preterm labor.

Some obstetricians find magnesium sulfate very beneficial with far fewer serious side effects than beta-sympathomimetics. If magnesium therapy is initiated early to bring about an elevation or correction in the serum magnesium level prior to cervical dilatation or rupture of membranes, it is effective in 92% to 95% of cases (Steer and Petrie, 1977). If used with intact or ruptured membranes at less than 5 cm of dilatation, delivery was effectively delayed for 24 hours or longer in 75% to 85% of cases (Petrie, 1981). Therefore its use may increase in the future except in the patient with a cardiac or renal disorder. Its use is contraindicated in these patients because it depresses cardiac contractility and is eliminated from the body by way of the kidneys.

A loading dose of 6 to 8 gm intravenous is usually recommended in the treatment of preterm labor followed by a maintenance dose of 2 gm/hr until one of the following occurs (Huddleston, 1982).

1. Uterine contractions cease
2. Signs of toxicity develop

Because magnesium relaxes skeletal as well as smooth muscle, respiratory and circulatory failure can occur if toxic levels are allowed to develop. The nurse must monitor the patient for signs of magnesium toxicity thus.

1. Checking the blood pressure and respirations every 15 minutes
2. Checking the knee jerk reflex hourly
3. Keeping record of hourly intake and output
4. Obtaining serum magnesium levels daily

If the patient becomes hypotensive, respirations drop below 12 breaths/min, or the knee jerk reflex is absent, toxicity is developing and the medication must be discontinued. Since magnesium is rapidly secreted from the mother's body by way of the kidneys, urinary output should be at least 30 ml/hr or magnesium will accumulate in the body and toxicity will develop. Therapeutic serum levels of 4 to 7.5 mEq/liter are effective in reducing uterine contractions. Toxicity can develop with levels of 10 mEq/liter. Calcium gluconate is an effective antidote against magnesium toxicity and should be available whenever a patient is receiving magnesium. The patient being treated for preterm labor can tolerate a much higher dose of magnesium than the preeclamptic patient. Kidney function is usually not compromised in the preterm labor patient as it can be in the preeclamptic patient (see Chapter 13).

The patient may complain of hot flushes, nausea, and vomiting during the loading dose. If these signs appear, the patient should be reassured that they will subside when the loading dose is completed. Pulmonary edema has been reported to occur in patients who have been treated with magnesium and betamethasone (Elliott et al., 1979). Petrie (1981) reports no correlation between administering magnesium with betamethasone and pulmonary edema. However, the nurse should observe any patient on magnesium and betamethasone closely for signs of pulmonary edema.

Narcotics or sedatives should not be administered to a patient on magnesium because of the potentiating effect of these drugs on respiratory depression. When the patient requires general anesthesia, smaller doses of muscle relaxants are usually needed. It would be helpful for a patient undergoing a general anesthesia to be taken off the magnesium at least 30 minutes prior to the introduction of anesthesia.

Neonatal side effects are rare as long as the mother's serum level is maintained below 8 mEq/liter and the mother does not receive morphine or meperidine hydrochloride (Demerol) for pain. According to Stone and Pritchard (1970) who studied 7,000 infants born to mothers who had received magnesium sulfate intravenously, there were no negative effects on the fetus. Only slight muscle flaccidity was noted.

Alcohol. Ethanol was the first drug to be used in the treatment of preterm labor. In 1965, Fuchs found that ethanol interferes with the release of oxytocin from the pituitary (Fuchs, 1965). Since the use of beta-sympathomimetics and magnesium sulfate began, ethanol has been demonstrated to be the least effective method with the most side effects (Steer and Petrie, 1977; Lauersen et al., 1977).

Pharmacologically, ethanol adversely effects nearly every body organ (Isselbacher, 1977). These side effects range from nausea, vomiting, urinary incontinence, restlessness, and disorientation to respiratory depression and aspiration pneumonia. Because alcohol inhibits gluconeogenesis, hypoglycemia can develop if IV glucose is not administered. It also promotes diuresis and can cause an electrolyte imbalance. The fetus is usually intoxicated and severe central nervous system depression and fetal acidosis can result. Therefore because of its limited effectiveness and severe side effects, ethanol is rarely used today in the treatment of preterm labor. The only situation where it might be useful is during a long transport from home to hospital; oral ethanol is easily available and other labor suppressants would not be accessible at that time.

Calcium antagonists. Because contraction of smooth muscle is dependent on the availability of calcium, calcium antagonists are being considered as a possible treatment for suppressing labor. Nifedipine is one calcium antagonist that has been used experimentally. Ulmsten, Andersson, and Wingerup (1980) gave nifedipine to 10 patients experiencing preterm labor prior to 34 weeks of gestation. Delivery was delayed in all 10 patients for 3 days or longer. No serious side effects were noted in the mothers or fetuses. From this limited study, a new approach for controlling uterine activity is being considered. Continuous research is being conducted regarding the use of calcium antagonists. Prior to its widespread use, an in-depth study with a larger sample size should be carried out to determine its safety and effectiveness as compared to beta-sympathomimetics and magnesium (Forman et al., 1981).

Prostaglandin inhibitors. Becuase prostaglandins are known to stimulate contractions at any time during pregnancy, studies are being conducted as to the effect of prostaglandin inhibitors in the treatment of preterm labor. Zuckerman, Reiss, and Rubinstein (1974) and Niebyl and Johnson (1980) found indomethacin, a prostaglandin inhibitor, very effective in stopping preterm labor.

Since animal studies have demonstrated fetal complications such as premature closure of the ductus arteriosus, pulmonary hypotension, and bleeding problems, prostaglandin inhibitors are used at present only as experimental therapy (Levin, 1980). However, in the limited study by Niebyl and Johnson (1980), no evidence of these side effects was found in the human fetus. Nevertheless, because further research has not been completed on this method of treatment, it is not commonly used today.

Intervention—drug therapy for stimulation of fetal lung maturity

Steroid therapy stimulates the production of a more stable lecithin, which is a surface-active phospholipid mainly responsible for facilitating normal alveolar function. It is thought to decrease the risk of neonatal respiratory distress in the fetus born between 28 and 34 weeks of gestation. This hypothesis was developed in 1972 when Liggins and Howie were able to demonstrate in a well-controlled study that glucocorticoid therapy administered to pregnant women 48 to 72 hours prior to delivery, and not longer than 7 days, reduced the incidence of respiratory distress in the neonate. Since that time, other research has supported these findings (Taeusch et al., 1979).

This hypothesis is not accepted by everyone in the field of obstetrics. In contrast, Quirk and associates (1979) did not find in their group of patients a significant reduction of respiratory distress syndrome (RDS) in the neonates who were exposed to glucocorticoid therapy prenatally. However, both the control group and the steroid group had a low incidence of RDS, which the authors attributed to the avoidance of intrapartum hypoxia and intrapartum stress, and to atraumatic deliveries. This study probably demonstrates another factor that decreases the risk of neonatal RDS and does not provide evidence that steroid therapy is ineffective. This is physiologically sound; lecithin is produced by two different pathways depending on gestational age. The premature fetus produces a very unstable lecithin that is affected negatively by hypoxia and hypothermia. As the fetus matures, the lecithin becomes more stable and is less affected by hypoxia and hypothermia.

The use of glucocorticoids is not without risk even though evidence appears to favor their therapeutic effect. Animal studies have demonstrated a relationship between glucocorticoid therapy and retardation of physical, mental, and neurologic growth (Johnson and Dubin, 1980). The question is, "Can this be applied directly to the human?" Liggins (1976) followed the neonates who had received steroids in utero for 4 years and found no deficiencies in mental, verbal, or visual maturation.

The effects on the mother include increased risk of infection and delayed wound healing. If she has diabetes or pregnancy-induced hypertension, steroids can aggravate these disorders. Garite (1981) and Taeusch and associates (1979) have demonstrated an increased risk of maternal endometritis if steroids are administered in the presence of premature rupture of membranes.

Because the use of steroids carries potential risks, the medical team must evaluate each patient individually to determine the risk to benefit ratio. The patients should be informed of the advantages and the risks involved with steroid therapy and allowed to participate in the choice of treatment.

When steroids are used, betamethasone or dexamethasone are the two drugs of choice because they cross the placenta unchanged whereas other steroids do not. Betamethasone (Celestone) has short- and long-term activities and is usually favored. The routine dose is 2 doses of 12 mg 24 hours apart.

Any time a patient is receiving steroid therapy, the fetus should be monitored closely to detect fetal distress early, because a hypoxic and stressed fetus has an increased risk for RDS. A premature infant should be kept warm; hypothermia can influence the development of hypoxia. A neonatologist should be available for the delivery and the neonatal intensive care unit should be notified of the coming neonate.

If the patient on steroids does not deliver within 1 week, the treatment should be repeated if the fetus is less than 34 weeks of gestation. Steroid therapy appears to have a transient effect on lecithin. Brown and associates (1979) and Liggins and Howie (1974) found that, 7 days following treatment, the surfactant levels dropped to their original levels.

Following delivery the neonate should be observed closely for signs of hypoglycemia and the mother observed for signs of infection because these complications can accompany steroid therapy. If steroids are used in the diabetic patient, she should receive IV insulin and her blood sugar levels should be evaluated frequently for hyperglycemia because of the effect of steroids on blood sugar.

Intrapartum intervention

If delivery is inevitable, it is best for the patient, if possible, to be transferred to a hospital with a neonatal intensive care unit. The fetus should be monitored closely for the development of fetal distress. The parents will need a lot of support at this time. They will be very fearful of the outcome for their baby and question what they did to initiate this early labor. Usually they have been unable to complete their prenatal classes and will therefore need extra support through the labor and delivery. Minimal to no analgesia is used during the labor to avoid compounding the problem of neonatal respiratory depression. If pain relief is required, epidural anesthesia is preferred; it does not interfere with the infant's own ability to initiate respirations at birth. During the second stage of labor, the nurse should instruct the mother not to bear down. This will help to slow the expulsion process and decrease the risk of trauma to the fragile premature infant since excessive pressure might cause a subarachnoid hemorrhage. An episiotomy is usually done and forceps are avoided to further decrease the risk of trauma.

The delivery room should be prepared early because labor will probably be shorter. The resuscitation equipment should be checked and made ready. The radiant warmer should be turned on. The neonatal intensive care nursery should be notified of the high-risk patient.

If the fetus is in a breech presentation or if signs of fetal distress develop, it will be less harmful to the fetus if delivery is by cesarean birth. The nurse should be prepared for this type of delivery and should prepare the patient.

Postpartum intervention

The postpartum patient who received a glucocorticoid during pregnancy to stimulate fetal lung maturity is at a greater risk for an endometrial infection. Therefore this patient should be assessed very closely for an infection by check-

---

S U G G E S T E D   P L A N

Preterm labor

Potential patient problem	*Outcome criteria*
Antepartum care	
A. Potential preterm labor related to:	Maintenance of pregnancy through 36 weeks of gestation or until fetal lungs are mature as indicated by an L/S ratio of $2:1$ or PG present in the amniotic fluid
Previous preterm labor	
Low socioeconomic status	
Low maternal weight gain	Mother infection-free
Smoking	
Maternal age less than 18 or greater than 40 years	
Performing heavy work	
Commuting long distances	
Having a chronic disease	
Multiple gestation	
Exposure to DES in utero	

ing her temperature and assessing the odor of the lochia every 4 hours for the first 2 postpartum days.

If an endometrial infection develops, treatment with antibiotics is usually effective. Ampicillin or cephalosporin are usually the drugs of choice. There is no need to isolate these patients if the infected organism is one normally present in the vaginal flora. The patient should be taught good hand washing prior to handling her infant and instructed to keep the infant on the top covers of her bed rather than on the bottom sheet, which can be contaminated with organisms.

Glucocorticoids can also delay wound healing, especially if the patient had to have a cesarean delivery. Therefore these patients should be instructed to eat foods high in protein and continue to take their prenatal vitamins to facilitate tissue repair.

O F   N U R S I N G   C A R E

Assessment and intervention

Dx.   Obtain a detailed prenatal history to determine the patient at risk for preterm labor
Screen throughout pregnancy for
infections
preeclampsia
abruptio placentae/placenta previa

Ed.   Teach all high-risk patients early warning signs of preterm labor such as
low back discomfort
menstruallike cramps
rhythmic pelvic pressure
a change in vaginal discharge
abdominal cramps with or without diarrhea
Teach all high-risk patients how to differentiate a true contraction from Braxton-Hicks contractions
Teach all high-risk patients how to feel for a uterine contraction
Teach all high-risk patients to lie down and drink several glasses of fluid if they experience any warning signs or any uterine contractions
Teach all high-risk patients that if warning signs do not ease in 1 hr or if they experience five contractions in 1 hr while at rest to notify their health care provider

Dx., diagnostic; Th., therapeutic; Ed., education; Ref., referral.   *Continued.*

Preterm labor—cont'd

Potential patient problem	Outcome criteria
Antepartum care—cont'd	
B. Preterm labor related to: Premature myometrial activity (treatment if suppressing labor)	Maintenance of pregnancy through 36 weeks or until fetal lungs are mature as indicated by an L/S ratio of 2:1 or PG present in the amniotic fluid
C. Potential side effects related to: Beta-sympathomimetic drugs (treatment with tocolytic agents)	Minimal side effects so a therapeutic dose of the medication can be administered No signs of fetal distress Maintenance of pregnancy to at least 37 weeks of gestation

Dx. Monitor FHR and UC with fetal monitor
Assess for signs of fetal distress
Assess for signs of bleeding
Collect urine for culture and sensitivity as ordered
Check TPR and BP as indicated
Assess for signs of PROM
Determine EDC

Th. Bed rest in the lateral position
Encourage 8 to 10 glasses of fluid daily
Assist with diagnostic procedures such as ultrasound and amniocentesis
Provide diversional activities of interest to the patient

Ed. Instruct as to the importance of bed rest
Instruct not to kneel or sit in bed

Ref. Notify physician if
signs of fetal distress develop
signs of bleeding develop
temperature is greater than 38° C
signs of PROM occur

Dx. *Prior to IV therapy:*
Obtain FHR and UC strip with external monitor
Check vital signs
Check history for cardiovascular disease, hyperthyroidism, or migraine
headaches
Obtain weight
Refer to lab studies such as
CBC with differential, blood glucose, urea nitrogen, serum electrolytes,
EKG

During IV therapy:
Monitor FHR and UC with external monitor continuously
Check VS every 15 min until 1 hr after maximum rate is reached, then
every 30 min
Check weight daily
Monitor I&O
Refer to such lab tests as blood glucose, serum potassium, hematocrit, hemoglobin, and ECG
Assess for signs and symptoms of hyperglycemia such as
weakness
nausea/vomiting
abdominal cramping
excessive thirst
frequent urination
glucosemia
ketonuria

Continued.

Preterm labor—cont'd

Potential patient problem	*Outcome criteria*

Antepartum care—cont'd
  C. Potential side effects related to:
      Beta-sympathomimetic drugs
        (treatment with tocolytic
        agents)—*cont'd*	

Assessment and intervention

Assess for signs of hypokalemia such as
    muscle weakness
    nausea/vomiting
    abdominal distension
    flatulence
    decreased respiratory rate
Assess for signs of pulmonary edema such as
    dyspnea
    wheezing
    coughing
Assess for other signs such as
    headache
    light-headedness
    tremors
    flushed feeling
    heart palpitations
    nausea/vomiting
During oral therapy:
    Check vital signs every 2 hr for first 24 hr, then every 4 hr
    Assess for uterine contractions with vital signs by
        palpating for uterine contractions
        asking about back pain and cramping
    Assess vaginal discharge
    Assess for side effects

Th. Obtain consent for terbutaline
    Start IV infusion with NS and an 18-gauge intracatheter
    Encourage a lateral recumbent position
    While administering IV therapy, restrict fluid intake to 2,000 ml/24 hr
    Test double voided urine specimen four times daily for glucose and ketone
        (must use testape, clinistix, or diastix for glucose-specific results)
    Monitor blood glucose two or more times daily as ordered (use B-G chem-
        strip or dextrometer)
    Piggyback intravenous medication with infusion pump
Terbutaline administration:
    Prepare terbutaline by diluting 5 mg in 500 ml of IV fluid such as NS or
        RL as ordered (concentration yields 10 µg/ml)
    Start IV terbutaline at 10 µg/min or as ordered
    Increase 5 µg/min every 10 min until
        uterine contractions cease
        intolerable side effects develop
        a maximum dose of 80 µg is reached

Continued.

Preterm labor—cont'd

Potential patient problem	*Outcome criteria*
Antepartum care—cont'd	
C. Potential side effects related to: Beta-sympathomimetic drugs (treatment with tocolytic agents)—*cont'd*	

Assessment and intervention

Maintain an effective dose for 8 hr, then taper off at a rate of 5 μg/min
  every 10 min
Start administering the subcutaneous injection or oral medication 30 min
  prior to discontinuation of the IV infusion
Administer oral medication with meals or a snack to lessen side effects
If chest pain, severe hypotension (less than 90/60), or tachycardia (greater
  than 140) develops:
  discontinue the medication
  increase mainline intravenous infusion
  administer oxygen by mask
  place patient in modified Trendelenburg position
Have available CPR equipment and propranolol (Inderal) 1 mg

Ritodrine administration
Prepare ritodrine by diluting 150 mg in 500 ml of intravenous fluid such
  as NS or RL as ordered (concentration yields 300 μg/ml)
Start ritodrine at 50 to 100 μg/min or as ordered
Increase 50 μg/min every 10 min until
  uterine contractions cease
  intolerable side effects develop
  a maximum dose of 350 μg is reached
Maintain an effective dose for 12 to 24 hr, then taper off at a rate of 50
  μg/min every 10 min
Start administering oral medication 30 min prior to discontinuation of the
  IV infusion
Administer oral medication with meals or a snack to lessen side effects
If chest pain, severe hypotension (less than 90/60), or tachycardia (greater
  than 140) develops:
  discontinue the medication
  increase the mainline intravenous infusion
  administer oxygen by mask
  place patient in modified Trendelenburg position
Have available CPR equipment and propranolol (Inderal) (1 mg)

Continued.

Preterm labor—cont'd

Potential patient problem   *Outcome criteria*

Antepartum care—cont'd
  C. Potential side effects related to:
        Beta-sympathomimetic drugs
        (treatment with tocolytic
        agents)—*cont'd*

Assessment and intervention

Ed. Explain treatment protocol
Explain that no treatment has been consistently proven effective but even a
few days of additional time for the fetus to grow is beneficial
Explain that there have been no detrimental effects manifested in the fetus or
mother from the medication
If discharged home on oral therapy, instruct to
stay on bed rest as much as possible
refrain from preparing the breast for nursing until 2 weeks prior to the
due date
avoid sexual intercourse
check pulse prior to taking medication, if greater than 130 to 140 beats/
min call physician
Check temperature daily
Report signs of regular contractions, low back pain, cramping or increased
vaginal discharge, vaginal bleeding, PROM, or signs of infection
Return for weekly obstetrician visits and ordered antepartum fetal testing
Ref. Notify attending physician if any of the following develop
maternal tachycardia greater than 140
fetal tachycardia greater than 180
BP less than 90/60
cardiac arrhythmias
output less than 30 ml/hr
If on oral therapy notify attending physician if uterine contractions reoccur

Continued.

Preterm labor—cont'd

Potential patient problem	Outcome criteria

Antepartum care—cont'd
   D. Potential side effects related to:
       Magnesium toxicity
	Respiratory rate greater than 12
	 +2 DTR; negative clonus
	 Urinary output greater than 30 ml/hr or greater than 120 ml/4 hr
	 Serum magnesium levels between 4 and 7.5 mEq/liter
	 No signs of fetal distress
	 Maintenance of pregnancy to at least 37 weeks of gestation

Assessment and intervention

Dx. Assess for MgSO$_4$ toxicity every 30 min to 1 hr by:
    checking DTR and clonus
    checking respirations
    checking urinary output
    observing for signs such as hot feeling, flushing, or sweating
    Assess serum magnesium levels as ordered
    Assess P and BP as indicated (15 to 30 min)
    Monitor FHR and UC with external monitor

Th. Start IV with 18-gauge intracatheter
    Encourage lateral recumbent position
    Administer IV loading dose IV push over 10 to 20 min for every 4 gm
    Administer IV maintenance dose piggyback into mainline by infusion pump
      (Imed, IVAC) (usual dose 2 gm/hr until uterine contractions cease)
    Discontinue MgSO$_4$ and notify physician if:
      DTR is absent
      respiratory rate is less than 12 to 14/min
      urinary output is less than 30 ml/hr or 120 ml/4 hr
      significant drop in P or BP occurs

Ed. Explain treatment protocol
    Explain that no treatment has been consistently proven effective but even a
      few days of additional time for the fetus to grow is beneficial
    Explain that there have been no detrimental effects manifested in the fetus or
      mother if monitored closely (The neonate may be hypotonic at birth but
      this is not related to neurological problems and will resolve itself in a day
      or two.)

Ref. Notify physician if any of the following develop:
    absence of DTR
    respiratory rate less than 12/min
    urinary output less than 30 ml/hr or 120 ml/4 hr
    significant drop in pulse or blood pressure occurs
    signs of fetal distress develop

Continued.

Preterm labor—cont'd

Potential patient problem	*Outcome criteria*
Antepartum care—cont'd	

E. Potential family stress and anxiety related to:
    Unknown outcome of preterm labor
    Long-term hospitalization
    Potential fetal deformity or neonatal death
	Parent(s) express fears and anxieties
	Parent(s) participate in decisions regarding care

F. Preterm labor related to: Uncontrollable myometrial activity (treatment if delivery is inevitable)	Labor and delivery without fetal distress

Assessment and intervention

Dx. Assess family resources, knowledge, and coping ability
Th. Encourage parent(s) to express their fears and anxieties
Assess for problems related to hospitalization such as
    work
    child care
    household duties
    finances
Discuss possible outcomes of preterm labor
Provide diversional activities
Ref. To social worker if problems are identified
Notify chaplain on parent(s) request

Dx. Monitor uterine activity
Assess clean-catch or catheterized urine specimen for bacteria and WBCs
Assess for signs of infection by
    checking temperature every 4 hr
    refering to WBC
    assisting with amniocentesis for amniotic fluid cultures if ordered
Assess for signs of bleeding
Assess for signs of PROM
Assess for signs of fetal distress with continuous fetal monitor
Determine EDC
Assist with ultrasound if ordered
If membranes intact, check amount of cervical dilatation
Assist with assessment of fetal maturity by amniotic fluid studies for L/S or
    PG if ordered
Th. Apply external monitor
Try not to use any analgesics
Instruct not to push during second stage of labor
Prepare delivery room early, check resuscitation equipment, turn on warmer,
    and notify NICU
Be prepared for possible cesarean delivery
Do not leave patient alone
Ed. If unable to attend prepared childbirth classes, instruct regarding breathing
    and relaxation techniques
Prepare for possible cesarean delivery
Explain reason for minimal to no analgesia
Ref. Notify physician of signs of fetal distress

Psychologic needs are great during this time, especially if the neonate was born prematurely. The parents should be encouraged to visit the neonatal nursery often to spend time with their baby. The nurse should point out reassuring characteristics and encourage the parents to participate in the care of their infant as much as possible. The parents will also need time to talk about their feelings regarding the birth experience; they may feel cheated, especially if they had planned a birthing room delivery with rooming-in.

Evaluation

The ultimate goal of treatment for preterm labor is delivery of a healthy neonate. It is known that neonatal outcome is greatly improved when intrauterine life can be extended until the fetal lungs have a mature surfactant. It is therefore suggested that delaying labor for even a few days can be beneficial. Early diagnosis is the key to treating preterm labor because medical management and labor-suppressing drugs are most effective when administered prior to any dilatation and effacement. The nurse can have a great impact on lowering fetal and neonatal mortality by educating all patients at risk for preterm labor. The patient can be instructed in how to interpret early uterine activity and other subtle signs of preterm labor and to report the development of any of these signs immediately. Treatment is much more successful when initiated early.

REFERENCES

Anderson, K.E., and others: The relaxing effect of terbutaline on the human uterus during term labor, Am. J. Obstet. Gynecol. **121**:602, 1975.

Aumann, G.M., and Blake, G.D.: Ritodrine hydrochloride in the control of premature labor: implications for use, JOGN Nursing **11**(2):75, 1982.

Barden, T.P.: Sympathomimetic drugs to inhibit preterm labor, Contemp. Obstet. Gynecol. **7**:56, 1976.

Bejar, R., and others: Premature labor. II. Bacterial sources of phospholipase, Obstet. Gynecol. **57**:479, 1981.

Benedetti, T.J.: Maternal complications of parenteral β-sympathomimetic therapy for premature labor, Am. J. Obstet. Gynecol. **145**:1, 1983.

Bieniozz, J., and others: Inhibition of uterine contractility in labor, Am. J. Obstet. Gynecol. **111**:874, 1971.

Bills, B.: Nursing considerations administering labor-suppressing medications, MCN **5**(4):252, 1980.

Bratlid, D., and Lindback, T.: Bacteriolytic activity of amniotic fluid, Obstet. Gynecol. **51**:63, 1978.

Brengman, S.L., and Burns, M.: Ritodrine hydrochloride and preterm labor, AJN **83**:537, 1983.

Brown, E.R., and others: Reversible induction of surfactant production in fetal lambs treated with glucocorticoids, Pediatr. Res. **13**:491, 1979.

Caritis, S., Edelstone, D., and Mueller-Heuback, E.: Pharmacologic inhibition of preterm labor, Am. J. Obstet. Gynecol. **133**:557, 1979.

Carsten, M.E.: Regulation of myometrial composition, growth, and activity. In Assali, N.S., editor: Biology of gestation. Vol. I. The maternal organism, New York, 1968, Academic Press, Inc.

Challis, J.R., and Mitchell, B.F.: Hormonal control of preterm and term parturition, Sem. Perinatol. **5**(3):192, 1981.

Chard, T.: The role of the posterior pituitaries of mother and fetus in spontaneous parturition. In Comline, K.S., Cross, K.W., and Dawes, G.S., editors: Foetal and neonatal physiology, Cambridge, 1973, Cambridge University Press.

Chez, R.A., and Creasy, R.K.: How to detect premature labor early, Contemp. Obstet. Gynecol. **19**(5):203, 1982.

Christensen, K., and others: A study of complications in preterm deliveries after prolonged premature rupture of the membranes, Obstet. Gynecol. **48**:670, 1976.

Chung, H.: Arresting preterm labor, AJN **76**:810, 1976.

Creasy, R.K., Gummer, B.A., and Liggins, G.C.: System for predicting spontaneous preterm birth, Obstet. Gynecol. **55**:692, 1980.

Creasy, R.K., and others: Oral ritodrine maintenance in the treatment of preterm labor, Am. J. Obstet. Gynecol. **137**:212, 1980.

Creasy, R.K., and Herron M.A.: Prevention of preterm birth, Sem. Perinatol. **5**:295, 1981.

Elliott, J.P., and others: Pulmonary edema associated with magnesium sulfate and betamethasone administration, Am. J. Obstet. Gynecol. **134**:717, 1979.

Fedrick, J.: Antenatal identification of women at high risk of spontaneous pre-term birth, Br. J. Obstet. Gynaecol. **83**:351, 1976.

Forman, A., Andersson, K.E., and Ulmsten, U.: Inhibition of myometrial activity by calcium antagonists, Sem. Perinatol. **5**(3):288, 1981.

Freyse, H., and others: A long term evaluation of infants who received a beta-mimetic drug while in utero, J. Perinatal. Med. **5**:94, 1977.

Fuchs, A.R., and others: Plasma levels of oxytocin and 13, 14-dihydro-15-keto prostaglandin F_{2a} in preterm labor and the effect of ethanol and ritodrine, Am. J. Obstet. Gynecol. **144**:753, 1982.

Fuchs, F.: Treatment of threatened premature labour with alcohol, J. Obstet. Gynaecol. Br. Commonwealth **72**:1011, 1965.

Fuchs, F.: Prevention of prematurity, Am. J. Obstet. Gynecol. **126**:809, 1976.

Fuller, W.: Management of premature labor, Clin. Obstet. Gynecol. **21**:533, 1978.

Garite, T.: Prevention and control of premature labor. Paper presented at the Western Symposium of Maternal-Infant Health, Anaheim, Calif., March 7, 1981.

Gillibrand, P.N.: Premature rupture of the membranes and prematurity, J. Obstet. Gynaecol. Br. Commonwealth **74**:678, 1967.

Gluck, L.: Administration of corticosteroids to induce maturation of fetal lung, Am. J. Dis. Child. **130**:976, 1976.

Grospietsch, G., and others: The renin angiotensin aldosterone system, antidiuretic hormone levels and water balance under tocolytic therapy with fenoterol, Int. J. Gynaecol. Obstet. **17**:590, 1980.

Guilliams, S., and Held, B.: Contemporary management and conduct of preterm labor and delivery: a review, Obstet. Gynecol. Surv. **34**(3):248, 1979.

Gustavii, B.: Labour: a delayed menstruation? Lancet **2**:1149, 1972.

Haesslein, H.: Premature labor. In Niswander, K., editor: Manual of obstetrics, Boston, 1980, Little Brown & Co.

Hemminki, E., and Starfield, B.: Prevention and treatment of premature labor by drugs: review of controlled clinical trials, Br. J. Obstet. Gynaecol. **85**:411, 1978.

Herron, M.A., Katz, M., and Creasy, R.K.: Evaluation of a preterm birth prevention program: preliminary report, Obstet. Gynecol. **59**:452, 1982.

Huddleston, J.F.: Preterm labor, Clin. Obstet. Gynecol. **25**:123, 1982.

Huszar, G.: Biology and biochemistry of myometrial contractility and cervical maturation, Sem. Perinatol. **5**(3):216, 1981.

Ingemarsson, I.: Effect of terbutaline on premature labor: a double-blind placebo-controlled study, Am. J. Obstet. Gynecol. **125**:520, 1976.

Ingemarsson, I.: Use of β-receptor agonists in obstetrics, Obstet. Gynecol. Surv. **38**(4):193, 1983.

Isselbacher, K.J.: Metabolic and hepatic effects of alcohol, N. Engl. J. Med. **296**:612, 1977.

Jacobs, M., Knight, A., and Arias, F.: Maternal pulmonary edema: a composition of premature labor therapy with betamimetics and glucocorticoids, Obstet. Gynecol. **56**:56, 1980.

Johnson, J.: Betamethasone: do side effects outweigh benefits? Contemp. Obstet. Gynecol. **15**(5):195, 1980.

Johnson, J., and Dubin, N.: Prevention of preterm labor, Clin. Obstet. Gynecol. **23**:51, 1980.

Johnson, J., and others: Efficacy of 17a hydroxyprogesterone caproate in the prevention of premature labor, N. Engl. J. Med. **293**:675, 1975.

Jones, M.: Respiratory distress syndrome and the induction of fetal lung maturity by the use of glucocorticoids, JOGN Nursing **6**(4):21, 1977.

Kaufman, R., and others: Upper genital tract changes and pregnancy outcome in offspring exposed in utero to diethylstilbestrol, Am. J. Obstet. Gynecol. **137**:299, 1980.

Keirse, M.J.: Epideminology of preterm labor. In Keirse, M.J., and others, editors: Human parturition, London, 1979, Martinus Nijhoff Publishers.

Lauersen, N.H., and others: Inhibition of premature labor: a multicenter comparison of ritodrine and ethanol, Am. J. Obstet. Gynecol. **127**:837, 1977.

Levin, D.L.: Effects of inhibition of prostaglandin synthesis on fetal development, oxygenation, and the fetal circulation, Sem. Perinatol. **4**(1):35, 1980.

Liggins, G.C.: Fetal influences on myometrial contractility, Clin. Obstet. Gynecol. **16**:148, 1973.

Liggins, G.C.: Adrenocortical related maturational events in the fetus, Am. J. Obstet. Gynecol. **126**:931, 1976.

Liggins, G.C., and Howie, R.N.: The prevention of RDS by maternal steroid therapy. In Glick, I., editor: Modern perinatal medicine, Chicago, 1974, Year Book Medical Publishers, Inc.

Liggins, G.C., and Howie, R.N.: A controlled trial of antepartum glucocorticoid treatment on prevention of the respiratory distress syndrome in premature infants, Pediatrics **50**:515, 1972.

Lipshitz, J.: Beta-adrenergic agonists, Sem. Perinatol. **5**(3):252, 1981.

MacDonald, P.C., and others: Initiation of parturition in the human female, Sem. Perinatol. **2**:273, 1978.

MacDonald, P.C., and others: Initiation of human parturition. I. mechanisms of action of arachidonic acid, Obstet. Gynecol. **44**:629, 1974.

Merkatz, I.R., and Barden, T.P.: Ritodrine reaches US clinicians, Contemp. Obstet. Gynecol. **16**(11):185, 1980.

Niebyl, J., and Johnson, J.: Inhibition of preterm labor, Clin. Obstet. Gynecol. **23**:115, 1980.

Niebyl, J., and others: The pharmacologic inhibition of premature labor, Obstet. Gynecol. Surv. **33**:507, 1978.

Niebyl, J.R., and others: The inhibition of premature labor with indomethacin, Am. J. Obstet. Gynecol. **136**:1014, 1980.

Oxorn, H.: Human labor and birth, ed. 4, New York, 1980, Appleton Century Crofts, Inc.

Petrie, R.H.: Tocolysis using magnesium sulfate, Sem. Perinatol. **5**:266, 1981.

Quirk, J.A., and others: The role of glucocorticoids, unstressful labor, and a traumatic delivery in the prevention of respiratory distress syndrome, Am. J. Obstet. Gynecol. **134**:768, 1979.

Ricke, P.S., Elliott, J.P., and Freeman, K.: Use of corticosteroids in pregnancy-induced hypertension, Obstet. Gynecol. **55**:206, 1980.

Rosene, K.A., Featherstone, A.J., and Benedetti, T.J.: Cerebral ischemia associated with parenteral terbutaline use in pregnant migraine patients, Am. J. Obstet. Gynecol. **143**:405, 1982.

Rush, R.W., and others: Contribution of preterm delivery to perinatal mortality, Br. Med. J. **2**:965, 1976.

Schutte, M.F., and others: The influence of betamethasone and oriprenaline on the influence of respiratory distress syndrome in the newborn after preterm labor, Br. J. Obstet. Gynaecol. **87**:127, 1980.

Schwarz, B.E., and others: Progesterone binding protein in human chorion and amnion, Gynecol. Invest. **7**:46, 1976a.

Schwarz, B.E., and others: Initiation of human parturition. IV. Demonstration of phospholipase A_2 in lysosomes of human fetal membranes, Am. J. Obstet. Gynecol. **125**:1089, 1976b.

Schwarz, B.E., and others: Progesterone binding and metabolism in human fetal membranes, Ann. N.Y. Acad. Sci. **286**:304, 1977.

Seppala, M., and others: Radioimmunoassay of oxytocin in amniotic fluid, fetal urine and meconium during late pregnancy and delivery, Am. J. Obstet. Gynecol. **114**:788, 1972.

Shortridge, L.A.: Using ritodrine hydrochloride to inhibit preterm labor, MCN **8**(1):58, 1983.

Sica-Blanco, Y., Rozada, H., and Remedio, M.R.: Effect of meperidine on uterine contractility during pregnancy and prelabor, Am. J. Obstet. Gynecol. **97**:1096, 1967.

Steer, C., and Petrie, R.: A comparison of magnesium sulfate and alcohol for the prevention of premature labor, Am. J. Obstet. Gynecol. **129**:1, 1977.

Stone, S., and Pritchard, J.: Effect of maternally administered magnesium sulfate on the neonate, Obstet. Gynecol. **35**:574, 1970.

Sweet, R.: Bacteriuria and pyelonephritis during pregnancy, Sem. Perinatol. **1**:25, 1977.

Taeusch, H.W., and others: Risks of respiratory distress syndrome after prenatal dexamethosome treatment, Pediatrics **63**:64, 1979.

Thornfeldt, R., and others: The effect of glucocorticoids on the maturation of premature lung membranes, Am. J. Obstet. Gynecol. **131**:143, 1978.

Tye, K., Desser, K., and Benchimol, A.: Angina pectoris associated with terbutaline for premature labor, JAMA **244**:692, 1980.

Ulmsten, U., Andersson, K.E., and Wingerup, L.: Treatment of premature labor with the calcium antagonist nifedipine, Arch. Gynecol. **229**:1, 1980.

Unbebann, V.: Effects of sympathomimetic tocolytic agents on the fetus, J. Perinatal Med. **2**:17, 1974.

Wallace, R., and others: Inhibition of premature labor by terbutaline, Obstet. Gynecol. **51**:387, 1978.

Zuckerman, H., Reiss, U., and Rubinstein, I.: Inhibition of human premature labor by indomethacin, Obstet. Gynecol. **44**:787, 1974.

CHAPTER 15

Premature rupture of membranes

Premature rupture of membranes (PROM) is defined as rupture of the amniotic sac surrounding the fetus prior to the onset of labor.

INCIDENCE

PROM occurs in 10% to 12% of all pregnancies, and approximately 20% of these cases occur before 36 weeks of gestation. Approximately 20% of all preterm deliveries are associated with PROM (Naeye, 1977).

ETIOLOGY

The cause of PROM is essentially unknown in most cases. Incompetent cervix, multiple gestation, multiple amniocentesis, and polyhydramnios are infrequent causes of PROM. It was once felt that an inherently weak fetal membrane might be a cause of PROM. However, when fetal membranes were tested following premature rupture by Polishuk, Kohane, and Hadar (1964), they were found to be just as strong as membranes from normal term deliveries. Current information reveals that an intrauterine infection can often precede and may possibly be the cause of PROM in a significant number of the cases (Cederqvist et al., 1979). According to Garite (1981), a local vaginitis or endocervicitis may be the cause of a large percentage of PROM. The presence of the bacteria may cause rupture by locally dissolving the membranes, or transversing the membrane, causing a chorioamnionitis that then dissolves the membrane.

The risk of PROM is increased in lower socioeconomic groups, sexually promiscuous teenagers, patients who smoke, and in any patient with decreased immunity.

PHYSIOLOGY
Normal

The developing fetus is protected from the outside world by two fetal membranes, the amnion and the chorion, which form a sac around the fetus. These membranes are thin but tough. They contain no blood vessels or nerve endings. Amniotic fluid is produced within the amniotic sac allowing the developing fetus to float freely. The fluid is slightly alkaline, with a pH of 7.0 to 7.5. In early pregnancy, the primary source of the fluid appears to be the amnion. As pregnancy advances, fetal urine makes an increasingly important contribution. This fluid is constantly being formed and reabsorbed with replacement about every 3 hours. At 12 weeks, the average volume is 50 ml; at 20 weeks the average volume is 400 ml. The maximum volume of 1,000 ml is reached between 36 and 38 weeks.

Amniotic fluid serves many functions. It provides a medium in which the fetus can move, grow, and develop symmetrically without pressure on its delicate tissue. Blood flow is also unrestricted as it is transported through the umbilical cord. The fluid also helps to maintain an even environmental temperature for the fetus.

Normal amniotic fluid contains an antibacterial substance, which gradually increases with gestational age until term and then decreases (Schlievert et al., 1975). The level of this antibacterial substance varies with individuals. According to Appelbaum and associates (1980), a diet deficient in protein and zinc may decrease the antibacterial substance in amniotic fluid.

Pathophysiology

According to Blanco and associates (1982), there are two possible mechanisms that cause an intraamniotic infection, called *chorioamnionitis*. Some patients have normal inhibitory activity of the amniotic fluid, but, when large volumes of bacteria enter the amniotic cavity, they are unable to overpower the inhibitors. In other patients, there may be a lack of inhibitory activity in the amniotic fluid. These patients are susceptible to chorioamnionitis if any bacteria enter the amniotic fluid.

The most common route of bacterial entry into the amniotic cavity is by way of the vagina. The normal vaginal bacterial flora varies with individuals and at different stages during pregnancy. There is a decreased amount of gram-negative anaerobic bacteria as gestational age nears 40 weeks (Ledger, 1977). According to Braun and associates (1971) and Walsh, Hildebrandt, and Prystowsky (1966), there is an increase in vaginal bacterial flora in women of a lower socioeconomic status, with increased sexual contacts, poor hygiene, and an inadequate nutritional state. There are several physiologic factors that provide a barrier to organisms reaching the uterine cavity from the vagina during pregnancy: (1) the cervical mucous plug and (2) intact chorionic and amnionic fetal membranes.

If the membranes rupture, one of the barriers is broken. At times, chorioamnionitis causes the membranes to rupture. However, if chorioamnionitis is not the cause of the rupture, the patient's risk of developing it appears to be related to (1) the location of the tear in the fetal membrane, (2) the patient's amniotic fluid immunity, *(3)* the amount of cervical dilatation, *(4)* the nutritional and hygenic state of the patient, and *(5)* the gestational age of the fetus.

If any of the following apply the patient will be less likely to develop chorioamnionitis.

1. The tear is above the cervical os
2. The cervix is closed
3. The patient has a high amniotic fluid immunity
4. No pelvic examinations or intercourse have taken place since the rupture
5. The gestational age is earlier than 28 weeks

If chorioamnionitis does not occur, fibrin may be laid down to form a clot that can close the tear. Since amniotic fluid is continuously being produced, the normal volume will return within 2 days.

When fetal membranes rupture there is also a potential risk of preterm labor. According to Garite (1981), 50% of all patients with a gestational age of less than 36 weeks at the time of the rupture of membranes will go into labor within 48 hours and over 85% will deliver within 1 week.

Signs and symptoms

A rupture can be signaled by a sudden gush of clear fluid from the vagina. However, more often it is a small leakage of clear fluid, which may be confused with urinary incontinence.

Maternal effects

If chorioamnionitis develops as a result of rupture of membranes, it can very quickly cause a serious maternal septicemia. This can lead to septic shock and death if not treated promptly. The risk of chorioamnionitis following PROM after 36 weeks of gestation appears to be related to the duration of membrane rupture. However, prior to 36 weeks of gestation, maternal infection following PROM is not related to the duration of membrane rupture (Johnson and Barnes, 1970; Johnson et al., 1981).

Fetal and neonatal effects

According to Naeye (1977), 10% of all perinatal deaths are associated with PROM. Prior to 36 weeks of gestation, respiratory distress syndrome is the main cause of morbidity and mortality of the neonate (Schreiber and Benedetti, 1980). The reason is that PROM usually triggers preterm labor and the fetus is born prematurely. Infection appears to play a very minor role in morbidity and mortality, and it does not correlate directly with the length of time the membranes are ruptured. However, if chorioamnionitis develops, the risk of infection increases fourfold (Garite, 1981). After 36 weeks of gestation, infection is the major risk factor to the fetus and there is a direct positive correlation between risk and the length of time the membranes are ruptured (Mead, 1980; Berkowitz, 1982).

PROM can also cause fetal distress. This is the result of *(1)* prolapsed cord, *(2)* decreased amniotic fluid, or *(3)* chorioamnionitis. The cord can prolapse if the presenting part is not well engaged. If the amniotic fluid volume is affected to a large degree, pressure can be applied on the cord as the fetus moves about, thereby causing fetal distress. If fetal distress is allowed to persist for any length of time, fetal hypoxia will result causing the anal sphincter to relax and release meconium into the amniotic fluid. Deep, gasping respiratory movements are triggered, which moves the meconium-stained amniotic fluid deep into the alveoli. Then the neonate is at risk of developing aspiration pneumonia.

MEDICAL DIAGNOSIS

When PROM is suspected, a sterile speculum examination is done. If amniotic fluid is observed leaking from the cervix and collecting in the posterior fornix of the vagina, an accurate diagnosis of PROM can be made. A digital vaginal examination should *never* be done if any attempt is to be made in delaying the labor for more than 12 hours. This is because vaginal bacteria could be transported into the cervical canal, thereby increasing the risk of chorioamnionitis.

If there is no visual sign of loss of amniotic fluid from the cervix, then the secretions of the posterior fornix of the vagina should be tested with nitrazine paper to determine the pH. Because amniotic fluid is alkaline and vaginal secretions are acidic, the nitrazine paper will turn blue in the presence of amniotic fluid. Blood, cervical mucus, and Betadine should not be allowed to contaminate the specimen; they are alkaline also. A small amount of the fluid should then be spread on a slide and allowed to dry. Microscopic examination of dried amniotic fluid shows a fernlike pattern because of the fluid's concentration of salt.

USUAL MEDICAL MANAGEMENT

The treatment of PROM is one of the most controversial subjects in obstetrics today because of conflicting scientific research. Therefore only general principles will be presented.

Most patients whose membranes rupture after 34 to 36 weeks of gestation are delivered within 12 to 24 hours by induction if spontaneous labor does not ensue because of the increased risk of chorioamnionitis. Some obstetricians, however, recommend a conservative approach of waiting for spontaneous labor while observing for signs of an infection in the presence of an uninducible cervix, providing no signs of chorioamnionitis are present. Kappy and associates (1982) have found this approach to decrease the occurrence of cesarean deliveries without increasing the risk of infection. Before 28 weeks of gestation, expectant management without amniocentesis is usually the choice of treatment if no signs of infection are present. The risk of prematurity in the neonate far outweighs the risk of chorioamnionitis. When the gestational age is over 28 weeks and under 34 to 36 weeks, care must be individualized, weighing the risk of interference against the risk of an infection. To determine whether expectant management or delivery should be the choice of treatment, an assessment must be made for *(1)* fetal maturity, *(2)* fetal distress, and *(3)* chorioamnionitis.

Gestational age is usually verified with ultrasound. If the biparietal diameter (BPD) cannot accurately be determined because the head is low in the pelvis, then femur length or abdominal circumference is used. Fetal lung maturity can be determined in one of two ways. First, amniotic fluid from the vaginal pool can be tested for phosphatidylglycerol (PG), and, if present, fetal lung maturity is indicated (Brame and MacKenna, 1983). Second, fetal lung maturity can be determined by collecting amniotic fluid by way of an amniocentesis and evaluating it for L/S ratio. An L/S ratio of from 1.8:1 to 2:1 indicates fetal lung maturity. It may be difficult at times for the physician to obtain amniotic fluid by an amniocentesis if the leak is large. If there is only a small amount of amniotic fluid, the procedure can be facilitated by encouraging the patient to drink fluids and placing the patient in a Trendelenburg position for 1 hour prior to the procedure. Then, with the aid of ultrasound, a pocket of amniotic fluid can often be found. The L/S ratio may be elevated if the amniotic fluid is contaminated by blood. Because amniotic fluid in the vagina is frequently contaminated with blood from the mucous plug, the L/S ratio is rarely done on vaginal pool amniotic fluid. Should blood contaminate the specimen during amniocentesis, fetal lung maturity should be determined by the presence of phosphatidylglycerol (PG); it is not affected by blood.

At the same time, the patient should be evaluated for chorioamnionitis. The only effective way of determining chorioamnionitis early is by taking a culture of the amniotic fluid by way of an amniocentesis since chorioamnionitis is usually asymptomatic in its early state. When the amniotic fluid is positive, chorioamnionitis will most likely develop (Garite et al., 1979). This fluid can also be tested for antibacterial properties, and, if present, the risk of an infection is less.

If chorioamnionitis is supected, fetal maturity is indicated by the presence of PG or an L/S ratio of 2:1, or fetal distress is assessed, then delivery is the choice of treatment. An induction is usually attempted unless obstetrical complications are present such as malpresentation, uterine dysfunction, or an unripe cervix in the presence of chorioamnionitis. In these cases a cesarean delivery is performed. If fetal distress is present, immediate delivery is imperative. Fetal hypoxia or a traumatic delivery will only increase the risk of perinatal mortality and morbidity associated with prematurity.

If there are any indications that an intrauterine infection is present, antibiotics may or may not be used until delivery. Many obstetricians have found them ineffective until the uterus is emptied. A few obstetricians will use antibiotics prophylactically. However, prophylactic antibiotics are not recommended in most cases because fetal infections are not reduced by maternal antibiotics, the early clinical signs of chorioamnionitis can be masked by their use, and this can foster the growth of resistant organisms that would be difficult to treat in the newborn. Following delivery, antibiotics such as ampicillin or penicillin are usually started.

If chorioamnionitis does not occur, fibrin can be laid down to form a clot that may close the tear. This process is more often effective when the patient is on bed rest because of the decreased trauma to the clot. Therefore if the fetus is not mature, there are no signs of infection, and no fetal distress is indicated, many physicians use expectant management consisting of bed rest and observation for signs of infection or fetal distress. This is done in the hopes that, by lengthening the pregnancy, fetal lungs may mature and decrease the risk of respiratory distress in the neonate. It is postulated by some that PROM also accelerates fetal lung maturity by stimulating the production of glucocorticoids by the fetal adrenals and that this stimulates an increased production of lecithin by the fetal lungs. However, whether or not rupture of membranes accelerates fetal lung maturity is undergoing much debate. Mead's (1980) literature review from 1972 through 1979 reveals an approximately equal amount of evidence supporting both sides.

Some are using glucocorticoids in an endeavor to enhance fetal lung maturity. If preterm labor ensues, they may use a tocolytic agent to attempt delay of labor until 48 hours of glucocorticoid therapy has been completed. Whether or not steroid therapy should be used in the presence of PROM is another controversial issue. The study of Mead and Clapp (1977) suggests that steroid therapy is beneficial in stimulating fetal lung maturity after PROM. When Taeusch and associates (1979) did a specific, randomized study on the use of glucocorticoids in PROM patients, they found no decreased incidence of respiratory distress in the neonates when steroids were used. However they found an increased incidence of maternal infection during the postpartum period. Garite (1981) conducted a similar study and obtained similar results. He was specific in identifying the maternal infection to be postpartum endometritis.

Because of these existing controversies and the increased risk of chorioamnionitis, there are other physicians who deliver every fetus after PROM. No matter which plan is decided on, 95% of patients will deliver within 2 weeks.

NURSING PROCESS
Prevention

Because the actual cause of PROM is unknown, prevention is difficult. However, it may be helpful to look at the risk factors and guard against these during pregnancy. Statistics indicate that lower socioeconomic group patients and teenagers have an increased risk of PROM. The reason for this is unknown, but nutrition probably plays an important role. Therefore these patients should be instructed early in pregnancy regarding a healthful diet for pregnancy and should be provided with reasons to follow this diet. They may also need referral to financial assistance programs and instruction in how to prepare these foods.

Cleanliness can also be a factor in decreasing the risk of PROM; the vaginal bacterial flora should be kept to a minimum. Daily bathing and wiping the perineum from front to back are important prenatal instructions. Multiple sexual relationships also increase the vaginal bacterial count and should be avoided.

Any attempt to facilitate as much immunity against infection as possible is beneficial. Therefore drinking six to eight glasses of fluid per day, daily exercise with adequate rest to avoid fatigue, an adequate diet high in protein and zinc, and cleanliness are all beneficial in guarding against PROM.

Underwood and associates (1967) demonstrated in their study a relationship between smoking and PROM. Therefore prenatal patients who smoke should be instructed regarding its effect on pregnancy and should be supported in their attempt to stop smoking.

All pregnant women should be instructed regarding the danger signs in pregnancy, and PROM should be pointed out as one of these signs. The signs of membrane rupture and the necessity of prompt notification if these signs occur should be explained early in prenatal care.

Assessment

When a patient comes in leaking amniotic fluid, the nurse should assess closely for fetal distress, signs of chorioamnionitis, and signs of labor. Fetal distress is usually the result of a prolapsed cord or decreased amniotic fluid with subsequent cord compression. This can be determined by placing the patient on a fetal monitor for at least the first 12 to 24 hours after PROM. The presence of either of these two problems would be seen on the fetal monitor strip as variable decelerations. The amount and color of amniotic fluid should also be assessed. Normal amniotic fluid is straw colored. Greenish brown amniotic fluid usually indicates fetal hypoxia with meconium passage. However, this may be normal in a breech presentation. At the same time, the patient's uterine activity should be monitored to detect signs of preterm labor. The patient should also be instructed to notify the nurse if she experiences any cramplike pain.

The classic symptoms of chorioamnionitis are fetal tachycardia or a maternal temperature of 38° C (100.4° F) or greater if no other cause can be determined for the fever. Other signs that can indicate chorioamnionitis are maternal tachycardia, leukocytosis, uterine tenderness, or foul, purulent amniotic fluid. However, these are late signs and are not manifested in the early stages of the infection. Patients in labor can also have an elevated white blood cell count without any infection. Nevertheless the patient's temperature, pulse, and respirations should be taken and fetal heart tones recorded every 4 hours. Blood for a WBC and differential should be drawn daily. The vaginal discharge should be observed for color and odor. To help determine the patient's potential risk of chorioamnionitis, the following data should be determined.

1. Exposure to disease during pregnancy
2. Nutritional habits
3. Activities since rupture of membranes

To help verify the EDC, the nurse should ask the patient whether her menstrual periods were regularly spaced and the length of her ovulatory cycles. If they were regularly spaced, 28 day cycles, the EDC is usually quite accurate. However, if her cycles were longer or shorter than 28 days, the EDC can be off several weeks.

Patients will have varied ideas as to what might have caused PROM and what this means to the outcome of their pregnancy and their unborn child. The nurse should identify these anxieties so that appropriate education can be given.

Antepartum intervention

Any patient leaking amniotic fluid is going to be very anxious. The earlier the gestation, the more fearful the parents will be of what will happen to their infant. The parents may feel that they did something to cause the rupture, especially if a fall, hard knock, or intercourse occurred just prior to the event. Even though the reason for the rupture is usually unknown, the nurse must reassure the parents that these events did not cause the membrane to rupture. The fetal membranes can withstand pressures that far exceed those of normal uterine contractions (MacLachlan, 1965). When fetal membranes were tested by Polishuk, Kohane, and Hadar (1964), following premature rupture, they were found to be just as strong as membranes from normal, term deliveries. Even though a cause of PROM cannot normally be given, the patient should be kept informed about each step of treatment and the possible outcome in an attempt to allay anxiety.

The patient should be placed on complete bed rest to facilitate clot formation over the tear and to decrease the risk of infection. An explanation to the patient as to the reason for this treatment would be beneficial. After 12 to 24 hours, some obstetricians will allow their patients bathroom privileges. They feel that the increased flow of amniotic fluid might wash the vaginal bacteria away from the cervix (Schwarz, 1980). Pericare should be given each shift and the bed linen changed each day and as needed. The patient should be instructed regarding proper perineal hygiene so organisms will not be transferred from the rectal area to the vagina. No vaginal examinations should be done until labor is in full progress and delivery is imminent within 12 hours because of the risk of introducing bacteria from the vagina into the cervix. Constipation should be prevented to avoid straining with stools. This can be accomplished by having the patient drink six to eight glasses of fluid each day and eat high-roughage and high-fiber foods such as whole grains, fruits, and vegetables. No enemas should be given because they can stimulate labor. The patient should also be instructed to report any uterine contractions, cramps, or tenderness.

Most patients are observed in the hospital for as long as they continue to leak fluid. If the leakage of fluid stops and all other parameters are stable, the patient may be discharged home. If discharged, the patient should be given the following instructions.

1. No intercourse or douching
2. Take temperature at least twice per day
3. Call physician if temperature is over 38° C (100.4° F), vaginal discharge becomes foul-smelling, or there is an increase in amniotic fluid loss
4. Showers only, no tub baths
5. If labor starts, come to the hospital
6. Return to the clinical laboratory for a WBC twice each week
7. Return for weekly nonstress tests and doctor's visit
8. Monitor fetal activity to indicate fetal well-being

The mother can monitor fetal well-being by noting fetal activity. If fetal activity seems decreased, the mother should be instructed to lie down for 1 hour. If fetal movement is not felt during this time, or is felt less than four times, this is an indication of some fetal problem. If fetal movement is felt four or more times within the hour, it is a good indication of no fetal distress (Rayburn, 1983).

Intrapartum intervention

Whether labor begins spontaneously or is medically induced, the nurse should monitor the patient as any other labor patient. If the fetus is less than 37 weeks of gestation, maternal hypotension, fetal hypoxia, and infection increase the neonatal risk of respiratory distress. Therefore these patients should be assessed more closely than the normal labor patient.

1. For an elevated temperature
2. For hypotension
3. For signs of fetal distress

This can be accomplished by checking the blood pressure and pulse every 15 to 30 minutes depending on the phase of labor, checking the temperature every hour, and monitoring the fetal heart rate with an external or internal monitor continuously. Any deviation from the patient's baseline should be brought to the physician's attention immediately. The patient should be encouraged to lie in a lateral recumbent position, not on her back, to decrease the risk of hypotension.

These patients will need added emotional support. They may not have had

S U G G E S T E D   P L A N

Premature rupture of membranes

Potential patient problem	*Outcome criteria*
A. Potential chorioamnionitis related to: PROM	Temperature below 38° C (100.4° F) FHR between 120 and 160 No foul vaginal discharge White blood count below 16,000 mm³ Negative amniotic fluid cultures

the opportunity to finish their prepared childbirth class, and they will be very concerned about the outcome for their neonate. They may also be concerned about a "dry labor" and should be reassured that there is no such thing; amniotic fluid is constantly being produced.

Postpartum intervention

The postpartum patient who had PROM is at a greater risk for developing an endometrial infection. If she was treated with glucocorticoids to stimulate

O F   N U R S I N G   C A R E

Assessment and intervention

Dx. Check TPR every 4 hr
Monitor fetal heart rate every 4 hr
Check vaginal discharge for foul odor or color change
Refer to such laboratory studies as WBCs and differential
Determine exposure to disease during pregnancy
Determine nutritional habits
Determine activities since PROM

Th. Bed rest unless otherwise ordered
Give pericare every shift
No vaginal exams
Change bed linen every day and as needed
Assist with diagnostic procedures such as amniotic fluid cultures

Ed. Teach proper pericare
Explain benefit of bed rest
No vaginal exams until labor is in full progress
If discharged home, instruct regarding
  no intercourse or douching
  take temperature twice per day
  notify physician if temperature is greater than 38° C (100° F) or if amnionic fluid loss increases or becomes foul-smelling
  shower only
  return to the clinical laboratory for a WBC twice weekly

Ref. Notify physician if
  temperature is greater than 38° C
  fetal or maternal tachycardia develops
  foul-smelling amnionic fluid develops
  amniotic fluid changes from straw colored

Dx., diagnostic; Th., therapeutic; Ed., education; Ref., referral.   *Continued.*

Premature rupture of membranes—cont'd

Potential patient problem	*Outcome criteria*

B. Potential fetal distress related to:
    Prolapsed cord
    Decreased amniotic fluid
	FHR between 120 and 160
	Beat to beat variability present
	No variable decelerations
	At least four fetal movements per hr

C. Potential preterm labor related to: PROM	Continuation of pregnancy to at least 37 weeks of gestation or until fetal lungs are mature as indicated by an L/S ratio of 2:1 or PG present in the amniotic fluid

D. Potential anxiety related to:
    Cause of rupture
    Risk of preterm delivery
    Risk of immature neonate
    Risk of maternal fetal infection
	Parent(s) express fears and anxieties
	Parent(s) participate in decisions regarding care

Assessment and intervention

Dx. Monitor FHR
Monitor mother's blood pressure
Monitor beat to beat variability
Monitor fetal activity
Observe amount of amniotic fluid that is being lost
Th. Reposition mother and administer oxygen by mask if variable decelerations
occur
Ed. Instruct to report any decrease in fetal activity
If discharged home, instruct regarding
return for weekly nonstress tests and physician's visit
monitor fetal activity
Ref. Notify physician if signs of fetal distress occur such as variable or late decel-
erations, fetal bradycardia, or tachycardia
Notify physician if hypotension develops

Dx. Monitor uterine activity
Determine EDC
Th. Encourage complete bed rest
Encourage patient to drink six to eight glasses of fluid every day and eat a
high-roughage and high-fiber diet to prevent constipation
No enemas (may stimulate labor)
Ed. Instruct to report any cramplike pain or uterine tenderness
Instruct regarding the therapeutic reasons for fluid and dietary needs
Instruct not to strain with bowel movements
If discharged home instruct regarding
if labor starts return to hospital
notify physician if uterine cramping occurs

Dx. Identify concerns and fears
Th. Allow patient to express concerns and fears
Allay false ideas of what might have caused PROM
Keep patient informed of treatment and possible outcome
Ed. Explain that the cause is usually unknown

fetal lung maturity, research indicates an even higher risk of endometrial infection. Therefore these patients should be assessed very closely for an infection by checking their temperature and assessing the odor of the lochia every 4 hours for the first 2 postpartum days.

If an endometrial infection develops, treatment with antibiotics is often effective. Ampicillin or cephalosporin are usually the drugs of choice. There is no need to isolate these patients if the infected organism is one normally present in the vaginal flora. The patient should be taught good hand washing prior to handling her infant and should be instructed to keep the infant on the top of the covers of her bed rather than on the bottom sheet, which can be contaminated with the organisms.

The patient who had premature rupture of membranes and was delivered by a cesarean because of signs of chorioamnionitis has an increased risk of septic pelvic thrombophlebitis. Therefore these patients should be observed closely for signs of thrombophlebitis.

Psychologic needs are great during this time, especially if the neonate was premature. The parents should be encouraged to visit the neonatal nursery often to spend time with their baby. The nurse should point out reassuring characteristics and encourage the parents to participate in the care of their infant as much as possible. The mother will also need time to think about her feelings regarding the birth experience. She may feel cheated, especially if the parents had planned a birthing room delivery with mother and infant recovery.

Evaluation

Because infections and lower amniotic fluid immunity play a significant role in PROM, the ultimate goal of the nurse should be education. Prenatal education should cover the need for adequate fluids and nutrition, appropriate hygiene, and the significance of reporting any signs of an infection immediately. This would decrease the risk of PROM. Once the membranes rupture, the goal of treatment is to maintain the pregnancy to allow for fetal maturity as long as the uterine environment is healthy. If the uterine environment becomes infected or causes fetal distress, the fetal outcome may be improved by premature delivery.

REFERENCES

Appelbaum, P.C., and others: The effect of amniotic fluid on bacterial growth in three population groups, Am. J. Obstet. Gynecol. **128:**868, 1977.

Appelbaum, P.C., and others: Studies on the growth-inhibiting property of amniotic fluids from two United States population groups, Am. J. Obstet. Gynecol. **137:**579, 1980.

Bada, H.S., Alojipan, L.C., and Andrews, B.F.: Premature rupture of membranes and its effect on the newborn, Ped. Clin. North Am. **24:**491, 1977.

Barrett, J.M., and Boehm, F.H.: Comparison of aggressive and conservative management of premature rupture of fetal membranes, Am. J. Obstet. Gynecol. **144:**12, 1982.

Bergman, N., Bercovici, B., and Sacks, T.: Antibacterial activity of human amniotic fluid, Am. J. Obstet. Gynecol. **114:**520, 1972.

Berkowitz, R.L.: Management of premature rupture of the membranes. In Queenan, J.T., and Hobbins, J.C., editors: Protocols for high-risk pregnancies, Oradell, N. J., 1982, Medical Economics Books, Inc.

Blanco, J.D., and others: The association between the absence of amniotic fluid bacterial inhibitory activity and intraamniotic infection, Am. J. Obstet. Gynecol. **143:**749, 1982.

Brame, R.G., and MacKenna, J.: Vaginal pool phospholipids in the management of premature rupture of membranes, Am. J. Obstet. Gynecol. **145:**992, 1983.

Bratlid, D., and Lindback, T.: Bacteriolytic activity of amniotic fluid, Obstet. Gynecol. **51:**63, 1978.

Braun, P., and others: Birth weight and genital mycoplasmas in pregnancy, N. Engl. J. Med. **284:**167, 1971.

Breese, M.W.: Spontaneous premature rupture of the membranes, Am. J. Obstet. Gynecol. **81:**1086, 1961.

Cederqvist, L., and others: The relationship between prematurely ruptured membranes and fetal immunoglobulin production, Am. J. Obstet. Gynecol. **134:**784, 1979.

Cherry, S.H., Filler, M., and Harvey, H.: Lysozyme content of amniotic fluid, Am. J. Obstet. Gynecol. **116:**639, 1973.

Christensen, K., and others: A study of complications in preterm deliveries after prolonged premature rupture of the membranes, Obstet. Gynecol. **48:**670, 1976.

Garite, T.: Premature rupture of membranes: current management methods. Paper presented at the Western Symposium of Maternal-Infant Health, Anaheim, Calif., March 7, 1981.

Garite, T.: What's the best care in preterm PROM? Contemp. Obstet. Gynecol. **19:**178, 1982.

Garite, T., and others: The use of amniocentesis in patients with premature rupture of membranes, Obstet. Gynecol. **54:**226, 1979.

Gibbs, R.S.: How to manage acute chorioamnionitis, Contemp. Obstet. Gynecol. **14:**69, 1979.

Gibbs, R.S., and Blanco, J.D.: Premature rupture of the membranes, Obstet. Gynecol. **60:**671, 1982.

Gunn, G., Mishell, D., and Morton, D.: Premature rupture of the fetal membranes, Am. J. Obstet. Gynecol. **106:**469, 1970.

Johnson, J.W.C., and Barnes, N.C.: Premature rupture of the membranes: 14 years experience, Int. J. Obstet. Gynecol. **8:**251, 1970.

Johnson, J.W.C., and others: Premature rupture of the membranes and prolonged latency, Obstet. Gynecol. **57:**547, 1981.

Kappy, L., and others: Premature rupture of the membranes: a conservative approach, Am. J. Obstet. Gynecol. **134:**655, 1979.

Kappy, K., and others: Premature rupture of the membranes at term: a comparison of induced and spontaneous labors, J. Reprod. Med. **27:**171, 1982.

Koh, K.S., Chang, F.H., and Ledger, W.J.: When chorioamnionitis threatens mother and offspring, Contemp. Obstet. Gynecol. **13**(6):147, 1979.

Larsen, B., Snyder, I.S., and Galask, R.P.: Bacterial growth inhibition by amniotic fluid. I. In vitro evidence for bacterial growth inhibiting activity, Am. J. Obstet. Gynecol. **119:**492, 1974.

Larsen, J.: Can amniotic fluid analyses predict infection? Contemp. Obstet. Gynecol. **14**(9):53, 1979.

Ledger. W.: Premature rupture of membranes and the influence of invasive monitoring techniques upon fetal and newborn infection, Sem. Perinatol. **1**(1):79, 1977.

MacLachlan, T.: A method for investigation of the strength of the fetal membranes, Am. J. Obstet. Gynecol. **91:**309, 1965.

Martin, J.E.: Management of premature rupture of the membranes, Clin. Obstet. Gynecol. **16**(4):213, 1973.

Mead, P.: Management of the patient with premature rupture of the membranes, Clin. Perinatol. **7:**243, 1980.

Mead, P.B., and Clapp, J.E.: The use of betamethasone and timed delivery in management of premature rupture of the membranes in the preterm pregnancy, J. Reprod. Med. **19:**3, 1977.

Naeye, R.: Causes of perinatal mortality in the U.S. collaborative perinatal project, JAMA **238:**228, 1977.

Polishuk, W., Kohane, S., and Hadar, A.: Fetal weight and membrane tensile strength, Am. J. Obstet. Gynecol. **88:**247, 1964.

Rayburn, W.: Fetal activity patterns in hypertensive pregnancies, Obstet. Gynecol. Surv. **38**(3):142, 1983.

Schlievert, P., Johnson, W., and Galask, R.: Bacterial growth inhibition by amniotic fluid, Am. J. Obstet. Gynecol. **127:**607, 1977.

Schlievert, P., and others: Bacterial growth inhibition by amniotic fluid. III. Demonstration of the variability of bacterial growth inhibition by amniotic fluid with a new plate count technique, Am. J. Obstet. Gynecol. **122:**809, 1975.

Schreiber, J., and Benedetti, T.: Conservative management of preterm premature rupture of the fetal membranes in a low socioeconomic population, Am. J. Obstet. Gynecol. **136:**92, 1980 .

Schwartz, R.: Premature rupture of the membranes: a symposium. In Queenan, J.T., editor: Management of high-risk pregnancy, Oradell, N.J., 1980, Medical Economics Books, Inc.

Shubeck, F., and others: Fetal hazard after rupture of the membranes, Obstet. Gynecol. **24:**22, 1966.

Spence, M.: Infection and prematurity: is there an interrelationship? Contemp. Obstet. Gynecol. **14:**87, 1979.

Taeusch, H.W., and others: Risk of respiratory distress syndrome after prenatal dexamethasome treatment, Pediatrics **63:**64, 1979.

Underwood, P., and others: Parental smoking empirically related to pregnancy outcome, Obstet. Gynecol. **29:**1, 1967.

Walsh, J., Hildebrandt, R.J., and Prystowsky, H.: Further observations on the microbiologic flora of the cervix and vagina during pregnancy, Am. J. Obstet. Gynecol. **96:**1129, 1966.

Wilson, J.C., Levy, D.L., and Wilds, P.L.: Premature rupture of membranes prior to term: consequences of nonintervention, Obstet. Gynecol. **60:**601, 1982.

CHAPTER 16

Hemolytic incompatibility

Hemolytic incompatibility occurs when a pregnant woman is sensitized to produce immunoglobulin G (IgG) antibodies against fetal red blood cells usually from the Rh or ABO blood systems. The antibodies, returning to the fetal circulation, can cause erythrocyte destruction in the fetus and subsequent fetal anemia with liver failure and congestive heart failure (hydrops).

INCIDENCE

Despite routine use of postpartum Rh immunoglobulin, 1% to 2% of all Rh-negative women who are pregnant continue to become sensitized. Although Rh incompatibility is the most common and usually the most serious, other hemolytic incompatibilities do occur. Hemolytic disease is seen in 10% of the ABO blood group incompatibilities. ABO and Rh incompatibilities account for 98% of all hemolytic disease in the fetus. Of the remaining 2%, rare antibodies such as Kell or Duffy antibodies are implicated. The pathophysiologic processes for all incompatibilities are similar.

ETIOLOGY

ABO incompatibility occurs when the mother's blood type is O and the fetal blood type is A, B, or AB. Rh incompatibility occurs when the mother is Rh-negative and the fetus is Rh-positive.

PHYSIOLOGY

Normal

The fetus receives his blood type as a result of his father's and mother's blood factors. Most blood factor systems carry antigenic properties to other factors within the system. This evokes antibody formation. The ABO system has the following antigens.

A has antigen A.

B has antigen B.

AB has both antigens A and B.

O has none.

The Rh system has two factors.

Rh positive has Rh antigen.

Rh negative has no Rh antigen.

Compared to the Rh system, the ABO system is weakly antigenic to its own factors. Other factors in the red blood cells occur so rarely that it is unlikely to have father-mother combinations resulting in incompatibilities.

Each father and mother, having received their blood type half from each parent, can be said to be homozygous or heterozygous. Thus, in the ABO system, combinations occur. All persons with type O blood are homozygous. When the mother is type O, she is homozygous, having received an O from both parents. If the father is type O also, there are no antigenic possibilities for the fetal ABO system; the fetus must be type O. If father is type A, he could be AO heterozygous or AA homozygous. If the father is type B he could be BB homozygous or BO heterozygous. If father is type AB he is heterozygous. To understand the possible fetal blood types from heterozygous fathers with types A, B, or AB and homozygous O mothers or from homozygous types A or B fathers and homozygous O mothers, the following examples may be helpful.

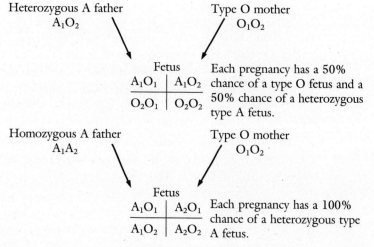

Heterozygous A father A_1O_2 — Type O mother O_1O_2

Fetus

A_1O_1	A_1O_2
O_2O_1	O_2O_2

Each pregnancy has a 50% chance of a type O fetus and a 50% chance of a heterozygous type A fetus.

Homozygous A father A_1A_2 — Type O mother O_1O_2

Fetus

A_1O_1	A_2O_1
A_1O_2	A_2O_2

Each pregnancy has a 100% chance of a heterozygous type A fetus.

The heterozygous type A fetus carried by a type O mother has an antigen A which can evoke antibody formation in the type O mother. Type B works the same way.

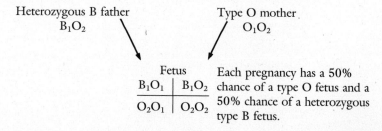

Heterozygous B father B_1O_2 — Type O mother O_1O_2

Fetus

B_1O_1	B_1O_2
O_2O_1	O_2O_2

Each pregnancy has a 50% chance of a type O fetus and a 50% chance of a heterozygous type B fetus.

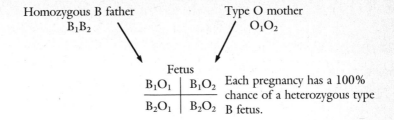

Homozygous B father
B_1B_2

Type O mother
O_1O_2

Fetus

B_1O_1	B_1O_2
B_2O_1	B_2O_2

Each pregnancy has a 100% chance of a heterozygous type B fetus.

The heterozygous type B fetus has the B antigen, which can evoke antibody formation in the type O mother.

Type AB fathers are always heterozygous. Their children from a type O mother have the following chances.

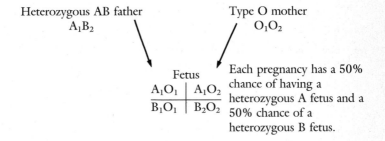

Heterozygous AB father
A_1B_2

Type O mother
O_1O_2

Fetus

A_1O_1	A_1O_2
B_1O_1	B_2O_2

Each pregnancy has a 50% chance of having a heterozygous A fetus and a 50% chance of a heterozygous B fetus.

Because type AB fathers, having children with type O mothers, will always produce heterozygous A or heterozygous B children, each fetus has the potential of antigenic factors evoking antibody formation by the type O mother. All have antigenic factors that are relatively weak compared to the Rh blood system.

If a mother is Rh-negative, she is always homozygous, having received the Rh-negative from both parents. The Rh-positive father may be Rh-positive heterozygous or Rh-positive homozygous. The following examples demonstrate this.

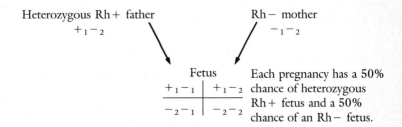

Heterozygous Rh+ father
$+_1-_2$

Rh− mother
$-_1-_2$

Fetus

$+_1-_1$	$+_1-_2$
$-_2-_1$	$-_2-_2$

Each pregnancy has a 50% chance of heterozygous Rh+ fetus and a 50% chance of an Rh− fetus.

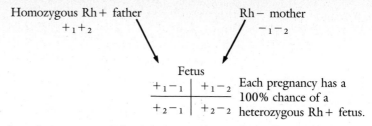

The Rh+ fetus has a strong Rh antigen on the surface of each red blood cell. These antigens will evoke antibody formation in the Rh− mother. The degree of sensitivity to the fetal Rh+ antigen varies but is assumed to be related to the total number of Rh+ fetal red blood cells entering the maternal circulation.

The placenta provides a large area in which exchange of nutrients and waste can take place across the placental membrane. This membrane consists of fetal tissues that separate maternal and fetal blood. As the pregnancy advances, the placental membrane, which also serves as a barrier, becomes progressively thinner. Because of the thinning of this membrane, some fetal blood cells may pass into the maternal blood in the intervillous space. It has been established that small numbers of fetal erythrocytes pass into the maternal circulation normally throughout pregnancy. Typically a greater amount enters at the time of delivery when the separation of the placenta traumatically forces entry of cells through the ciliated, open maternal vessels. However, small separations of the placenta can occur during pregnancy or with any potentially traumatic procedure such as amniocentesis. In most instances the fetal-maternal transfusion is small enough to evoke no sensitivity or involves no incompatibilities such as Rh or ABO.

Pathophysiology

The pathophysiology for all the hemolytic incompatibilities is similar. Rh incompatibility, being the most common, will be used to describe the process of isoimmunization. Isoimmunization occurs when the mother is sensitive to the fetal cells; it is also called *sensitization.*

Fetal erythrocytes, with the paternal Rh antigen, gain entry across the placental membrane into the intervillous blood, which is made up entirely of maternal blood. The fetal erythrocytes mix with the maternal blood and are then carried into the mother's circulation.

The breakthrough of fetal erythrocytes carrying the Rh antigen into the maternal circulation requires certain conditions favorable to sensitization of the mother and antibody formation. The widely dilated uteroplacental vessels facilitating blood flow also facilitate this process. Maximum maternal blood volume increasing between 28 and 32 weeks further facilitates dilatation of these vessels. Changes in fetal blood pressure are responsive to changes in blood flow in the maternal circulation and presumably could increase the chance of a few fetal erythrocytes, under increased pressure, breaking into the intervillous space. For this reason, the second most likely time for Rh isoimmunization to occur in the mother is at approximately 28 weeks of gestation.

The most likely time for fetal erythrocytes to escape into maternal circulation is at the time of delivery. The wide open vessels at the site of placental separation allow rapid back pressure as the uterus relaxes, and large numbers of fetal erythrocytes can escape into maternal circulation.

The formation of antibodies is gradual in the mother. Conditions favoring small areas of placental separation such as placenta previa, marginal abruption, or trauma to the placenta during amniocentesis can also favor the entry of increased numbers of fetal erythrocytes carrying the Rh antigen into maternal circulation.

Signs and symptoms

Evidence of antibody formation in the Rh-negative woman can be detected with an indirect Coombs and positive identification of the specific antibody on a screen. A titer of 1:4 or greater is significant and indicates maternal sensitization.

In the fetus, signs of anemia and impending hydrops include the following.
1. A baseline heart rate of 180 or greater
2. Late decelerations or loss of short-term variability (sinusoidal pattern)
3. Decreased fetal activity
4. Ascites or congestive heart failure on ultrasound examination

Maternal effects

There are no physiologic negative effects on the well-being of the mother other than discomfort if polyhydramnios occurs with fetal hydrops. If the mother is sensitized and desires future pregnancies, she may experience significant psychologic difficulties. The various feelings evoked will depend on the circumstances leading to the isoimmunization.

Fetal and neonatal effects

Harmful effects of Rh isoimmunization of the mother are seen as hemolysis of fetal erythrocytes. If the sensitization process begins at the time of delivery and Rh immune globulin is not given postpartum, the effects will be seen in future pregnancies.

The current pregnancy may be in jeopardy if the process of sensitization is undetected. This can occur if minute placental tissue fragments enter maternal circulation during an amniocentesis, at 28 weeks, or because of placental previa or abruption. The current pregnancy may also be jeopardized because sensitization occurred inadvertently with a previous pregnancy.

Hemolysis of fetal erythrocytes can lead to various degrees of fetal anemia. When anemia becomes severe, large amounts of bilirubin, resulting from hemolysis of the erythrocytes, place an overwhelming burden on the fetal liver. As a result, swelling occurs in the liver and portal pressure increases causing abdominal ascites and congestive heart failure. This phenomena is called *hydrops fetalis* and can be fatal to the fetus if not corrected by intrauterine transfusion or by delivery so that exchange transfusion of the neonate can occur.

Because of excessive bilirubin breakdown from rapid, increased hemolysis of fetal erythrocytes, the fetus makes an attempt to excrete as much bilirubin as possible. It is excreted in abnormally large amounts into the amniotic fluid and gives it a characteristic yellow-brown appearance.

A fetal sign of hypoxia unique to hemolytic anemia or anemia from fetal-maternal hemorrhage is loss of short-term variability in the FHR. The pattern is that of regular smooth oscillations resembling a sine wave and is called a *sinusoidal* pattern. There are no accelerations or variation from the regular smooth oscillations around the baseline. A sinusoidal pattern (Fig. 16-1) is often a terminal event and is indeed ominous for neonatal outcome.

MEDICAL DIAGNOSIS

Diagnosis in the Rh-negative mother is made by routine prenatal screening, which should be done in all patients, regardless of Rh factor, to screen for other hemolytic incompatibiliti⁀s. The test that detects this is an indirect Coombs.

If the patient is not sensitized at the beginning of the pregnancy, at approximately 28 weeks of gestation another screen should be done. Transplacental transfusion at 28 weeks is the second most common time for sensitization to occur; the placental membrane becomes thin enough by this time for fetal red blood cells to cross. To prevent this in an unsensitized woman, many obstetricians will give Rh immune globulin at 28 weeks to an unsensitized woman. Rh immune globulin is also given any time a traumatic fetal-maternal bleed is likely to occur such as after a genetic amniocentesis (Queenan, 1982).

If the mother has been Rh isoimmunized from a previous pregnancy, fetal erythroblastosis must be detected early to promote optimal fetal outcome either by early delivery or by intrauterine transfusions. Unless previous obstetric history indicates earlier involvement, the fetal erythroblastosis is followed by serial amniocentesis beginning at 26 to 28 weeks of gestation. Bilirubin, a breakdown product of red blood cells, can be measured in the amniotic fluid.

Liley, of Aukland, New Zealand, developed a graph for measuring the optical density of indirect bilirubin in the amniotic fluid. He divided the levels of bilirubin optical density into "zones" of safety based on gestation. Levels of indirect bilirubin should decrease with increasing gestation.

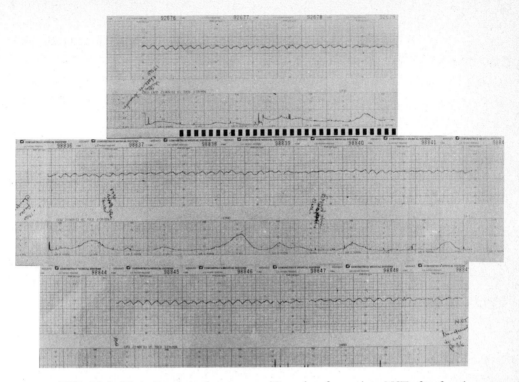

FIG. 16-1. Rh isoimmunized woman at 30 weeks of gestation. NST after fourth amniocentesis (*top*); the following day with obvious sinusoidal pattern (*middle and bottom*). (Courtesy John Elliott, Good Samaritan Medical Center, Phoenix, Ariz.)

In the unsensitized Rh-negative woman at other times of potential fetal hemorrhage into maternal circulation other tests may be done. A Kleihauer-Betke blood test on the mother is one means of determining fetal hemorrhage into the maternal circulation. It detects fetal blood cells in maternal circulation. If traumatic entry is suspected, greater than normal amounts may have entered, and the usual Rh immune globulin dose of 300 μg may not be sufficient. This test aids determination so that an increased amount of Rh immune globulin can be administered if necessary.

USUAL MEDICAL MANAGEMENT

To prevent sensitization in unsensitized Rh-negative women, the usual dose of Rh immune globulin is 300 μg at 28 weeks, at the time of any amniocentesis, and within 72 hours after delivery. If a test such as the Kleihauer-Betke indicates greater than 30 ml of fetal blood having entered the maternal circulation, a higher dose may be required to prevent sensitization. First trimester abortion, whether spontaneous or induced, requires a minidose of 30 μg within 72 hours (Virgilio and Simon, 1977). There are no immune globulins for prevention of other blood group sensitization incompatibilities.

If a hemolytic incompatibility is present, the usual medical management depends on levels of bilirubin optical density in the amniotic fluid, which are obtained by serial amniocenteses. When levels are low for a particular gestational age, the amniocentesis is repeated in 3 weeks. If levels rise, the amniocentesis may be repeated in 1 to 2 weeks. Extremely high levels for a particular gestation indicate a need for intrauterine transfusion in the very immature fetus. Delivery by cesarean may be necessary when this occurs after 34 weeks of gestation (Queenan, 1982).

By 26 weeks fetal heart rate monitoring should be started. A nonstress test may be done biweekly or a contraction stress test may be done weekly. Between heart rate monitoring, daily fetal activity charts should be kept by the mother. At the time of each amniocentesis, an ultrasound evaluation or biophysical profile should be done to further assess the fetus for presence of hydrops.

Although an intrauterine transfusion is not a common procedure, in some tertiary care centers it is a possible means of treatment and allows more time in utero for the immature or nonviable fetus. It must be done by a specially skilled physician, usually a perinatologist, who has learned the procedure during postgraduate training in maternal-fetal medicine.

The procedure is done under ultrasound direction. Approximately 50 to 150 ml of negative blood, cross matched to the mother, is used. It is spun down to increase the hematocrit to 70% to 80%. Rh-negative blood from a donor must be used because it contains no antibodies to the fetal Rh-positive blood.

The mother is given a narcotic or tranquilizer to quiet the baby for the procedure. After an abdominal scrub of the amniocentesis site, and with the direction of ultrasound, a large-gauge intracath is inserted through the maternal abdomen, into the uterus, and into the fetal abdomen, just under the fetal diaphragm. The intracath tubing, the attached intravenous tubing, and the syringe for the blood are all preflushed with normal saline. A small amount of normal saline can be injected to view on ultrasound and confirm placement. The syringe with the specially prepared blood is connected to an infusion pump designed for constant speed infusion via syringe. Depending on fetal gestation, 50 to 150 ml of blood is infused over a 1- to 2-hour period. The fetus is monitored before and during the procedure if the fetus is 26 weeks or more of gestation. If the fetus is less than 26 weeks, frequent auscultation of the fetal heart rate is usually done. Over the next 3 to 4 days, the fetal diaphragmatic lymph system absorbs the blood, and improvement in fetal anemia can be expected.

Success of intrauterine transfusion generally depends on a number of factors. If the fetus is extremely immature or there is significant liver and congestive heart failure, the potential for improved fetal well-being is unlikely, and death in utero can ensue in a matter of a few days.

The earlier the transfusions must be started, the greater the number required to gain maturity while maintaining fetal well-being. This puts the fetus at higher risk for intrauterine infection or premature rupture of membranes (Larkin et al., 1982) and therefore interferes with the potential successful outcome for the fetus.

NURSING PROCESS
Prevention

The nurse caring for the pregnant woman prenatally must recognize the importance of antibody screening in all pregnant patients for not only Rh incompatibility but for any blood system incompatibility. Education of the patient regarding necessary prenatal laboratory work should include the need for antibody screening. Patients can be given this information in early bird prenatal classes as well as during early office visits.

In addition, the nurse should advocate screening of Rh-negative women at 28 weeks of gestation for sensitization at that time. Regardless of the setting, the care giver must be cognizant of the fetus of the Rh-negative woman. For instance, if an Rh-negative woman presents to a labor and delivery setting in premature labor at 28 weeks, the nurse must, in addition to caring for her preterm labor, remember to care for her potentially Rh-positive fetus. Rh immune globulin should be given if the patient is Rh-negative and unsensitized.

At the time of delivery all Rh-negative women should be screened for sensitization if the baby is Rh-positive. Unsensitized patients should receive Rh immune globulin within 72 hours after delivery. The nurse caring for the woman during this time is responsible for assuring that the workup for eligibility has been done and that the patient is educated regarding indications for the injection. Even when permanent sterilization is expected, the woman should be instructed regarding potential future problems should sterilization fail or should she ever choose to have a reversal of the sterilization after becoming sensitized with this pregnancy. If an Rh-negative woman becomes sensitized, she must know that emergency transfusions of Rh-positive blood when Rh-negative is not available will be impossible and would be dangerous to her well-being.

Assessment

Part of the history elicited from an Rh-negative woman includes whether or not Rh immune globulin was received after each pregnancy, including any spontaneous or therapeutic abortions. If a woman has been sensitized, it may be from a previous pregnancy or an accidental transfusion of Rh-positive blood. If from a previous pregnancy, it is important to know at what gestation fetal problems occurred so that earlier assessment and intervention can be instituted with this pregnancy. If a previous infant had neonatal problems, it is important to elicit specific information about the extent and treatment needed.

Accurate information is needed regarding last menstrual period. All other dating information available, such as the date of a positive pregnancy test, regularity of menstrual cycles, type of birth control used, and ultrasound, may aid in correctly assigning a due date and in counting gestational weeks. These will be invaluable in determining when necessary interventions should be instituted.

Assessment of the psychosocial impact of Rh sensitization is also necessary. If the Rh-sensitized woman became sensitized because of the omission of Rh immune globulin injection, various feelings may be unresolved. If the injection was overlooked or mistaken Rh results were reported with a previous pregnancy, anger may be unresolved. This can be true especially if the matter is under litigation. If the injection was omitted after a therapeutic abortion, guilt regarding the abortion may be overriding other feelings. When a previous pregnancy occurred before the routine use of Rh immune globulin, feelings of frustration with an event that could not be controlled and anxiety for the future or the present pregnancy will interact. The serial amniocenteses, ultrasounds, and possible intrauterine transfusions will place an added financial burden on many couples because of the extreme expense involved. Discussion of their resources, such as insurance, can aid in the assessment of psychosocial needs.

In the unsensitized woman, it is unusual to find the awareness that there is a potential for sensitization occurring at any times other than delivery. Assessment of the patient's understanding of this process is a must if the nurse is to be able to educate the patient in a reassuring rather than alarming manner regarding the use of Rh immune globulin at the other recommended times. As public awareness increases with the change in medical management, the nurse must also assess for degrees of anxiety.

Because of the varying feelings of unresolved guilt, anger, frustration, anxiety, or fear, the nurse should assess for coping mechanisms previously used successfully by the couple. During the discusssion of events leading to sensitization, questions specifically related to how they felt then and now and what means they utilized to cope can aid in formulating plans to help in the present situation.

Physical assessment parameters indicating adequate fetal oxygenation should also be made. These include the following.

Antepartum

1. Fundal height measurements in centimeters should be consistent with weeks gestation from 20 weeks on. Fundal measurements should also show growth from one week to the next. Concern for fetal growth should occur if fundal growth stops or decreases. If the fetus becomes anemic, the decreased oxygenation can lead to decreased growth rate. If the fetus becomes hydropic, fundal height can be abnormally large due to associated polyhydramnios.

2. Maternal report of fetal activity should be queried at each visit. Daily records after 26 weeks of gestation should be kept. An active fetus can be assumed to be adequately oxygenated.

3. Prior to an amniocentesis a baseline FHR should be determined. When an amniocentesis is performed after 26 weeks of gestation, a 20- to 30-minute fetal monitoring strip should be run to assess fetal heart rate for signs of hypoxia, such as tachycardia, late decelerations, or decreased short-term variability (sinusoidal pattern, Fig. 16-1). During an intra-uterine transfusion, the fetal heart rate should be continuously monitored to document a normal baseline rate and absences of periodic changes suggestive of hypoxia. Because of maternal sedation during intrauterine transfusion, baseline variability can be decreased and should be compared to the strip prior to premedication and to the strip 1 hour after. Routine office visits should assess fetal heart rate for tachycardia.

4. Amniotic fluid color should be observed for signs of bilirubin breakdown products. If present, the amniotic fluid takes on a characteristic yellow-brown cast. It should also be inspected for evidence of meconium staining, which might cause a yellow-green cast.

5. The mother should be assessed for anxiety related to fear for her infant and potential outcome.

Intrapartum. Intrapartum assessment will depend on the mode of delivery. Labor can stress the fetus and cause distress if anemia has developed. Therefore the fetus should be closely monitored for signs of hypoxia such as tachycardia, late decelerations, and loss of variability, or meconium-stained amniotic fluid.

A cesarean delivery may be necessary with a severely compromised infant. Little warning or preparation may be possible. In addition to anxiety over an emergent surgery, there can be great fear for the infant. Rapid assessment for signs of unrealistic fears must be made.

Postpartum. Routine physical assessment of the mother is dependent on mode of delivery. Assessment for appropriate mothering attachment behaviors with a premature or sick neonate are important for Rh-sensitized mothers. They should be assessed for the usual early positive behaviors of frequent vis-itation, early touching and stroking, calling the infant by he or she appropriately, and attempting good eye contact. Assessments of the couple's support of each other and of significant others will also be important for the plan of care.

Because of prematurity, the neonate may have other problems causing parental concern. All areas should be explored and close contact maintained with nursery personnel for explanations.

Antepartum intervention

The nurse caring for the patient in the outpatient setting should ensure that the following diagnostic screening be completed.

1. Antibody screen should be drawn on the first prenatal visit as well as blood and Rh type. If the antibody screen is positive, specific identification and titers should be determined.
2. All Rh-negative women who are not sensitized should be rescreened at 28 weeks and Rh immune globulin given if unsensitized.
3. All Rh-negative sensitized women or women with other incompatibilities should have arrangements made for serial amniocenteses with ultrasound as ordered by the physician. Appropriate antepartum fetal heart monitoring beginning at 26 to 28 weeks should be ordered and scheduled. Fetal activity charts should be utilized as a nursing intervention to encourage daily monitoring of fetal well-being after 26 to 28 weeks.

Rh immune globulin should be administered with explanations given to the patient if she is unsensitized at 28 weeks, following a genetic amniocentesis, and at any time a placental accident (previa or abruption) is ascertained.

Education regarding all tests is necessary when the mother is sensitized. The nurse must allay unrealistic fears and encourage participation of the mother in planning for care of other family members during any necessary hospitalizations. Giving adequate education can help the family plan financially for the additional expense and help the couple cope with the prospect of a sick neonate.

When assisting with an intrauterine transfusion, the nurse must provide pain relief by careful positioning for comfort during the considerable immobilization. Side tilt, intravenous fluids, and oxygen at 10 liters by tight face mask may be necessary if signs of fetal distress are present.

Fetal monitoring with fetal activity charts should be explained in such a way as to provide reassurance rather than fear. Focusing on the preventive aspects of maternal attention to fetal signs of well-being often accomplishes this. When fetal distress is detected during monitoring, by ultrasound or amniocentesis, support by the nurse is important. Remaining with the mother and giving simple, honest explanations aid the couple's coping mechanisms. Lengthy or detailed explanations confuse them in times of crisis and should be avoided.

Signs of fetal distress require rapid nursing response. Being prepared for an emergency cesarean delivery can aid in providing a reassuring atmosphere while also effecting optimal outcome for the neonate.

Referrals in the antepartum period may be made to tertiary care centers because of the few physicians with skill in intrauterine transfusion available elsewhere. When clinical nurse specialists, nurse clinicians, or antepartum testing personnel are available, nursing referrals should be made. A brief summary of nursing diagnoses identified, interventions such as diagnostic testing scheduled, and educational materials and resources used can be helpful in maintaining continuity of care. Referral to a social worker for obtaining financial assistance when family resources are inadequate may be helpful.

Intervention—drug therapy

Rh immune globulin is a specially prepared gamma globulin that contains a specific concentration of Rh antibodies. These antibodies neutralize the Rh-positive fetal antigens that have entered the maternal circulation. For this reason it cannot correct sensitization but can prevent it from occurring. Research has shown it to be effective if given within 72 hours of the potential fetal-maternal red blood cell infusion. However, there is no research evidence that time intervals greater than 72 hours are not effective.

Because the antibody formation in the mother is gradual, it is also apparently effective in preventing sensitization during pregnancy. When it is given at 28 weeks of gestation to unsensitized women, the incidence of Rh isoimmunization may be further reduced.

Rh immune globulin is injected intramuscularly. Sometimes a patient experiences temporary soreness at the site of injection. Occasionally a low-grade fever develops. In rare instances, an anaphylactic reaction occurs. It is for this reason that the patient should remain in the health care setting for 15 to 30 minutes following the injection.

The nurse must instruct the patient regarding indications for Rh immune globulin. An identification card confirming the injection should be filled out at the time of injection and given to the woman. She should be instructed to keep it with her identification papers for emergency verification of protection if Rh-positive transfusion should be necessary when Rh-negative blood is unavailable in an emergency.

The blood bank form with the ampule should be filled out appropriately by the nurse and returned with the empty container. In the event of an allergic reaction, the blood bank needs the information these provide.

Intrapartum intervention

The interventions in labor and delivery center around prevention of fetal distress. Response to late decelerations or loss of variability by the provision of optimal oxygenation for the fetus should be provided if readying for emergency delivery. These measures include left side tilt, oxygen by tight face mask, and intravenous fluids. If a sinusoidal pattern evolves, rapid cesarean delivery may proceed within minutes. If the pattern is present when the monitor is first connected, there is great controversy regarding a cesarean delivery for a fetus who will very likely not survive. In this case, the nurse should exercise great caution against alarming others, especially the parents, and in giving any conflicting information. Simple, direct information reaffirming the physician's stated plan to the parents can enhance their ability to cope.

SUGGESTED PLAN

Hemolytic incompatibility

Potential patient problem	Outcome criteria
A. Potential isoimmunization in Rh-negative woman related to: Failure to receive Rh immune globulin at prescribed times Fetal RBCs crossing into maternal circulation at unpredicted times	No Rh isoimmunization in unsensitized Rh-negative woman; titer less than 1:4 Detection of other hemolytic incompatibilities through routine antibody screening Good neonatal outcome at time of delivery when isoimmunization has previously occurred No evidence of sinusoidal FHR pattern
B. Potential fetal distress or poor neonatal outcome related to: Fetal RBCs crossing into maternal circulation in large numbers especially Rh+ cells into Rh− woman or type A or B cells into type O mother	

Referral to neonatal intensive care personnel should occur prior to delivery especially when signs of fetal distress have been present. A neonatal team should be available in the delivery room.

Postpartum/postoperative intervention

Interventions for care of the Rh-sensitized patient are not unique to this condition. They frequently depend on mode of delivery and neonatal well-being. The nurse should encourage early and frequent parental contact to foster attachment behaviors. Acceptance of their feelings of grief can assist the

O F   N U R S I N G   C A R E

Assessment and intervention

Dx. Assess antibody screen in all pregnant women
   Refer to laboratory data: do antibody screen in prenatal screen, at 28 weeks of gestation, at time of delivery, and at any other time of potential fetal cells transfusion to maternal circulation

Th. Give Rh immune globulin at all appropriate times to unsensitized Rh-negative women
   Prepare for ultrasound examination, amniocentesis, and potential intrauterine fetal transfusion in the Rh-isoimmunized woman
   Continous fetal monitoring during labor

Ed. Instruct all Rh-negative pregnant women in all of the appropriate times for screening and Rh immune globulin administration
   Explain all special evaluation examinations or procedures if isoimmunization has occurred.

Ref. Any signs of fetal distress to physician
   Any laboratory data suggesting isoimmunization to physician
   Tertiary obstetric care center if intrauterine fetal transfusion necessary
   Neonatal intensive care personnel if neonate is compromised from isoimmunization

Dx. Assess for sinusoidal FHR pattern if mother is Rh sensitized
Th. Antepartum FHR testing (NST or CST) as ordered

Dx., diagnostic; Th., therapeutic; Ed., education; Ref., referral.

parents in moving on to attachment. Referral for spiritual support may be helpful if religious affiliation is valued by the couple.

For the unsensitized Rh-negative mother, the Rh immune globulin injection should be adminstered by the nurse after she ensures that the appropriate eligibility workup had been done (see Intervention—drug therapy).

Evaluation

For the unsensitized Rh-negative woman, prevention is the primary goal. This is best accomplished through antibody screening at the first prenatal visit and at 28 weeks and giving Rh immune globulin at 28 weeks, postdelivery, with potential placental accidents, and postabortion. Education regarding indications for Rh immune globulin and times of greatest risk can improve the future protection of Rh-negative women from sensitization. As yet, there is no preventive therapy for other hemolytic incompatibilities.

For the sensitized woman, the primary goal is providing optimal neonatal outcome through close monitoring of fetal well-being.

Nurses providing information to Rh-sensitized women, should encourage them to seek new, proven improvements in care of the Rh-sensitized mother and fetus such as those described under Usual Medical Management.

REFERENCES

Berkowitz, R.L., and Hobbin, J.C.: Intrauterine transfusion utilizing ultrasound, Obstet. Gynecol. **57**:33, 1981.

Brewer, C., and others: Comparative risks of rhesus autoimmunisation in two different methods of mid-trimester abortion, Br. Med. J. **282**:1929, 1981.

Chard, T.: Human placental lactogen in the monitoring of high-risk pregnancy, Ric. Clin. Lab. **12**(1):207, 1982.

Eklund, J.: Embryonic rhesus-positive red cells stimulating a secondary response after early abortion (letter), Lancet **2**:748, 1981.

Elias, S.: The role of fetoscopy in antenatal diagnosis, Clin. Obstet. Gynecol. **7**:73, 1980.

Hammer, R., Bower, E., and Messina, L.: The prenatal use of Rho (D) immune globulin, MCN **9**(1):29, 1984.

Hensleigh, P.A.: Preventing rhesis isoimmunization: antepartum Rh immune globulin prophylaxis versus a sensitive test for risk identification, Am. J. Obstet. Gynecol. **146**:749, 1983.

Hughes, G., Bischof, P., and Klopper, A.: Relation between pregnancy-associated plasma protein A and fetal sex and blood group, Hum. Hered. **33**:69, 1983.

Kirkinen, P., Jouppila, P., and Eik-Nes, S.: Umbilical vein blood flow in rhesus-isoimmunization, Br. J. Obstet. Gynaecol. **90**:640, 1983.

Kochenour, N.K., and Beeson, J.H.: The use of Rh-immune globulin, Clin. Obstet. Gynecol. **25**:283, 1982.

Laferla, J.J., and Butch, S.: Fetal Rh blood group determination in pregnancy termination by dilatation and evacuation, Transfusion **23**:67, 1983.

Larkin, R.M., Knochel, J.Q., and Lee, T.G.: Intrauterine transfusion: new techniques and results, Clin. Obstet. Gynecol. **25**:303, 1982.

Lloyd, L.K., and others: Intrapartum fetomaternal bleeding in Rh-negative women, Obstet. Gynecol. **56:**285, 1980.

Powell, S.B., Howell, P., and Renton, P.H.: Automated screening of antenatal samples using a low ionic strength polybrene system, Clin. Lab. Hematol. **3:**343, 1981.

Queenan, J.T.: Current management of the Rh-sensitized patient, Clin. Obstet. Gynecol. **25:**293, 1982.

Ramzy, I., Vilos, G.A., and DesRosiers, P.A.: Antenatal assessment of fetal age and maturity using fetal fat staining cells in amniotic fluid, Acta Cytol. **22:**105, 1978.

Scott, J.R., and Warenski, J.C.: Tests to detect and quantitate fetomaternal bleeding, Clin. Obstet. Gynecol. **25:**277, 1982.

Sebring, E.S., and Polesky, H.F.: Detection of fetal hemorrhage in Rh immune globulin candidates: a rosetting technique using enzyme-treated Rh_2Rh_2 indicator erythrocytes, Transfusion **22:**468, 1982.

Sistonen, P.: A phenotypic association between the blood group antigen nea and the Rh antigen D, Med. Biol. **59**(4):230, 1981.

Virgilio, L.A., and Simon, N.V.: Measurement of fetal cells in the maternal circulation, Obstet. Gynecol. **50:**364, 1977.

White, C.A., Stedman, C.M., and Frank, S.: Anti-D antibodies in Du-negative and Du-positive women: a cause of hemolytic disease of the newborn, Am. J. Obstet. Gynecol. **145:**1069, 1983.

UNIT V

ALTERATIONS
IN THE MECHANISM
OF LABOR

Successful termination of pregnancy heralded by labor requires the harmonious interplay of the uterus, placenta, fetus, and pelvis. Disruptions can result if labor is not stimulated on time, the uterus contracts ineffectively, the fetus is larger than the pelvis, or the fetus is in a presentation that makes it impossible to accommodate the pelvis. When a disruption in the mechanism of labor develops, early detection and appropriate management are important to facilitate the best maternal and fetal outcome. These can be accomplished by augmenting the labor with a labor stimulant or delivering the fetus by a cesarean delivery.

CHAPTER 17

Dysfunctional labor

Labor does not always progress within the normal labor curve. Conditions can exist or develop that interfere with normal progress. An abnormal or difficult labor is usually termed *dysfunctional labor* or *dystocia*.

INCIDENCE

Dysfunctional labor occurs in approximately 8% of all deliveries (Friedman, 1978a). Malpresentations account for approximately 5% of these abnormal labors. Uterine dystocia accounts for approximately 1%, and pelvic disproportion, without an associated fetal factor, accounts for 2% (Seeds and Cefalo, 1982).

ETIOLOGY

Dysfunctional labor is caused by three main factors: uterine dystocia, fetal dystocia, and pelvic dystocia. Uterine dystocia is related to ineffective uterine activity. Some of the causes that appear to increase one's risk for developing uterine dystocia are listed below.

1. Thirty pounds or more overweight
2. Infertility difficulties
3. Masculine characteristics
4. A congenitally abnormal uterus, an overdistended uterus as in the case of a multiple pregnancy, or polyhydramnios
5. Lack of reflex stimulation of the myometium related to malpresentations such as posterior positions, face, brow, or breech presentations, or transverse lie
6. Fetopelvic disproportion; uterine activity usually slows if the pelvis is too small for fetal descent
7. Overstimulation of the uterus with oxytocin
8. Extreme maternal fear or exhaustion
9. Dehydration
10. Electrolyte imbalance
11. Administration of an analgesic too early in labor

Fetal dystocia is usually related to one of the following.

383

1. An abnormal fetal presentation or position, such as face, brow, or breech, posterior occiput presentation, or transverse lie
2. Fetal anomalies such as hydrocephalus, abdominal enlargement, tumors, or conjoined twins
3. Excessive fetal size, usually greater than 4,000 gm (9 pounds)

Pelvic dystocia is usually related to one of these conditions.

1. A small pelvic inlet, midpelvis, or pelvic outlet as the result of heredity, previous pelvic fracture, or disease
2. An immature pelvis; the growth of the bony pelvis is not complete until approximately age 18 (Moerman, 1982)

PHYSIOLOGY
Normal

Normal uterine contractions have a contraction (systole) and relaxation (diastole) phase. The contraction phase is initiated by a pacemaker situated at the uterine end of the right fallopian tube. The contraction, like a wave, moves downward to the cervix and upward to the fundus of the uterus. At the acme (peak) of the contraction the entire uterus is contracting, with the greatest intensity in the fundal area. The relaxation phase follows and occurs simultaneously in all parts of the uterus. The round ligaments contain muscle and are stimulated to contract as the uterus contracts, thereby anchoring the uterus and promoting a downward force on the presenting part (Oxorn, 1980). The most effective uterus is one that maintains a low resting tone of 8 to 12 mm Hg but can contract in intensity to 50 or 60 mm Hg amniotic pressure during a contraction.

Pathophysiology

Uterine dystocia. There are two types of abnormal uterine activity leading to uterine dystocia. First, there is hypotonic uterine activity in which the rise in uterine pressure during a contraction is insufficient (less than 25 mm Hg) to promote cervical effacement and dilatation. The force provided by voluntary contractions of the abdominal musculature, facilitated by the urge to push, may be insufficient to facilitate fetal descent and delivery. Second, there are hypertonic or incoordinated uterine contractions in which the contractions are frequent and painfully strong but ineffective in promoting effacement and dilatation. They can be ineffective because the uterine pacemakers arise in other areas of the uterus. This causes the myometrium to contract spasmodically and frequently but ineffectively, and the presenting part is not forced downward.

Fetal dystocia. The fetus can move through the birth canal with the greatest ease when the head is sharply flexed so that the chin rests on the thorax and the occipital area of the skull (vertex) is presenting anteriorly to the mother's pelvis. Thus the smallest diameter of the fetal head enters the mother's pelvis and the most flexible part of the fetal body, the back of the neck, adapts to the curve of the birth canal. At times, the fetus will assume other presentations making labor difficult or impossible. These presentations are discussed in the next section.

OCCIPUT POSTERIOR PRESENTATION. This occurs in approximately 10% to 15% of labors when the occiput of the fetus is in the posterior portion of the pelvis instead of in the anterior portion (Fig. 17-1) As the fetus moves through the birth canal, the occiput bone presses on the mother's sacrum. This usually causes severe back pain. The occiput must also rotate 135°. This rotation can occur during fetal descent, but most often it does not occur until the occiput reaches the pelvic floor. Therefore the second stage of labor is usually prolonged.

FACE PRESENTATION. Face presentation, or mentum, occurs approximately once in every 500 to 600 deliveries (Seeds and Cefalo, 1982) when the fetal head is in extension instead of flexion as it enters the pelvic inlet (Fig. 17-2). If the mentum is in an anterior position, the labor usually progresses very closely to normal and vaginal delivery results without much difficulty. This is because the widest diameter of the presenting part is similar in size to an

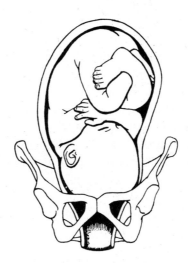

FIG. 17-1. Occiput posterior presentation. (Reproduced with permission from The Normal Female Pelvis [Clinical Education Aid No. 18], Ross Laboratories, Columbus, Oh.)

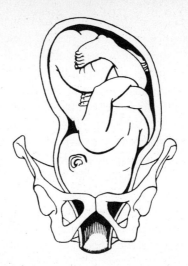

FIG. 17-2. Face presentation. (Reproduced with permission from The Normal Female Pelvis [Clinical Education Aid No. 18], Ross Laboratories, Columbus, Oh.)

occupit presentation and the neck can glide around the short symphysis pubis with ease. When the mentum is in a posterior position, approximately 70% of the time it will rotate to an anterior face presentation making vaginal delivery possible but causing the labor to be prolonged. If the posterior position persists, delivery by cesarean will be necessary because the neck is too short to stretch the long distance of the sacrum.

BROW PRESENTATION. This occurs approximately once in every 1,500 deliveries (Abell, 1973) when the fetal head presents in a position midway between full flexion and extreme extension (Fig. 17-3). This causes the largest diameter of the fetal head to engage. However, Cruikshank and White (1973) found that approximately 66% of these presentations converted to a vertex or face presentation and could be delivered vaginally. In 33% of the cases, the brow presentation persisted and had to be delivered by cesarean. A brow presentation may be present when descent of the presenting part is prolonged or is arrested early in active labor.

SHOULDER PRESENTATION. This occurs approximately once in every 300 deliveries (Cruikshank and White, 1973) when the fetal spine is lying vertical to the mother's spine (Fig. 17-4). Because of the high mortality risk due to prolapsed cord, cesarean delivery is usually the best management. However, if placenta previa and fetopelvic disproportion (FPD) are not present, external cephalic version has been successful in very controlled circumstances.

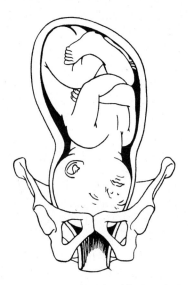

FIG. 17-3. Brow presentation. (Reproduced with permission from The Normal Female Pelvis [Clinical Education Aid No. 18], Ross Laboratories, Columbus, Oh.)

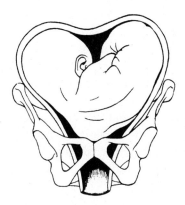

FIG. 17-4. Shoulder presentation. (Reproduced with permission from The Normal Female Pelvis. [Clinical Education Aid No. 18], Ross Laboratories, Columbus, Oh.)

COMPOUND PRESENTATION. This occurs approximately once in every 1,000 deliveries (Cruikshank and White, 1973) when one or more of the fetal extremities accompanies the presenting part. An arm with the head is the most common compound presentation. Vaginal delivery is usually possible unless cord prolapse occurs or labor fails to progress. Then an immediate cesarean delivery is done. Attempts should not be made to replace the prolapsed fetal part (Seeds and Cefalo, 1982).

BREECH PRESENTATION. Breech presentation occurs in approximately 4% of all deliveries (Collea, 1980) when the buttocks of the fetus present. The breech can present in three different attitudes. It is termed a *frank breech* when the thighs are flexed and the legs lie alongside the fetal body, a *complete breech* when the fetus's legs are flexed at the thighs allowing the feet to present with the buttocks, and a *footling breech* when one foot (single footling) or both feet (double footling) present before the buttocks (Fig. 17-5). Prematurity is the main cause of breech presentation. Other causes are placenta previa, multiple gestation, polyhydramnios, and hydrocephaly, with an increased incidence in women who jog.

A breech presentation is considered high-risk for the following reasons.
1. Prolapse of the cord is more likely to occur, especially in a footling breech, because the buttocks do not fit as snugly into the cervix as does the fetal head.
2. Dysfunctional labor is much more likely to result because the buttocks are soft and make a poor dilating wedge against the cervix.
3. Birth trauma is more likely to occur because the head does not have time to mold and it must pass through the birth canal quickly. If the fetus is premature, it is even more prone to birth trauma from fetal pelvic disproportion.

Therefore vaginal delivery is rarely attempted unless it is a frank breech, without hyperextension of the head, with a gestational age greater than 36 weeks, and an estimated fetal weight between 2,500 and 3,500 gm (Main et al., 1983; Seeds and Cefalo, 1982; Jaffa et al., 1981). Theoretically, only 25% to 28% of all breeches will be delivered vaginally if this protocol is followed (Quilligan, 1980; Gimovsky and Paul, 1983).

Pelvic dystocia. Pelvic dystocia is related to a contraction of one or more of the three planes of the pelvis.

INLET CONTRACTION. The pelvic inlet is considered contracted when the widest part of the brim, the transverse diameter, is less than 12 cm and the anteroposterior diameter is less than 10 cm. The anteroposterior diameter can be approximated by measuring the diagonal conjugate, the distance from the lower portion of the symphysis pubis to the middle of the promontory of the

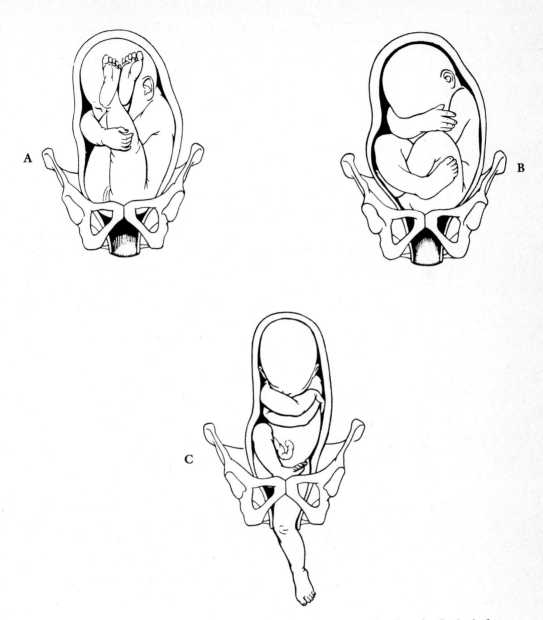

FIG. 17-5. Breech presentation. **A,** Frank breech; **B,** complete breech; **C,** single footling breech. (Reproduced with permission from The Normal Female Pelvis [Clinical Education Aid No. 18], Ross Laboratories, Columbus, Oh.)

sacrum and subtracting 1.5 cm. The transverse diameter can be measured only by x-ray studies or ultrasound.

If the contraction is pronounced, a cesarean birth will be planned. If the contraction is borderline, the decision of treatment will depend on fetal size. Descent and engagement of the fetal head would indicate an adequate pelvic inlet.

MIDPELVIS CONTRACTION. Contraction of the midpelvis is three to four times more prevalent than a contraction of the inlet or outlet and more difficult to determine manually. Possible indicators are (1) prominent ischial spines, (2) convergent pelvic side walls, and (3) a narrow sacrosciatic notch. Usually, a contraction of the outlet accompanies a midpelvis contraction.

OUTLET CONTRACTION. The outlet of the pelvis can be approximated by measuring the transverse diameter, the distance between the inner aspects of the ischial tuberosities. If it is 8 cm or less, the outlet is considered contracted. With the use of a Thoms' retractor, the anteroposterior diameter can also be approximated by measuring from the middle of the lower margin of the symphysis pubis to the tip of the sacrum, not the coccyx; the fetal head can usually push the coccyx back. Normally, the anteroposterior diameter is 14 cm.

When the medical team is determining whether a vaginal delivery can be attempted or delivery should be by cesarean, the pelvic and the fetal size must be considered. If the fetus is too large to pass through the pelvis, or the pelvis is too small for the fetus to pass through, the condition is usually referred to as *fetopelvic disproportion* (FPD) or *cephalopelvic disproportion* (CPD).

Signs and symptoms

Cervical dilatation, effacement, and fetal descent should occur progressively during labor. In an abnormal labor (1) contractions slow or fail to advance in frequency, duration or intensity; (2) the cervix fails to respond to the uterine contractions by dilating and effacing; or (3) the fetus fails to move downward. Thus labor does not progress normally.

Normal labor usually begins with a latent phase, which is characterized by the cervix slowly dilating to about 4 cm. The average duration of this phase for the nullipara is 6.4 hours, and for the multipara it is 4.8 hours (Koontz and Bishop, 1982). An active phase follows and is identified as the time when dilatation takes place more rapidly. It is characterized by a period of acceleration, then a period of maximum slope, followed by a period of deceleration (Fig. 17-6).

The deceleration phase, often referred to as *transition,* is not associated with decreased uterine activity, but during this phase the cervix is being retracted around the fetal presenting part. The normal rate of cervical dilatation during active phase should be at least 1.2 cm/hr in nulliparas and 1.5 cm/hr in multi-

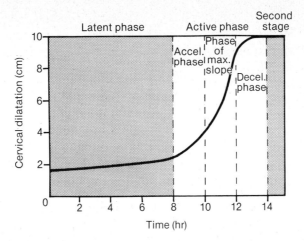

FIG. 17-6. Average dilatational curve. Composite of the average dilatation curve for nulliparous labor based on analysis of the data derived from the patterns traced by a large, nearly consecutive series of primigravidas. The first stage is divided into a relatively flat latent phase and a rapidly progressive active phase. The active phase has three identifiable component parts, an acceleration phase, a linear phase of maximum slope, and a deceleration phase. (Reproduced with permission from Friedman, E.A.: Labor: clinical evaluation and management, ed. 2, New York, 1978, Appleton-Century-Crofts, Inc.)

paras (Friedman, 1982a). Except for prelabor engagement, fetal descent does not generally begin until the active phase of dilatation and starts to reach its maximum slope during the deceleration phase of active labor, which continues throughout the second stage of labor. The normal rate of descent is at least 1 cm/hour in nulliparas and 2 cm/hr in multiparas (Friedman, 1982a).

Maternal effects

Any time the birth canal is too small to accommodate the presentation of the fetus, uterine rupture can result. This can lead to maternal death related to hemorrhage. However, the incidence is rare; an obstructed labor is not usually allowed to continue. The greatest risk to the mother with a dysfunctional labor is associated with a cesarean delivery; 40% of all primary cesarean deliveries are the result of dysfunctional labor. These risks include postoperative complications of hemorrhage, hematoma, thrombophlebitis, pneumonia, endometrial infections, and bowel and bladder trauma (Monheit and Resnik, 1981).

Fetal and neonatal effects

Infant mortality ranges from 0.6% to 40% when a dysfunctional labor develops. The highest rate of mortality is associated with such labor patterns as a protracted disorder or a secondary arrest of dilatation. There is no increased mortality associated with a prolonged latent phase disorder (Friedman, 1978a).

Fetal and infant mortality is usually related to hypoxia or birth trauma. Hypoxia is often the result of intense, uterine contractions, which lead to uteroplacental insufficiency or cord prolapse related to malpresentation. A malpresentation can also cause such birth traumas as cranial or neck compression; fracture of the trachea, larynx, or shoulder; and traumatic injury of the spinal cord during an attempted vaginal delivery. The various interventions to facilitate delivery also increase the risk of the fetus for hypoxia and trauma. For instance, if midforceps are used following an abnormal labor, perinatal mortality increases to 28.5%. Those infants who live have four to six times the rate of neurological developmental defects (Friedman, 1983).

MEDICAL DIAGNOSIS

During the prenatal period the health care provider will determine general pelvic size and configuration and fetal position and presentation. This is done by abdominal palpation and vaginal examinations. If a deviation from normal is suspected, ultrasound will be carried out. The value of x-ray pelvimetry in predicting the outcome of labor is limited by the difficulty of assessing fetal weight (Joyce et al., 1975). Laube, Varner, and Cruikshank (1981) report that x-ray pelvimetry findings changed the plan of medical treatment in only 2% of patients. Therefore its usefulness is being critically evaluated and many obstetricians are concluding that the risks of exposing the fetus to harmful radiation outweigh the benefits of x-ray pelvimetry (Barton et al., 1982).

Diagnostic prediction of the outcome of labor is not always possible prior to labor. Many causes of dysfunctional labor do not develop until labor has started. These will be diagnosed based on such clinical findings during labor as the uterine contraction pattern or the progression of labor as indicated by cervical dilatation and effacement and fetal descent.

USUAL MEDICAL TREATMENT

If a very small or deformed pelvis is determined clinically or fetal malpresentation is confirmed by ultrasound contraindicating a vaginal delivery, a cesarean delivery is planned. The specific date is set when fetal lung maturity is established by amniocentesis. All other patients are given a trial labor to determine if a vaginal delivery will be possible and safe for the fetus.

Progress during the trial labor should be evaluated according to Friedman's normal labor curves (Fig. 17-7). Significant slowing of any phase of labor indicates dysfunctional labor and should be treated according to the cause of the disorder.

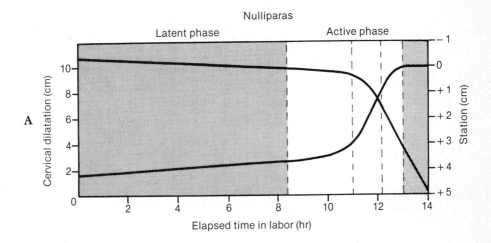

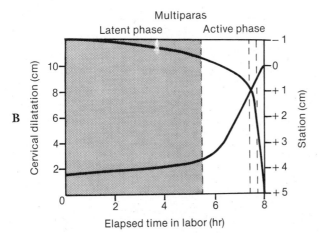

FIG. 17-7. Normal labor patterns. **A,** Normal labor pattern for the nullipara; **B,** normal labor pattern for the multipara. (Reproduced with permission from Friedman, E.: An objective method of evaluating labor, Hospital Pract. **5**(7):82, 1970; Artist, Albert Miller.)

Dysfunctional labor disorders

Friedman (1978a) has classified the various disorders thus.

1. Prolonged latent phase disorders
2. Protraction disorders, which include protracted active phase dilatation and protracted descent disorders
3. Arrest disorders, which include secondary arrest of dilatation, arrest of descent, and failure of descent disorders.
4. Precipitous labor disorders

Prolonged latent phase (Fig. 17-8). The latent phase of labor begins with the onset of regular uterine contractions and ends when dilatation starts to take place more rapidly. This phase of labor becomes prolonged when it continues for 20 hours or longer in the nullipara and 14 hours or longer in the multipara (Friedman, 1978a). However, diagnosis of a prolonged latent phase labor can be made long before the patient has spent that much time in labor. After 6 to 8 hours of little progress, an assessment should be made. False labor should be considered as a possible cause, because it can be mistakenly diagnosed as this disorder. Emotional stress such as fear and anxiety can cause the adrenal medulla to secrete catecholamines that interfere with uterine contractibility. Also during this phase of labor the uterus appears to be very sensitive to extraneous influences such as early heavy sedation, narcotic analgesics, or conduction anesthesia. Therefore these conditions can cause this type of labor pattern often characterized by hypertonic uterine contractions.

The best treatment, according to Dr. Friedman (1980), is to sedate the pa-

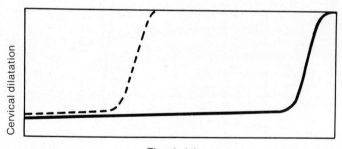

Time in labor

FIG. 17-8. Prolonged latent phase pattern (solid line) is the only disorder thus far objectively diagnosable in the preparatory division of labor. It is an abnormality characterized by latent phase duration exceeding established critical limits, shown with typical elongation of the lower initial arm of the sigmoid curve of cervical dilatation. It is followed by a normal active phase here, as is usually the case. The average dilatation curve for nulliparas *(broken line)* is shown for comparison. (Reproduced with permission from Friedman, E.A.: Labor: clinical evaluation and management, ed. 2, New York, 1978, Appleton-Century-Crofts, Inc.)

tient. If the mother is in false labor, the contractions will cease. If she is overly anxious, this will calm her and decrease the release of catecholamines and she will awaken in active, effective labor. In only 5% of patients will the contractions continue to be ineffective and a labor stimulant be needed. Other obstetricians evaluate the condition of the cervix as to whether it is closed and thick or soft and inducable and treat it accordingly. If it is thick, they will administer a narcotic analgesic such as morphine to induce a therapeutic rest, and if it is soft they will administer a labor stimulant (Koontz and Bishop, 1982). In any case, most patients who experience prolonged latent phase abnormal labors will progress to active labor and deliver vaginally.

Protraction disorders (Fig. 17-9). Protracted active phase labor can be characterized by either a slowing in the dilatation or the descent pattern once the labor has become active. In the nullipara, the dilatation rate is less than 1.2 cm/hr and the rate of descent is less than 1 cm/hr. In the multipara the dilatation rate is less than 1.2 cm/hr and the rate of descent is less than 2.0 cm/hr.

According to Friedman (1978a), about one third of these patients experience fetopelvic disproportion and develop an arrest of labor. Other causative factors such as a posterior occiput presentation, excessive sedation, early administration of conduction anesthesia, or early rupture of membranes will usually slow the labor but do not prevent a vaginal delivery.

Treatment will depend on whether or not FPD is present. If severe FPD is diagnosed, a cesarean will be performed as soon as possible. If FPD cannot be documented, the labor will be allowed to continue. There are two schools of

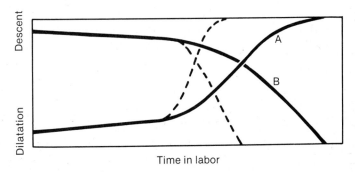

FIG. 17-9. Protraction disorders of labor. **A,** Protracted active phase dilatation pattern with abnormally slow maximum slope of dilatation; **B,** protracted descent pattern with maximum slope of descent less than prescribed critical limits of normal. These labor aberrations are similar to each other in many ways and frequently occur together in the same patient. They are clearly different from the average normal dilatation and descent patterns *(broken lines)*. (Reproduced with permission from Friedman, E.A.: Labor: clinical evaluation and management, ed. 2, New York, 1978, Appleton-Century-Crofts, Inc.)

thought as to how to manage the labor continuation. According to Friedman (1978a) and O'Brien and Cefalo (1982a), labor stimulants such as oxytocin are of no benefit, and they recommend treating the patient with IV fluid to prevent dehydration and electrolyte imbalance, providing emotional support, and monitoring closely for arrest of descent. Other obstetricians recommend the use of a labor stimulant, especially if the contractions are hypotonic. According to Oxorn (1980), in about 70% of these patients the cervix will dilate slowly but the labor will proceed, and they will deliver spontaneously or with the use of low forceps. About 20% will require midforceps, and only 10% will have to be delivered by cesarean.

Arrest disorders (Fig. 17-10). Secondary arrest of dilatation is characterized by cessation of dilatation in active labor before full dilatation occurs and continues for at least 2 hours. This abnormal labor pattern is frequently associated with hypotonic uterine contractions.

Arrest of descent is characterized by cessation of descent in active labor but most often in the second stage of labor for longer than 1 hour in the multipara and 2 hours in the nullipara. Failure of descent occurs when the onset of descent fails to occur during the deceleration phase of active labor.

According to Friedman (1978a), approximately 45% of these patients experience fetopelvic disproportion (FPD). Excessive sedation, early conduction anesthesia, uterine exhaustion, and fetal malpresentations such as persistent

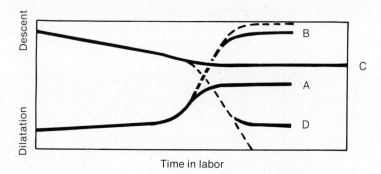

FIG. 17-10. Arrest disorders of labor. **A,** Secondary arrest of dilatation pattern with documented cessation of progression in the active phase; **B,** prolonged deceleration phase pattern with deceleration phase duration greater than normal limits; **C,** failure of descent in the deceleration phase and second stage; **D,** arrest of descent characterized by halted advancement of fetal station in the second stage. These four abnormalities are similar in etiology, response to treatment, and prognosis, being readily differentiated from the normal dilatation and descent curves *(broken lines)*. (Reproduced with permission from Friedman, E.A.: Labor: clinical evaluation and management, ed. 2, New York, 1978, Appleton-Century-Crofts, Inc.)

occiput posterior, occiput transverse, face, or brow presentations are other causes.

If FPD is present, delivery is always by cesarean. If FPD cannot be documented, it is fairly well agreed upon that the treatment of choice is to stimulate labor with oxytocin and monitor the labor and fetus closely. The prognosis is good that the patient will be able to deliver vaginally if the postarrest slope is as great or greater than the prearrest slope. According to O'Brien and Cefalo (1982a), 80% of these patients will deliver vaginally. If arrest persists or fetal distress develops, the patient should be delivered by a cesarean immediately.

Precipitous labor (Fig. 17-11). On the other side of the spectrum is precipitous labor. In the nullipara, diagnosis is made when the cervix dilates faster than 5 cm/hr or the descent is faster than 1 cm every 12 minutes. In the multipara, diagnosis is made when the cervix dilates faster than 10 cm/hr or the descent is faster than 1 cm every 6 minutes.

Currently there is no effective treatment for slowing uterine contractions. Magnesium sulfate and terbutaline have been tried but have not proven effective. Treatment should center around preventing the possible complications such as fetal intracranial bleeding or maternal lacerations because the mother's body may not have time to stretch to accommodate the passage of the fetus. This is done by controlling and guiding the fetal head over the perineum. No attempt should be made, however, to forcibly slow the descent.

Table 17-1 summarizes the types, possible causes, and treatments for each of these dysfunctional labor patterns.

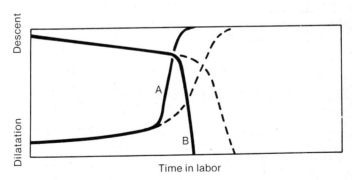

FIG. 17-11. Precipitate labor patterns. Precipitate dilatation **(A)** and precipitate descent **(B)** are defined by their excessively rapid rates of progressive cervical dilatation and fetal descent, respectively, which distinguish them from the course of normal labor *(broken lines)*. (Reproduced with permission from Friedman, E.A.: Labor: clinical evaluation and management, ed. 2, New York, 1978, Appleton-Century-Crofts, Inc.)

TABLE 17-1. *Summary of abnormal labor patterns*

Type	Definition	Cause in order of frequency	Treatment

Prolonged latent phase	Nullipara:
	  Latent phase of labor continues for longer than 20 hr
	
	Multipara:
	  Latent phase of labor continues for longer than 14 hr
		1. Inhibitory effect of early administration of a narcotic, analgesic, or sedatives
		2. Unripe cervix at onset of labor—thick, uneffaced, rigid cervix
		3. Anxiety or fear
		4. False labor
		5. Early administration of regional anesthesia
		6. Abnormal position of the fetus
		7. Fetopelvic disproportion
			After 12 hr of no progress:
			1. Reevaluate
			2. If cervix is closed and rigid, therapeutic rest will be attempted with administration of large doses of a narcotic analgesic such as morphine for the purpose of inhibiting contractions and providing a rest period of 4 to 6 hr.
			3. If the patient was in false labor, when she awakens her contractions will be gone; otherwise she will usually awaken in active labor; Only 5% awaken to the original problem
			4. If cervix is soft labor can be stimulated with a labor stimulant
			5. Outcome: most patients progress to active labor and deliver vaginally

Protraction disorders:
  Protracted active phase dilatation
  Protracted descent
	Nullipara:
	  Rate of dilatation in the active phase is less than 1.2 cm/hr or rate of descent is less than 1.0 cm/hr
	
	Multipara:
	  Rate of dilatation in the active phase is less than 1.5 cm/hr or rate of descent is less than 1.0 cm/hr
		1. Fetopelvic disproportion
		2. Excessive sedation
		3. Fetal malpresentation
		4. Early conduction anesthesia
		5. Rupture of membranes prior to the onset of labor
			1. Rule out fetopelvic disproportion (FPD)
			2. If FPD patient will be delivered by cesarean
			3. Expectant management consisting of a trial of labor and close assessment is the choice of treatment for all other patients as long as mother and fetus remain in good condition; this includes:
			  a. continuous monitoring of the labor progress and for fetal well-being
			  b. providing physical and emotional support
			  c. keeping patient informed and allaying anxiety

			d. assessing fluid and electrolyte needs and administering intravenous fluids as ordered
			4. A labor stimulant may or may not be used
			5. The use of excessive sedation or conduction anesthesia can inhibit or arrest the labor further
			6. Outcome: of these patients, two-thirds dilate the cervix slowly and proceed to vaginal delivery spontaneously or with use of low forceps; about 20% require midforceps and 10% require delivery by cesarean
Arrest disorders:		1. Fetopelvic disproportion (accounts for nearly 45%)	1. Assess for fetopelvic disproportion and fetal malpresentation
Secondary arrest of dilatation	Progressive dilatation during active labor stops before full dilatation occurs and continues for 2 hr or longer	2. Excessive sedation	2. Assess for other factors, such as excessive sedation and conduction anesthesia
		3. Fetal malpositions (persistent occiput, face, and brow)	3. If FPD delivery will be by cesarean
		4. Conduction anesthesia	4. If FPD is not indicated a labor stimulant will probably be used; the postarrest slope should be monitored closely; if FPD is not present the postarrest slope should be as great or greater than the prearrest slope
Arrest of descent	Progressive descent stops during the second stage of labor for longer than 1 hr in the multipara and longer than 2 hr in the nullipara	5. Exhausted uterus	5. Monitor fluid and electrolyte needs
			6. If arrest persists or fetal distress develops delivery must be by cesarean
Failure of descent	Onset of descent fails to occur during the deceleration phase of labor		7. If second stage arrest persists for more than 2 hr in the nullipara and 1 hr in the multipara usually delivery is by cesarean

Data from Friedman, E.: Labor: Clinical evaluation and management, ed. 2, New York, 1978, Appleton-Century-Crofts and Oxorn, H.: Human labor and birth, ed. 4, New York, 1980, Appleton-Century-Crofts.

Continued.

TABLE 17-1. Summary of abnormal labor patterns—cont'd

Type	Definition	Cause in order of frequency	Treatment
Failure of descent—cont'd			8. Outcome: a labor stimulant will be effective in facilitating dilatation and fetal descent in 80% of these cases; however, 30% of these cases will require forceps during the vaginal delivery and 20% will require a cesarean delivery
Precipitous labor	Nullipara: The cervix dilates faster than 5 cm/hr or the descent is faster than 1 cm/12 min Multipara: The cervix dilates faster than 10 cm/hr or the descent is faster than 1 cm/6 min	1. Abnormally low cervical resistance 2. Abnormally strong uterine or abdominal muscular contractions	No effective treatment is available; magnesium sulfate and terbutaline have been tried

Fetal malpresentations

The manner in which the fetus presents also influences the outcome and manner of treatment. Table 17-2 outlines the various fetal malpresentations and the appropriate treatments.

External cephalic version

External cephalic version is an old technique that is being considered once again as a possible treatment for abnormal presentations, especially breech presentations. It consists of converting an unfavorable presentation to a vertex presentation by an external maneuver prior to labor to avoid the need for a cesarean delivery.

Complications such as abruptio placentae or cord strangulation made this procedure unsafe in the past. Now with the use of (1) ultrasound to visualize the placenta site in order to avoid any force against it and to evaluate the adequacy of amniotic fluid, (2) a tocolytic agent such as terbutaline or ritodrine to relax the uterus and facilitate manipulation, and (3) a fetal monitor to detect any fetal distress immediately the technique is being reevaluated as to its usefulness.

The procedure is usually done between 37 and 40 weeks of gestation in a very controlled environment where a cesarean delivery could be performed immediately if indicated. An ultrasound examination is carried out, blood is drawn for a complete blood count and blood type, an intravenous infusion is started with an 18-gauge intracatheter, and a 15 to 30 minute fetal monitor strip is obtained to determine the baseline fetal heart rate prior to the version. The tocolytic agent should be prepared in the same manner and concentration as that used for tocolysis in preterm labor and piggybacked into the main IV line. The usual rate is 5 μg/min of terbutaline and 100 μg/min of ritodrine. Fetal heart rate should be monitored every 5 minutes, or as ordered, during the procedure. On completion of the procedure, the IV tocolytic drug should be discontinued and the external fetal monitor reapplied to assess the fetal heart rate pattern and to assess for the development of uterine contractions.

If the version is successful, greater than 90% of the fetuses will present in labor in a vertex presentation (Van Dorsten et al., 1981). This procedure decreases the rate of cesarean deliveries.

NURSING PROCESS
Prevention

False labor can easily be confused with true labor. Patients should be evaluated carefully when they come into the labor and delivery area to determine whether or not they are really in true labor. If the patient is in false labor and does not demonstrate any complications, she should be sent home and en-

TABLE 17-2. *Fetal malpresentations*

	Occiput posterior	Face	Brow	Shoulder	Compound presentation	Breech
Definition	When the fetal occiput lies in either the right or left posterior quadrant of the mother's pelvis	The presenting head is completely extended	The presenting head is midway between full flexion and extreme extension	When the fetal spine is lying vertical to the mother's spine	When one or more of the fetal extremities is accompanying the presenting part	When the buttocks of the fetus present in one of three attitudes: Frank: the thighs are flexed and the legs lie alongside the fetal body. Complete: the fetus's legs are flexed at the thighs allowing the feet to present with the buttocks. Footling: One or both thighs are extended and present before the buttocks
Presenting part	Occiput (vertex)	Chin (mentum)	Brow	Scapula		Sacrum
Incidence	10% to 15%	0.2%	0.1%	0.33%	0.1%	4%
Etiology	Narrow midplane of the pelvis. Anthropoid type of pelvis	Parity greater than 5. Pelvic contraction. Large for gestational age. Anencephaly. Prematurity	FPD (most common). Parity greater than 5. Large for gestational age. Prematurity. Pendulous abdomen	Parity greater than 5. FPD related to pelvic contraction. Placenta previa. Prematurity. Pendulous abdomen	Prematurity. Parity greater than 5. FPD related to pelvic contraction. Large for gestational age. Polyhydramnios. Placenta previa	Prematurity. Placenta previa. Anything that interferes with the fetal accommodation to the uterus such as hydrocephaly, hydramnios, and parity greater than 5

Diagnosis: Leopold's maneuver	The patient will often complain of severe back pain Differentiation by Leopold's maneuver is difficult	Absence of a smooth, flexed spine Prominent extremities and head	No differentiation	Abdomen may look wider than it does long The head can be palpated on one side of the mother's abdomen and the buttocks on the other side	No differentiation	Fetal heart tones heard best above the umbilicus; fetal head is palpated in the upper part of the uterus
Vaginal exam	Anterior fontanelle can be felt in the anterior quadrant of the mother's pelvis and the posterior fontanelle in the posterior quadrant	A nose, eyes, and mouth can be felt	Anterior fontanelle can be felt in the center of the cervical opening with the eyes on one side	The scapula can be felt or no presenting part reached since it is often high	Fetal extremity felt alongside the presenting part	A soft presenting part is felt
Treatment	Almost all fetuses rotate spontaneously to an anterior position and are delivered vaginally; in the 10% that do not rotate completely rotation is usually done with forceps. If a posterior position persists without progress, a cesarean delivery is done	Vaginal delivery if anterior rotation of the chin occurs. Cesarean delivery is done if chin is directed posterior and progress stops	Vaginal delivery if the brow presentation converts by flexion to an occiput presentation or by extension to a face presentation. Cesarean delivery if the brow presentation persists	Cesarean delivery is the best management; external cephalic version can be attempted under very controlled circumstances if placenta previa or FPD is not present	Vaginal delivery unless cord prolapses or labor fails to progress. Immediate cesarean delivery if prolapse cord develops or progress stops	Vaginal delivery in a frank breech, with adequate pelvis without hyperextension of the head, gestational age greater than 36 weeks, and estimated fetal weight between 2,500 and 3,500 gm; external cephalic version can be attempted under very controlled circumstances. Cesarean delivery for all others because of increased risk of cord prolapse, entrapment by the cervix due to small trunk to head ratio in a premature or small for gestational age infant, and FPD in a fetus over 3,800 gm

Data from Seeds, J., and Céfalo, R.: Malpresentation, Clinical Obstetrics and Gynecology 25(1):145, 1982; and Cruikshank, D., and White, C.: Obstetric malpresentations: Twenty years' experience, Am. J. Obstet. Gynecol. 116(8):1097, 1973.

couraged to maintain a balance between activity and rest. Once in true labor, the nurse should assist the patient with relaxation and in using effective distraction tools such as breathing and focal point. This will strengthen the patient's coping ability and prevent or put off the need for sedation and conduction anesthesia until labor has been well established. Thus arrest of labor related to early administration of a sedative or conduction anesthesia can be prevented.

Dehydration should be avoided; it can cause ineffective uterine activity. Since the gastrointestinal function is slowed or stopped during labor, an IV infusion should be started on all patients who are in labor for more than 6 hours to prevent a dysfunctional labor related to dehydration.

Any patient in labor should be encouraged to change her position at least every 30 minutes to 1 hour. Walking, sitting, or side lying are all positions that may enhance the effectiveness of uterine contractions and should be encouraged. When a patient is positioned on her back during labor, the frequency of contractions usually increases but the intensity decreases. If the patient maintains a standing, sitting, or side lying position during labor, the frequency of contractions usually decrease but the intensity increases (Roberts et al., 1983). This facilitates fetal oxygenation while enhancing labor. During second-stage labor, the mother's position and her method of breathing can also facilitate the progress and outcome of labor. The traditional supine position requires the woman to push against gravity, impairs the blood supply to the fetus and the mother's kidneys, and narrows the vaginal opening. Side lying, squatting, sitting on a birthing chair, or semisitting (in which the woman's body is in a C position with her legs bent, relaxed, and apart) avoids these hazards and decreases the risk of impaired fetal descent. While the woman utilizes these various positions, she should be encouraged to use the slow breath release method of pushing. This is done by taking two to three deep inhalations, then holding her breath for a few seconds to fix the abdominal muscles. This is followed by slowly exhaling through pursed lips. These steps are repeated until the urge to push is gone. The woman should also be instructed to use her abdominal muscles to push while relaxing her pelvic floor muscles. Tense facial muscles are a sign of a tight pelvic floor (McKay, 1981, 1984).

Because a full bladder or rectum can slow the descent of the fetus, the patient should be encouraged to empty her bladder every 30 minutes or at least every hour.

Assessment

The patient's progress in labor should be monitored continuously to detect early signs of dysfunctional labor. First, the uterine contraction pattern should be followed closely for frequency and duration with the use of a fetal monitor. The intraamniotic pressure is assessed if an internal fetal monitor is being used.

This adds helpful information as to the resting tone and intensity or strength of the uterine contractions. Uterine contractions of an intensity of 30 mm Hg or greater initiate cervical dilatation. During active labor, the intensity usually reaches 50 to 80 mm Hg. During the second stage of labor, the intensity can peak at 100 mm Hg. Resting tone is normally between 5 and 10 mm Hg in early labor and between 12 and 14 mm Hg in active labor.

Next the nurse must monitor the patient's progress through the stages of labor. To do this, the nurse should periodically assess the cervix for consistency and amount of dilatation and effacement. Fetal position, station, and status of the presenting part is determined by a sterile vaginal examination. Sterile vaginal examinations should be done as often as is consistent with the progress being made. If progress is rapid, every hour might be appropriate, but every 2 to 4 hours might be adequate if progress is slow. The amount of dilatation and the fetal station found on examination should be graphed on the normal labor curve. Friedman (1970) developed an evaluation tool after graphically plotting the relationship of time to station and dilatation of many patients in labor. He developed a normal labor curve for nulliparas and one for multiparas (see Fig. 17-7).

This method of evaluation can be instituted by using square ruled graph paper. Across the top, the nurse should number the hours the patient is in labor from left to right using hourly intervals. The vertical side should be numbered from 1 to 10 in ascending order to indicate dilatation in centimeters and from -1 to $+5$ in descending order to indicate station. According to Friedman (1980), dilatation is indicated by small circles and station by small Xs, each connected with a straight line. The normal labor curve for a nullipara and a multipara should appear on the graph for easy comparison (Fig. 17-12).

On admission, the patient is asked when regular contractions began and this time is the first time interval entered on the graph. Each time a vaginal exam is performed, the dilatation and station are recorded under that hour on the graph.

Once the nurse recognizes a deviation from the normal labor pattern, the patient should be immediately assessed for the possible cause and the attending health care provider should be notified. To determine a possible cause, the following data should be collected.

1. Whether or not the bladder or rectum is full
2. State of the cervix, whether soft or hard, effaced or long, dilatable or resistent, and amount of dilatation
3. Engagement of presenting part and presence of molding
4. Position of fetus
5. Uterine contractions as to type, strength, and coordination
6. Level of maternal anxiety and fatigue
7. Signs of dehydration

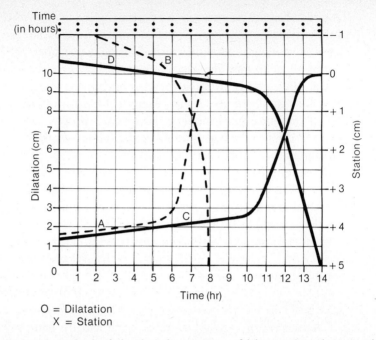

FIG. 17-12. A method of charting the progress of labor against the normal labor curves. **A,** Normal dilatation for the multigravida; **B,** normal fetal descent for the multigravida; **C,** normal dilatation for the primigravida; **D,** normal fetal descent for the primigravida. (Modified from Friedman, E.: An objective method of evaluating labor, Hospital Pract. **5**(7):82, 1970.)

The fetus should be monitored continuously throughout labor because uterine contractions actually decrease or stop intervillous blood flow. Whether or not this causes fetal hypoxia depends on the fetus's reserve going into labor and the strength, duration, and resting tone of the uterine contractions during labor. Therefore during a dysfunctional labor the risk of fetal distress is even greater. For example, hypertonic uterine contractions can lead to fetal hypoxia; the frequently and intensely contracting uterus prevents the placenta from filling adequately with oxygenated blood. Any malpresentation increases the risk of cord prolapse. Therefore in any patient who develops a dysfunctional labor the fetal heart rate should be monitored continuously, preferably with an internal monitor. The color of the amniotic fluid should also be noted because the passage of meconium indicates fetal distress. However, in a breech presentation meconium-stained amniotic fluid does not always indicate fetal distress; pressure on the buttocks may cause the anal sphincter to relax.

Complications that can develop during a dysfunctional labor are (1) a uterine infection, (2) fatigue and exhaustion, (3) dehydration, (4) hypoglycemia, and (5) uterine rupture. Any patient whose labor is prolonged for any reason has an increased risk of a uterine infection, especially if the membranes are ruptured. The patient's temperature should be assessed every 2 hours. The linen should be changed often and the perineal area kept clean. A prolonged difficult labor depletes the mother's energy and stores of glucose. Fatigue, exhaustion, dehydration, and hypoglycemia can result. Any of these factors can accentuate abnormal uterine activity and compound uterine dystocia. Therefore all patients experiencing a dysfunctional labor should receive IV glucose to prevent hypoglycemia and dehydration. They should also be supported in every way possible and be encouraged to rest between contractions to conserve their energy.

Uterine rupture should never occur when the labor is being monitored appropriately. If the passage of the fetus is impossible through the pelvis, it will be demonstrated by a persistent abnormal labor pattern. When this occurs, a cesarean delivery should be performed without delay. Impending rupture would be manifested as a pathologic retraction ring called *Bandl's ring*. Normally there is a physiologic retraction ring that develops during labor where the upper and lower uterine segments juncture. In the event of an obstruction, this normal physiologic retraction ring will develop into a pathologic retraction ring and be felt just below the umbilicus, or be seen as an abdominal indentation. An obstructed labor causes this ring due to increased thinning of the lower uterine segment and signifies impending rupture.

Intrapartum intervention

The most helpful method of detecting dysfunctional labor is to compare each phase of the patient's labor to the established labor pattern. Any significant deviation should be reported to the attending physician. If fetopelvic disproportion is known to be present, delivery by cesarean is the only treatment of choice and the nurse should prepare the patient. For all other patients, a trial labor will be the choice of treatment, and this should be explained to the patient. When a trial labor is being carried out to determine FPD, a definite time limit should be set. FPD should be suspected after 3 to 4 hours of no progress when a labor stimulant is being used or 6 to 12 hours of no progress if a labor stimulant is not being used. In these cases the nurse should notify the attending physician and be prepared for a cesarean delivery. If hypotonic uterine contractions are the cause without fetopelvic disproportion or a persistent fetal malpresentation, labor can be facilitated with a labor stimulant and the nurse should be prepared to carry this out.

When fetal presentation is the causative factor, many times the presentation converts to normal and a vaginal delivery is possible. With a face presentation, there is an 88% chance that the chin (mentum) will rotate anteriorly and vaginal delivery will be possible. For an early brow presentation, there is a 70%

chance it will convert to an anterior face or vertex presentation and vaginal delivery will ensue. Almost all occiput posterior presentations will convert to occiput anterior presentations making vaginal delivery possible (Cruikshank and White, 1973).

For these conversions to take place, time must be allowed. Labor is usually allowed to proceed as long as progress is being made. The maximum time a nullipara is allowed to labor in the second stage is usually 2 hours and 1 hour for a multipara. At that time the nurse should be prepared for a possible forceps or cesarean delivery. Because the labor will be longer than normal, the patient needs continous support and encouragement to promote uterine effectiveness and continuous fluids because dehydration can cause hypotonic contractions. Because a full bladder interferes with fetal descent, the nurse should encourage the patient to empty her bladder frequently, approximately every 30 minutes to 1 hour. When the patient is completely dilated, the nurse should encourage effective voluntary pushing with contractions accompanied with relaxation of the pelvic flood to facilitate the descent. As the head crowns and the patient experiences a burning, stretching sensation, she should push more gently (Simkin, 1982).

Severe back pain often accompanies an occiput posterior or transverse position as the fetus's head presses against the mother's sacrum. Back rubs or pressure low to the back are sometimes helpful. Placing the patient in a knee-chest position for several contractions and encouraging her to do the pelvic tilt or placing her on the side opposite to which the fetal occiput is directed can facilitate the internal rotation. Squatting and kneeling are other positions effective in promoting fetal head rotation (McKay, 1984; Andrews and Andrews, 1983).

In the event of a breech presentation, the following principles should be kept in mind.

1. The patient should understand the risks of a vaginal delivery such as cerebral hemorrhage (because the head must mold in a minute rather than taking hours) and a prolapsed cord. In a footling breech presentation, the risk for prolapsed cord is 20 times greater. However, in a frank breech presentation, the risk is not increased.
2. Cesarean birth is always a possibility even if a vaginal delivery is to be attempted, and the patient should be prepared for this.
3. Blood should be available for a possible transfusion.
4. An anesthesiologist or nurse anesthetist should be present in an attempted vaginal delivery as well as at a cesarean delivery in order to administer general anesthesia with uterine relaxants in case the fetal head becomes entrapped following the delivery of the body.
5. Right angle retractors should be included in the delivery room set up for

a breech vaginal delivery to facilitate fetal breathing if the fetal head does become entrapped.

During any long, difficult labor, the patient needs a lot of emotional support. Someone should be with the patient at all times, instructing her in an effective breathing technique, helping her to relax, eliminating such extraneous discomforts as dry lips and mouth, back pain, and feelings of hot and cold, and encouraging her frequently. The nurse should also encourage her to rest between contractions. These patients will wonder about what is going on, why the labor is taking so long, and how all this will affect their baby. Explanations should be given and the treatment plan outlined so that the patient and her significant other will be prepared for what might occur.

Postpartum intervention

The mother should be observed closely during the early postpartum period for hemorrhage. A uterus that does not contract effectively during labor often does not contract well after delivery either. At the same time, a difficult delivery can cause lacerations, which might manifest themselves as bright red bleeding during the postpartum period. Thus the amount of bleeding should be assessed by counting the number of perineal pads saturated and by appraising the pulse, respiration, and blood pressure. The vaginal discharge should also be evaluated as to color and the presence of clots or tissue.

There is an increased risk of infection following a long, difficult labor, especially if the membranes were ruptured for longer than 12 hours. The nurse should check the odor of the vaginal discharge every 8 hours and check the patient's temperature every 4 hours for the first 48 hours. The physician should be notified if the temperature rises above 38° C or 100.4° F.

A long, difficult labor that ended with a surgical intervention can leave the mother exhausted and feeling like she has failed. The nurse should allow the patient time to express these feelings and to discuss her labor and delivery experience. She should also be encouraged to rest. A sedative may help her to relax and get this much-needed rest.

Evaluation

The ultimate goal for any patient during labor is progression of labor within the normal labor curve with no fetal distress. The nurse can facilitate this by removing all extraneous variables that might hamper or interfere with labor progress. There are other factors, however, that can impede labor that the nurse has no control over. These the nurse must assess for, and she should report any signs of their development to the attending health care provider immediately. The medical team should then work together to facilitate the labor and delivery for the best maternal and neonatal outcome.

Dysfunctional labor

Potential patient problem	*Outcome criteria*
Intrapartum care	
A. Potential dysfunctional labor related to: Uterine dystocia Fetal dystocia Pelvic dystocia	Progression of labor according to the normal labor pattern

O F N U R S I N G C A R E

Assessment and intervention

Dx. Determine onset of true labor
Plot and compare the patient's labor with the normal labor pattern
Assess contractions as to frequency, intensity, duration, type, and coordination every 30 min
Assess state of cervix as to soft or hard, effaced or long, dilatable or resistant, and amount of dilatation as indicated (depending on phase of labor)
Assess for a malpresentation by doing a Leopold's maneuver
Assess for distended bladder every 2 hr
Assess level of anxiety
Assess for signs of discomfort and tension
Assess for signs of dehydration and electrolyte imbalance
Assess for signs of hypoglycemia

Th. Encourage patient to void every hour
Catheterize for distended bladder if unable to void
Encourage patient to verbalize anxieties and fears
Encourage patient to change positions every 30 min to 1 hr
Monitor for effective use of breathing and relaxation techniques
Be supportive of coping methods and provide help with new ones as needed
Provide support to labor coach
Encourage rest between contractions
Monitor intravenous fluids as ordered
Provide comfort techniques such as
    back rubs
    position with pillows
    cold cloth to neck
    treat chapped lips
Be prepared to administer a labor stimulant as ordered (see Suggested Plan of Nursing Care for labor stimulation)
If fetus is in an occiput posterior position:
    administer frequent back rubs
    apply pressure to low back
    position patient on her side opposite which the occiput is directed
    place patient in a knee chest position for a few contractions to encourage rotation

Ed. Explain all procedures
Keep patient and significant others informed of progress
Explain need for withholding analgesia and anesthesia in early labor
Explain need for empty bowel and bladder
Teach coach and patient breathing and relaxation techniques if needed
Teach patient the importance of not lying on her back during labor

---

Dx., diagnostic; Th., therapeutic; Ed., education; Ref., referral.   *Continued.*

Dysfunctional labor—cont'd

Potential patient problem	*Outcome criteria*
Intrapartum care **A.** Potential dysfunctional labor related to: 　　Uterine dystocia 　　Fetal dystocia 　　Pelvic dystocia—*cont'd*	Progression of labor according to the normal labor pattern
B. Potential uterine infection related to: 　　A long difficult labor	Temperature below 38° C No foul-smelling amniotic fluid WBC below 16,000 mm³
C. Potential anxiety related to: 　　A long, difficult labor 　　Fear of neonatal outcome	Verbalizes fears and concerns Participates in decisions affecting care
D. Potential fetal distress related to: 　　Uteroplacental insufficiency 　　Cord compression 　　Supine hypotension syndrome	FHR baseline remains between 120 and 160 No ominous periodic FHR changes Long- and short-term variability present

Assessment and intervention

Ref. Notify physician immediately of abnormal labor progress:
    Nullipara:
        no progress after 6 to 8 hr in the latent phase of labor
        rate of dilatation in the active phase less than 1.2 cm/hr
        rate of descent in the active phase less than 1 cm/hr
        arrest of progress for 2 hr or more
    Multipara:
        no progress after 6 to 8 hr in the latent phase of labor
        rate of dilatation in the active phase less than 1.5 cm/hr
        rate of descent in the active phase less than 1 cm/hr
        arrest of progress for 1 hr
    Notify physician of signs of hypoglycemia
    Notify nursery and pediatrician of possible high-risk neonate

Dx. Check temperature every 4 hr
    Assess amniotic fluid for foul odor
    Refer to such laboratory data as WBC
Th. Keep patient clean and dry
    Change linen as needed
    Use only sterile gloves when doing a vaginal exam
Ref. Notify physician if
        temperature develops over 38° C
        amniotic fluid develops a foul odor
        WBC is greater than 16,000 mm^3

Dx. Assess parent(s) level of fear, anxiety, and concerns
Th. Encourage parent(s) to express fears and concerns
    Keep parent(s) informed of the cause, if known, and the treatment plan

Dx. Assess FHR with external or internal fetal monitor; note changes in baseline, loss of beat to beat variability, or the presence of late or variable decelerations
    Assess amniotic fluid for meconium and blood stain
Th. Encourage patient to lie in a lateral recumbent or semi-Fowler position
Ref. Notify physician of any signs of fetal distress such as
        periodic late or severe variable decelerations
        increase or decrease in FHR baseline

Continued.

Dysfunctional labor—cont'd

Potential patient problem	Outcome criteria
E. Potential uterine rupture related to: A prolonged obstructed labor	No Bandl's ring develops

F. Potential surgical intervention related to:
    Persistent malpresentation
    FPD
	No surgical complications
	Mother expresses positive feeling of birth experience
	Physically and neurologically healthy newborn
	Apgar score of 7 to 10

G. Potential precipitous labor related to:
    Abnormally low cervical resistance
    Abnormally strong uterine contractions
	Delivery without lacerations
	Delivery without birth trauma

Assessment and intervention

Dx. Assess progress of labor
Assess for a Bandl's ring by observing for an indentation on the abdomen
Assess intensity of uterine contractions
Th. Compare labor progress according to the normal labor pattern
Ref. Notify physician of an abnormal labor progress

Dx. Assess parent(s) knowledge regarding cesarean delivery
Th. Prepare for cesarean delivery by:
    Shaving from the xiphoid process to the pubic area
    Inserting a Foley catheter and connecting it to continuous drainage when
        ordered
    Checking to see if lab work is done such as CBC, blood typed and cross
        matched for 2 units, and urinalysis
    Administering Maalox or other antacid as needed to prevent reflux of acid
        into lungs during surgery
    Starting an intravenous infusion with an 18-gauge intracatheter
    Completing routine preoperative protocol such as:
        NPO except medications
        remove dentures, contact lenses, and fingernail polish
        tape or remove rings
        lock up valuables
        obtain signed consent
        staying with patient to decrease feeling of abandonment
        allowing patient to ventilate fears
Ed. Instruct as to what to expect
Ref. Notify nursery and pediatrician of cesarean birth

Dx. Compare progress of labor to the normal labor curve
Th. Prepare for delivery
If physician is not in attendance:
    reassure patient
    support fetal head and perineal area
    instruct to pant, not push, on delivery of fetal head
Ref. Notify physician if labor is progressing faster than normal

Continued.

Dysfunctional labor—cont'd

Potential patient problem	Outcome criteria
Postpartum care	
A. Potential hemorrhage related to: Ineffective uterine contractions	Vital signs stable for patient No more than two pads saturated in 1 hr Fundus firm
B. Potential infection related to: A long, difficult labor	Temperature less than 38° C (100.4° F) No foul-smelling lochia

REFERENCES

Abell, D.: Brow presentation, South Afr. Med. J. **47:**1315, 1973.

Andrews, C., and Andrews, E.: Nursing, maternal postures, and fetal position, Nursing Res. **32**(6):336, 1983.

Arcarese, J., and Morrison, J.: The utilization of x-ray pelvimetry in the United States, Clin. Obstet. Gynecol. **25:**165, 1982.

Barton, J., and Garbaciak, J.: Is x-ray pelvimetry necessary? Contemp. Obstet. Gynecol. **13**(6):27, 1979.

Barton, J., Garbaciak, J., and Ryan, G.: The efficacy of x-ray pelvimetry, Am. J. Obstet. Gynecol. **143:**304, 1982.

Collea, J.: Current management of breech presentation, Clin. Obstet. Gynecol. **23:**525, 1980.

Collea, J., and others: The randomized management of term frank breech presentation: vaginal delivery vs. cesarean section, Am. J. Obstet. Gynecol. **131:**186, 1978.

Cruikshank, D., and White, C.: Obstetric malpresentations: Twenty years' experience, Am. J. Obstet. Gynecol. **116:**1097, 1973.

Currie, W.B.: Physiology of uterine activity, Clin. Obstet. Gynecol. **23:**33, 1980.

Friedman, E.: Use of labor pattern as a management guide, Hospital Topics **46**(8):57, 1969.

Friedman, E.: An objective method of evaluating labor, Hospital Pract. **5**(7):82, 1970.

Friedman, E.: Patterns of labor as indicators of risk, Clin. Obstet. Gynecol. **16:**172, 1973.

Assessment and intervention

Dx. Record blood pressure, pulse, and respiration every 15 min eight times, every
      30 min two times, every 4 hr two times, then routinely
     Check firmness of uterus and vaginal flow with each vital sign check
     Keep a pad count
Th. Encourage patient to empty bladder every 4 hr
     Manually massage a relaxed, boggy fundus very gently until firm
     Maintain oxytocics and intravenous fluids as ordered
Ref. Notify physician if uterus fails to contract or stay contracated with massage

Dx. Check temperature every 4 hr for 48 hr; if greater than 38° C (100.4° F)
     check every 2 hr
     Check lochia every shift for odor
Th. Use aseptic technique in care of patient
Ed. Explain perineal care and good hand washing
Ref. Notify physician if temperature elevated over 38° C (100.4° F) or if any
     other signs of infection develop

Friedman, E.: Labor: clinical evaluation and management, ed. 2, New York, 1978a, Appleton-Century-Crofts, Inc.

Friedman, E.: Labor management updated, J. Reprod. Med. **20**:59, 1978b.

Friedman, E.: Failure to progress in labor. In Queenan, J., editor, Management of high-risk pregnancy, Oradell, N.J., 1980, Medical Economics Books, Inc.

Friedman, E.: Assessing labor progression. In Friedman, E., editor: Obstetrical decision making, Saint Louis, 1982a, The C.V. Mosby Co.

Friedman, E.: Prolonged latent phase. In Friedman, E., editor, Obstetrical decision making, Saint Louis, 1982b, The C.V. Mosby Co.

Friedman, E.: Protraction disorders. In Friedman, E., editor: Obstetrical decision making, Saint Louis, 1982c, The C.V. Mosby Co.

Friedman, E.: Arrest disorders. In Friedman, E., editor, Obstetrical decision making, Saint Louis, 1982d, The C.V. Mosby Co.

Friedman, E.: Whither midforceps? its place in ob today, Contemp. Obstet. Gynecol. **17**(2):85, 1983.

Friedman, E., Sachtleben, M., and Bresky, P.: Dysfunctional labor, Am. J. Obstet. Gynecol. **127**:779, 1977.

Gimovsky, M., and Paul, R.: Singleton breech presentation in labor: experience in 1980, Am. J. Obstet. Gynecol. **143**:733, 1983.

Harbert, G.: Uterine contractions, Clin. Obstet. Gynecol. **25**:177, 1982.

Jaffa, A., and others: Management of term breech presentation in primigravidae, Obstet. Gynecol. Surv. **37**(4):243, 1981.

Joyce, D., Giwa-Osagie, F., and Stevenson, G.: Role of pelvimetry in active management of labour, Br. Med. J. **4:**505, 1975.

Karp, L., and others: The premature breech: trial of labor or cesarean section? Obstet. Gynecol. **53:**88, 1979.

Koontz, W., and Bishop, E.: Management of the latent phase of labor, Clin. Obstet. Gynecol. **25:**111, 1982.

Laube, D., Varner, M., and Cruikshank, D.: A prospective evaluation of x-ray pelvimetry, Obstet. Gynecol. Surv. **37**(6):399, 1981.

Main, D., Main, E., and Maurer, M.: Cesarean section versus vaginal delivery for the breech fetus weighing less than 1,500 grams, Am. J. Obstet. Gynecol. **146:**580, 1983.

Mann, L., and Gallant, J.: Modern management of the breech delivery, Am. J. Obstet. Gynecol. **134:**611, 1979.

McKay, S.: Maternal position during labor and birth: a reassessment, JOGN Nursing **9**(5):288, 1980.

McKay, S.: Second stage labor: has tradition replaced safety? AJN **81:**1016, 1981.

McKay, S.: Squatting: An alternate position for the second stage of labor, MCN **9**(3):181, 1984.

Moerman, M.: Growth of the birth canal in adolescent girls, Am. J. Obstet. Gynecol. **143:**528, 1982.

Monheit, A., Resnik, R.: Cesarean section: current trends and perspectives, Clin. Perinatol. **8:**101, 1981.

O'Brien, W., and Cefalo, R.: Abnormalities of the active phase: recognition and treatment, Clin. Obstet. Gynecol. **25:**115, 1982a.

O'Brien, W., and Cefalo, R.: Evaluation of x-ray pelvimetry and abnormal labor, Clin. Obstet. Gynecol. **25:**157, 1982b.

Ott, W.: Relationship of normal and abnormal late labor patterns to perinatal mortality, Clin. Obstet. Gynecol. **25:**105, 1982.

Oxorn, H.: Human labor and birth, ed. 4, New York, 1980, Appleton-Century-Crofts, Inc.

Phillips, R., and Freeman, M.: The management of the persistent occiput posterior position, Obstet. Gynecol. **43:**171, 1974.

Quilligan, F.J.: Response to discussant of the randomized management of term frank breech presentation: a study of 208 cases, Am. J. Obstet. Gynecol. **137:**242, 1980.

Roberts, J., Mendez-Bauer, C., and Wodell, D.: The effects of maternal position on uterine contractility and efficiency, Birth **10**(4):243, 1983.

Seeds, J., and Cefalo, R.: Malpresentations, Clin. Obstet. Gynecol. **25:**145, 1982.

Simkin, P.: Preparing parents for second stage, Birth **9**(4):229, 1982.

Van Dorsten, J., Schifrin, B., and Wallace, R.: Randomized control trial of external cephalic version with tocolysis in late pregnancy, Am. J. Obstet. Gynecol. **141:**417, 1981.

Ylikorkala, O., and Hartikoinen-Sorri, A.: Value of external version in fetal malpresentation in combination with use of ultrasound, Acta Obstet. Gynecol. Scand. **56:**63, 1977.

Yamazaki, H., and Uchida, K.: A mathematical approach to problems of cephalopelvic disproportion at the pelvic inlet, Am. J. Obstet. Gynecol. **147:**25, 1983.

CHAPTER 18

Postterm pregnancy

A postterm or prolonged pregnancy is one that has a gestational period of 42 weeks or more from the first day of the last menses. *Postmaturity* refers to the abnormal condition of the fetus or newborn resulting from a postterm pregnancy.

INCIDENCE

Postterm pregnancy has long been reported in humans (Ballantyne, 1902). Postmaturity in the fetus is listed by some as the second most common cause of intrapartum asphyxia (Dawkins et al., 1961). Others deny that there is a problem in prolonged pregnancy sufficient enough to warrant action, and controversy continues even at the present time.

Nwosw (1976) stated that approximately 10% of all pregnancies continue 14 or more days beyond term. Of these, 20% to 40% result in the delivery of postmature neonates with a perinatal mortality rate three times that of term newborns. Average mortality shows that about 35% of the deaths occur before the onset of labor, 47% during labor, and 18% in the neonatal period (Vorherr, 1975).

ETIOLOGY

Since the early 1900s, it has been widely accepted that postmaturity in the neonate is caused by placental insufficiency; however, this does not explain the cause of the prolongation of the pregnancy past term. The etiology of prolongation of a pregnancy is probably related to the causation of spontaneous labor.

The mechanism for the onset of spontaneous labor continues to be elusive. As early as 460 BC, Hippocrates proposed that the fetus determined in large part the initiation of labor. We seem to understand very little more. Although many theories have been suggested, there are several that interrelate and are currently accepted (see Chapter 14).

1. The progesterone block theory
2. The oxytocin theory
3. The fetal adrenocortical theory

Although no single theory fully explains the initiation of labor, it is probable that no single mechanism is responsible. Rather, multiple back-up mechanisms initiated and maintained by the mother and fetus together are more likely.

PHYSIOLOGY
Normal

The placenta is the primary organ implicated in problems associated with postterm pregnancy. The placenta normally has three main functions.
1. Metabolism
2. Transfer
3. Endocrine secretion

The placenta provides a large area in which materials can be exchanged across the placental membrane between the fetal and maternal circulations. From the maternal blood the fetus obtains nutrients and oxygen. Waste products formed by the fetus are transferred back across the placental membrane into the intervillous space.

The intervillous space is maternal blood that is temporarily out of the maternal circulation. Blood enters the intervillous space through 80 to 100 spiral arteries from the endometrium of the uterus. The blood slowly flows around and over the villi, which are fingerlike projections from the fetal side into the intervillous space. These villi allow an exchange of metabolic and gaseous products with the fetal blood. The maternal blood reaches the floor of the intervillous space and enters the endometrial veins to return wastes to the mother.

The welfare of the fetus depends on the adequate bathing of the chorionic villi by maternal blood. Acute reductions result in hypoxia of the fetus. Chronic reductions first affect the nutrition and growth of the fetus and eventually affect oxygenation.

Pathophysiology

As the pregnancy advances, the placental membrane becomes progressively thinner. The many capillaries come to be very close to the syncytiotrophoblast, which is the outer layer of fetal villi bathed by maternal blood in the intervillous space. Toward the end of the pregnancy, fibrinoid material forms on the surface of the villi and causes a natural aging of the placenta.

The placenta is a temporary organ, designed to provide the fetus with necessary nutrients for growth up to the time of delivery at term. Its maximum functioning is achieved between 36 and 38 weeks from the first day of the last period. After 36 to 38 weeks, the fibrinoid material begins to form on the surface of the villi. Because the placenta, in the absence of disease or complicating conditions such as PIH, is generally much larger in surface area than the fetus requires, this aging process does not usually affect fetal growth and oxygenation until approximately 42 weeks of gestation or later. At that point, fetal needs begin to compete with the rapidity of the placental aging process.

Certain diseases or complications can increase the rate of placental aging. These include diseases such as diabetes, chronic hypertension, and collagen vascular diseases. Complications such as PIH can also increase the rate of placental aging.

The fibrinoid material formed on the surface of the chorionic villi eventually decreases the available surface area that can be adequately bathed by maternal blood. At what exact point this results in fetal wastage or hypoxia cannot be precisely pinpointed. However, effects are usually observable by week 42 and progress thereafter.

The amniotic fluid volume is derived from maternal blood. Amniotic fluid quantity is contributed to by the fetus through excretion of urine and diminished through fetal swallowing of fluid into the gastrointestinal tract. In a postterm pregnancy the amount of maternal blood going into the intervillous space can diminish. The fetus presumably drinks a greater proportion than it excretes because of its own increased needs. These two factors may contribute to oligohydramnios and then reduce the cushioning effect the amniotic fluid would otherwise provide. As a result it becomes far more likely that the fetus will entrap its own cord, effectively shutting off the blood flow to or from itself for periods of time.

Signs and symptoms

A number of obstetric warning signs in conjunction with a pregnancy continuing past the estimated due date can alert care givers to potential problems. These include the following.

1. Maternal weight loss in the last weeks of pregnancy in excess of 3 pounds per week may warn of postterm pregnancy.
2. Oligohydramnios of less than 300 ml of amniotic fluid frequently correlates with maternal weight loss and with a decrease in uterine size. The decrease in uterine size reflects fetal growth retardation.
3. Meconium-stained amniotic fluid is invariably a sign of previous insult. The fetus responds to hypoxic episodes with hyperparastalsis of the intestines and relaxation of the anal sphincter.
4. Advanced bony maturation of the fetal head is associated with advanced gestational age. This can be detected by palpation of an excessively hard fetal head. It can lead to a lack of cephalic molding and a high arrest of the fetal head.
5. Prolonged labor can also be due to uterine inertia or failure of cephalic molding.

Maternal effects

The maternal effects of a postterm pregnancy are primarily emotional. Except for the increased incidence of cesarean delivery for failure to progress, the physical effects of a postterm pregnancy are seen in the neonate. Whereas most attention in the literature has been devoted to the impact of postmaturity on the fetus and neonate, the very specific psychological impact on the mother is frequently ignored.

Women express a great deal of frustration with the prolongation of the pregnancy and a feeling of total lack of control in being able to make the pregnancy end. Feelings of inadequacy and failure emerge because of the inability to complete the process of pregnancy "like everyone else." Women often blame themselves for prolonging the pregnancy.

Relationships with those people closest to them become strained. Resentment is expressed that friends and relatives repeatedly check on the woman's progress and condition. Physical discomfort becomes a burden, which decreases the ability to continue caring for the home and other family members in the accustomed manner. Physical discomforts are reported as feelings of having lost their "glow," being bulky, and feeling generally unattractive. A woman's negative feelings about herself may be projected to feelings of resentment toward the baby.

Realistic fears are commonly shared about the continued well-being of the baby. Women report fears that the baby is "stuck" and will somehow be harmed or that something is very wrong and that the baby has decided not to be born.

Finally, women commonly describe the belief that they are more likely to have a cesarean birth and express anger and feelings of potential loss of a less than desired "special" birthing experience. Plans for their birthing experience are viewed as being thwarted by just one more failure to control their situation.

Fetal and neonatal effects

Postmaturity is a syndrome that results because of certain effects of a prolonged pregnancy on the neonate. Of all prolonged pregnancies, 20% to 40% result in the delivery of a postmature neonate (Nwosw, 1976). In addition to the syndrome itself, there is a greater likelihood of fetal growth retardation and hypoxic-anoxic insults. The syndrome must be considered as an imbalance between continued placental capacity to function and fetal nutritive and respiratory demands. Postmaturity is clinically recognized by the following symptoms.

1. Failure of growth
2. Dehydration

3. Dry, cracked, wrinkled, parchmentlike skin due to reduction of subcutaneous fat
4. Long, thin arms and legs
5. Advanced hardness of the skull
6. Absence of vernix and lanugo
7. Skin maceration, especially in the folds and the external genitalia
8. Brownish green or yellowish discoloration of skin, umbilical cord, and membranes
9. An increased appearance of alertness

The placental deterioration in a prolonged pregnancy can lead to acute and extensive disturbances of oxygenation resulting in intrauterine fetal demise or can lead to chronic restrictions resulting in fetal malnutrition. Fetal hypoxia leads to anaerobic glycolysis, exhaustion of carbohydrate reserves, and fetal acidemia. Acidemia leads to inhibition of the metabolic enzyme systems and fetal circulatory collapse. Fetal passage of meconium can result from the circulatory collapse and lead to fetal aspiration of that substance and asphyxia. This may lead to central nervous system, cardiovascular, respiratory, and hepatic lesions, which can then result in fetal heart failure and intrauterine death (Vorherr, 1975).

MEDICAL DIAGNOSIS

A postterm pregnancy may or may not result in a postmature neonate. It becomes a challenge, therefore, to make postmaturity a prenatal rather than a postnatal diagnosis in an already compromised neonate.

Certain maternal factors are associated with an increased incidence of postterm pregnancy.

1. Parity, regardless of maternal age; prolonged pregnancy is common in primigravidas and in high-parity mothers
2. Maternal age; mothers under the age of 25 years have a higher rate of postterm pregnancy than do older mothers; however, older mothers past the age of 35 years more often have neonates with the more severe effects of postmaturity
3. Previous obstetrical history; positive history of prolonged pregnancy in preceding pregnancies is associated with a twofold increase in the prevalence of a repeat postterm pregnancy
4. Present obstetrical course; certain subgroups such as patients who are preeclamptic with potential uteroplacental insufficiency superimposed on a postterm pregnancy contribute to increased perinatal mortality figures.

At present, there is no single diagnostic test that accurately diagnoses a postmature fetus. However, a combination of evaluation tools has been found valuable.

Ultrasound

For really accurate dating, ultrasound measurements should be done prior to 20 weeks of gestation. An early crown-rump length offers the most accurate means. After 20 weeks, and particularly during the last 10 weeks of gestation, accuracy of estimating gestational age is progressively limited. For these reasons, in the presence of questionable LMP (last menstrual period), ultrasound should be used as early as possible and preferably before 20 weeks to prevent confusion regarding diagnosis of postterm pregnancy once the EDC is past.

Amniotic fluid volume

A noticeable decrease in abdominal girth may occur postterm as a result of a gradual decrease in amniotic fluid volume. The average amniotic fluid volume at 42, 43, and 44 weeks of gestation is estimated at 484 ml, 332 ml, and 162 ml, respectively. Ultrasound can be a useful means of measuring amniotic fluid volume serially and thus assisting in the diagnosis of postterm pregnancy.

Contraction stress test (CST)

Although the relationship between postmaturity and antepartal placental insufficiency is controversial, the oxytocin challenge test has been found useful in managing postterm pregnancy, especially if the patient's cervix is not conducive to induction. The CST gives the reassurance of continued fetal well-being and oxygenation, so unnecessary intervention is eliminated. (The CST is discussed in considerable detail in Chapter 3.) The CST should be done weekly after 41 weeks of gestation (Freeman and Garite, 1981).

USUAL MEDICAL MANAGEMENT

When a pregnancy extends beyond 7 days postterm, the prenatal chart should be reviewed for confirmation of due date. Parameters for review include uterine fundal height at the umbilicus at 20 weeks of gestation and 1 cm per week growth thereafter, audible fetal heart rate with a fetoscope at 18 to 20 weeks, and fetal movement noted at 18 to 20 weeks. Early ultrasound gestational age assessment before 20 weeks can be invaluable in confirming other dating information. It is extremely important that all parameters are clearly documented. In the absence of early prenatal evaluation, information obtained later from the patient is often confused or has been forgotten.

By 14 days past the due date, a pelvic exam should be performed to ascertain potential readiness for induction. If the cervix is not conducive to successful induction, CSTs should be scheduled. A negative CST indicates that the fetus is well and that no intervention need be planned. The pelvic examination is repeated biweekly for reassessment of cervical changes conducive to induction. Negative CSTs are continued weekly until the pelvic examination indicates readiness for induction or the patient goes into spontaneous labor. If the CST is positive in the presence of an unfavorable cervix, a trial labor can be attempted with the judicious use of oxytocin, artificial rupture of membranes oxygen at 10 liters by tight face mask, and the patient positioned on her left side if the fetal heart rate demonstrates adequate variability. If decreased or absent variability is present, a cesarean delivery should be performed.

During labor it is usually recommended that membranes be ruptured artificially if they have not spontaneously ruptured. Internal monitoring is the method of choice for optimal accuracy in recognizing potential late decelerations and loss of variability.

At the time of delivery, pediatric assistance should be present for any necessary resuscitation of the neonate. A DeLee suction should be in the delivery room set-up for probable suctioning of the neonatal nares and mouth while the baby's head is still on the maternal perineum.

NURSING PROCESS
Prevention

Prevention of postterm pregnancy, resulting in a postmature neonate with potential hypoxic compromise, should be a nursing goal and the goal of medical management. Those parameters that aid in accurate dating of the gestation of the pregnancy are essential in the history. These must include the following.

1. First day of last normal menstrual period
2. First fetal movement (quickening)
3. Review of fundal height measurements after 20 to 22 weeks as they correspond to weeks of gestation

Education of childbearing women regarding the very real dangers of postterm pregnancy and their responsibility in seeking early prenatal care, and in remembering dates, can also aid the pregnant patient. Finally, educating couples regarding testing for fetal well-being and what can be done to aid ripening of the cervix can also promote the mother's belief in a safe delivery and optimal neonatal outcome. Some studies have shown that, with careful selection of pregnant patients between 40 and 42 weeks, nipple stimulation for endogenous release of oxytocin three times daily for 1 hour each time can aid in cervical ripening within 4 days for greater than 80% of patients (Elliott and Flaherty, 1983). Careful selection includes accurate dating between 40 and 42 weeks, absence of other risk factors such as disease or complications with the present pregnancy, and daily reports of adequate fetal activity (more than four movements of the fetus detected per hour). Patients are taught to time each contraction caused and to cease stimulation for that hour if a contraction lasts longer than 60 seconds. They are also taught to lie on their left side, throughout the stimulation, to facilitate uterine blood flow.

Assessment

Nurses involved in prenatal care, regardless of the setting, can play an important role in screening and identifying those women at risk for prolonged pregnancy. Careful attention to asking questions regarding previous history, recognizing those groups vulnerable to postterm pregnancy, and recording information carefully can be valuable in planning the care as term approaches. Documentation of all important parameters for evaluating and confirming due date is vital.

The following areas of assessment should be included in the prenatal history and may be clues to detecting those patients particularly vulnerable to prolonged pregnancy.

1. Primipara older than 35 years or younger than 25 years
2. Previous history of postterm pregnancy
3. Grand multiparity
4. Present pregnancy history of potential uteroplacental insufficiency

During prenatal care, assessments that can provide information that aids in accuracy of dating include the following.

1. LMP (last normal menstrual period)
2. First fetal movement felt
3. First FHR by fetoscope
4. Fundal height measurements consistent with dates (at the umbilicus at 20 to 22 weeks and 1 cm per week thereafter)

During the last weeks of pregnancy all women should be assessed for such early warning signs as the following.

1. Maternal weight loss
2. Decelerated increase or actual decrease in uterine size (may indicate oligohydramnios or intrauterine growth retardation)
3. Decreased fetal activity (less than four increments in 1 hour of counting)

Warning signs that the nurse must assess for during labor are listed below.

1. Meconium in the amniotic fluid
2. Indications of advanced bony maturation of the skull such as palpation of a hard fetal head or high arrest of the fetal head during labor
3. Prolonged labor (longer than 24 hours for a primipara or 18 hours for a multipara)
4. Abnormal fetal heart rate or patterns such as bradycardia, tachycardia, late decelerations, and, especially, loss of beat to beat variability

Interventions

Nurses should carefully document the complete history and continue assessment information that can aid in the prenatal diagnosis of postmaturity. By aiding the physician with this information, it can be expected that good clinical judgment, for optimal timing of delivery, will prevent the adverse effects of hypoxia-anoxia on the fetus.

The nurse can advocate techniques for assessing fetal well-being such as ultrasound and contraction stress tests by educating those patients at risk regarding the use and value of these tests. This information can often best be presented during prenatal education classes when the information is presented for public awareness. When such tests are ordered for patients, specific information about the importance of the tests can reassure the patient that a careful watch is being kept and yet does not minimize the realistic aspects of fear for fetal well-being. In clinical settings and primary care centers, nurses can play an important role in establishing such testing as part of the care for patients at risk.

In the presence of a prolonged pregnancy, the psychologic impact on the mother and the family must be appreciated. The concerns for fetal well-being must not be ignored or minimized by false reassurance. Correct information regarding the value and efficacy of testing should be volunteered. A fetal activity chart can be started to aid in keeping the mother in tune with the fetal energy and activity and giving her a day to day means of providing a reliable report of changes. Emotional preparation for the possible cesarean birth and the selection of birthing centers giving family-centered cesarean birth experiences can generate more positive feelings about the experiences encountered.

Nurses working in labor and delivery settings, by being alert for the warning signs, can better prepare for the potential neonatal problems at the time of delivery. Continuous monitoring should be instituted early, and the nurse can advocate early artificial rupture of membranes for observation of fluid color and the use of the internal fetal scalp electrode for best assessment of fetal heart rate variability. In this way, early signs of fetal distress from the insults of labor in the presence of uteroplacental insufficiency can be treated and corrected before metabolic acidosis results. If signs of fetal distress necessitate an emergency cesarean birth, all necessary actions for activating the team of necessary people should have been thought out in advance.

At the time of delivery, the nurse should have pediatric assistance for possible resuscitation of the neonate. Preferably, this assistance will include a pediatrician or a neonatal nurse. DeLee suction should be made available for probable neonatal suction of the mouth and nares while still on the maternal perineum, if delivery is vaginal. All other equipment for tracheal suction and oxygen administration should be available and in working order.

Evaluation

Given modern techniques for detecting and monitoring fetal well-being, there is little excuse for parents being denied information aimed at aiding them

Postterm pregnancy

Potential patient problem	Outcome criteria
A. Potential postterm pregnancy related to: Inaccurate dating for EDC Unrecognized at-risk patients	Identification of patients at risk for prolonged pregnancy Prevention of a neonate with postmaturity syndrome
B. Potential uteroplacental insufficiency related to: Loss of optimal placental function after 38 weeks of gestation Gradual deterioration of the placental function reaching a marginal reserve status by 42 weeks of gestation Failure of spontaneous labor before 42 weeks of gestation	Continued adequacy of placental function as evidenced by: four fetal movements or more in any 1 hr negative, reactive CST no late decelerations, loss of variability, tachycardia, or bradycardia during labor clear, normal amount of amniotic fluid delivery of a neonate with Apgar scores of better than 7 at 1 and 5 min

Assessment and intervention

Dx. Determine date of last menstrual period
Record date when FHR was first heard with a fetoscope
Record date when mother first felt fetal movement
Measure fundal height at each prenatal visit
Assess for such risk factors as:
    primipara less than 25 or greater than 35 years old
    grand multiparity
    previous history of prolonged pregnancy
Th. Record all data
Prepare patient for ultrasound, especially when dates are questionable
Ed. To record such events as LMP and first fetal movement
Give information about ultrasound procedure, purpose, risks versus benefits

Dx. Assess for signs of intrauterine growth retardation and oligohydramnios such as:
    maternal weight loss of 3 pounds or more per week after 38 weeks of gestation
    fundal height loss greater than 2 cm per week
    amniotic fluid less than 300 ml
Assess for fetal activity
Assess for signs of cervical ripening such as effacement and dilatation
Assess for signs of fetal distress such as:
    CST that is equivocal, nonreactive, or positive
    meconium-stained amniotic fluid
    during labor: late decelerations, loss of variability, tachycardia, or prolonged bradycardia
Assess for signs of postmaturity such as:
    palpatation of a hard fetal head
    prolonged labor with high fetal head arrest
Th. If cervix is ripe after 40 weeks, expect an induction for medical indications
If cervix is unripe:
    expect weekly CST and biweekly assessment for cervical changes conducive to induction
    prepare for testing:
        CST
        ultrasound
If CST is positive:
    with reactivity can attempt labor induction with rupture of membranes, O_2 at 10 liters by mask, pitocin, left-side positioning
    continuous fetal monitoring preferably internal monitor
    without reactivity or variability, expect cesarean birth immediately
Prepare patient for potential medical interventions
Ref. Pediatric personnel for presence during delivery
Antepartum testing nurse when available

Dx., diagnostic; Th., therapeutic; Ed., education; Ref., referral.   *Continued.*

Postterm pregnancy—cont'd

Potential patient problem	Outcome criteria
C. Potential altered perception of self and fetus related to: 　Fatigue 　Anger and frustration over prolonged pregnancy 　Loss of control 　Fear for safety of baby 　Fear for potential loss of expected birth experience	Positive feelings expressed toward the neonate Positive feelings expressed toward the birth experience Positive relationships maintained with significant others

in their own best advocacy, nor is there good reason for professional obstetric care to result in poor neonatal outcome because of prolonged pregnancy. The nurse's role as patient advocate and patient educator is vital in the goal of prevention of postmaturity syndrome and neonatal hypoxic sequelae.

REFERENCES

Affonso, D., and Clark, A.: Childbearing: a nursing perspective, Philadelphia, 1979, F.A. Davis Co.

Ballantyne, J.: The problem of the postmature infant, Am. J. Obstet. Gynecol. **2:**521, 1902.

Assessment and intervention

Dx. Expressions of anger, frustration, fatigue, unattractiveness, fear for fetal well-being, loss of desired birth experience
Disruption of family and friends relationships:
 husband resentful, inattentive
 patient reclusive
 stress over potential inability of family or friends making arrangements for postpartal help
Th. Provide opportunity for expressions of negative feelings for patient and mate
Assist in alternative arrangements for help in the home for the present and postpartum
Examine the alternatives for coach in the cesarean delivery, mother/infant recovery, rooming-in if cesarean birth becomes necessary
Ed. Fear for fetal well-being is real
Control of situation can be enhanced through testing for fetal well-being and optimal timing of delivery by most judicious means
Alternatives for positive and satisfying birth experience
Ref. Prenatal educator
Support services for home help such as social service, home health aids if available, visiting nurse, church members—all as available and appropriate

Dawkins, M., Martin, J., and Spector, W.: Postterm pregnancy, Br. J. Obstet. Gynaecol., **68**:604, 1961.

Elliott, J., and Flaherty, J.: Breast stimulation and term pregnancies, MCH News (published by Arizona Department of Health Services) **1**(2): 1983.

Freeman, R., and Garite, T.: Fetal heart rate monitoring, Baltimore, 1981, Williams and Wilkins Co.

Mati, J., and others: Induction of labor in sheep and humans by single dose of corticosteroids, Br. Med. J. **2**:149, 1973.

Nwosw, U.: Postterm pregnancy, Obstet. Gynecol. **47**:137, 1976.

Vorherr, H.: Placental insufficiency in relation to postterm pregnancy and fetal postmaturity, Am. J. Obstet. Gynecol. **123**:67, 1975.

CHAPTER 19

Labor stimulation

Induction of labor is any attempt to initiate uterine contractions prior to their spontaneous onset to facilitate a vaginal delivery. There are two types of inductions, elective and therapeutic:

1. Elective induction is done for the convenience of the physician or patient, and there is no medical indication.
2. Therapeutic induction is done when there is a medical indication such as an aging placenta caused by diabetes, hypertensive disorders, Rh disease, or prolonged pregnancy; placental separation; premature rupture of membranes with delivery indicated; or intrauterine fetal death.

Elective inductions have been prohibited by the Food and Drug Administration (1978).

Augmentation of labor is any attempt to stimulate uterine contractions during the course of labor to facilitate a vaginal delivery. It is frequently used for certain types of uterine dysfunction. A labor should not be augmented until noninvasive interventions have been tried such as (1) making sure the bladder is empty, (2) changing positions, (3) providing comfort measures, and (4) making sure the patient is properly hydrated.

INCIDENCE

The use of a labor stimulant for either inducing or augmenting labor varies between countries, cities, and hospitals. Lumley (1983) gives a range between 5% and 50%.

CRITERIA

Criteria for an induction of labor are listed below.

1. An engaged presenting part
2. No previous uterine surgery or trauma
3. No fetopelvic disproportion
4. No fetal distress
5. Fetal weight estimated as less than 4,300 gm
6. No major bleeding from an abruptio placentae or placenta previa

Criteria for augmentation of labor are the same as for an induction. There should also be definite signs that the progress of labor is slowing down.

Labor is seldom induced or augmented *(1)* on a grand multipara over 5 parity, *(2)* on a multiple pregnancy, or *(3)* in the presence of polyhydramnios because of the increased risk of uterine rupture related to uterine overdistension.

The success of the induction or augmentation usually depends on a ripe cervix. A cervix is considered ripe when it is soft, anterior, effaced more than 50%, and dilated 2 cm or more. Bishop (1964) developed a 13-point scoring system to predict the responsiveness of a patient to an induction. He found that an induction is usually successful when the pelvic score totals 9 or more (Table 19-1). Breast stimulation is currently being used to facilitate cervical ripening and has been found to increase the success rate of an induction (Elliott and Flaherty, 1983). Vaginal prostaglandin E_2 and lamenaria tents are also being used to enhance cervical ripening (Jeeva and Dommisse, 1982; Norstrom, 1982). Good hydration also increases the chance of establishing an adequate labor pattern.

MATERNAL EFFECTS

Pain is reportedly more intense when labor is stimulated; therefore more pain medication is needed. According to Lumley (1983), 92% of all patients whose labors are stimulated need an analgesic, as opposed to 50% of the patients who have a spontaneous labor.

Oxytocin and prostaglandins can cause uterine overstimulation leading to uterine rupture, placental separation, amniotic embolism, and cervical lacerations. These complications are rare if the medication is administered properly and the patient's reactions to the drug are monitored continuously.

The risk of failed induction is as high as 50% if the cervix is not ripe and oxytocin is used (Shepherd and Knuppel, 1981). This increases the patient's risk of a cesarean delivery.

If an amniotomy is the method used to stimulate labor, the patient has an

TABLE 19-1. *Pelvic scoring system*

	Score			
	0	*1*	*2*	*3*
Dilatation (cm)	0	1-2	3-4	5-6
Effacement (%)	0-30	40-50	60-70	80
Station	−3	−2	−1/0	+1/+2
Consistency of cervix	Firm	Medium	Soft	
Cervical position	Posterior	Median	Anterior	

Reprinted with permission from The American College of Obstetricians and Gynecologists (Obstet. Gynecol. 24:266, 1964).

increased risk of infection. The membranes being ruptured longer and the greater number of vaginal exams both increase this risk.

When oxytocin or prostaglandin is used, the risk for such postpartum complications as hemorrhage and postpartum depression are increased. Oxytocin also increases the risk for water intoxication.

FETAL AND NEONATAL EFFECTS

Any time labor is induced, there is a risk of prematurity. Therefore fetal maturity should always be assessed prior to an induction unless it is being performed because of medical indications when the benefits of delivery outweigh the risks of prematurity.

Labor contractions normally impede uterine blood flow. A healthy fetus has an adequate oxygen reserve and can withstand this stress. However, if the frequency, intensity, duration, or resting tone of the contractions is increased by a labor stimulant, this can further impede the uterine blood flow and can cause fetal distress.

If an amniotomy is performed early in labor, there is a 10% increased risk of fetal distress (Simkin, 1983). Fetal distress is related to increased pressure applied to the fetal head in a cephalic presentation and can cause a caput succedaneum or cranial bone misalignment. When the membranes are intact, hydrostatic pressure distributes the pressure more evenly. If the presenting part is not well engaged at the time of the membrane rupture, the cord can prolapse and cause fetal distress. The decrease in amniotic fluid can increase the risk of cord compression and cause fetal distress as well. This is seen as variable decelerations on the fetal monitor (Gabbe et al., 1976).

Oxytocin or prostaglandins can predispose to hyperbilirubinemia in the neonate. This can occur if fetal hypoxia develops because of excessive uterine stimulation.

LABOR STIMULATED BY AMNIOTOMY

An amniotomy is done by artificially rupturing the fetal membranes with an amniotic hook. This procedure is commonly abbreviated as AROM. When the membranes are ruptured, arachidonic acid is incorporated into F_{2a} prostaglandin, a stimulator of smooth muscle, and this promotes uterine contractions.

Nursing assessment and intervention

The procedure should be explained to the patient first. This can effectively be accomplished by informing the patient that the procedure is done by way of a vaginal examination. The nurse can show her the amniohook and inform her that the hook simply nicks the fetal membrane, and she will not feel it because there are no nerve endings in the membrane. The only physical sensation she will feel will be a "gush" of warm fluid from the vagina. Following the rupture, she will continue to feel the fluid leaking throughout labor.

The presenting part must be engaged and the cervix must be soft and partially dilated for the membranes to be ruptured. This is because the medical team is committed to delivering the infant within 12 to 24 hours following the rupture because of the increased risk of intrauterine infection. To decrease this risk, the number of vaginal exams should be kept to a minimum. Following an AROM, the nurse should keep the patient as dry and comfortable as possible, since she will continue to leak amniotic fluid, and should check her temperature every hour.

There is always the risk of a cord prolapse following an amniotomy. Therefore the nurse should assess fetal heart rate prior to and immediately following the rupture of membranes. The amniotic fluid should also be assessed for color and odor. Foul-smelling amniotic fluid is a sign of an intrauterine infection. Black or green amniotic fluid usually indicates that the fetus has passed meconium. If blood is present in the amniotic fluid, the nurse should notify the obstetrician immediately; this can indicate a placental separation or vasa previa.

If the fetal heart rate reveals fetal distress after the rupture of membranes, a vaginal exam should be performed with a sterile glove to feel for a cord in the cervix or vagina. If a cord is felt and it is still pulsating, pressure should be applied and maintained to the presenting part to prevent pressure on the cord. Next the nurse should call for help and with the free hand push the abdomen up to elevate the uterus. When help arrives, the nurse should give instructions to (1) put the bed in a Trendelenburg position by elevating the foot of the bed or elevating the buttocks with pillows, (2) listen for fetal heart rate with a Doppler or fetoscopy, (3) start oxygen by mask at 7 liters/min, (4) apply warm, moist saline gauze over the cord if the cord is visible, and (5) notify the health care provider. The nurse should also attempt to keep the patient calm and prepare her for a cesarean delivery. If there is no intravenous in place, one should be started with an 18-gauge intracatheter.

If fetal distress develops and a prolapsed cord cannot be determined, the nurse should reposition the patient and determine whether or not the fetal distress is related to the fetus lying on the cord. Oxygen by mask should be administered at 7 liters/min to increase the oxygen saturation of the blood, and the health care provider should be notified immediately.

LABOR STIMULATED WITH OXYTOCIN

Oxytocin, a normal body hormone excreted from the posterior pituitary gland, is chemically related to vasopressin/ADH. It promotes smooth muscle contractions of the uterus by activating the myometrium. The effect of oxytocin is enhanced in the presence of high levels of estrogen. This is the reason why oxytocin has very little effect on the pregnant uterus until near term when estrogen levels are high. Because oxytocin has a weak antidiuretic property, large doses can cause the kidneys to increase the reabsorption of water. Bolus IV injections can have a generalized relaxing effect on vascular smooth muscle, which can lead to hypotension and tachycardia. High infusion rates can cause hypertension (O'Brien and Cefalo, 1982).

Oxytocin is administered in synthetic form as Pitocin or Syntocinon. It is available in solution form for intravenous or intramuscular injections, in a nasal spray, or in buccal tablets for sublingual use. It cannot be administered orally because the digestive enzyme trypsin inactivates it.

Intravenous administration of dilute oxytocin is the preferred route of administration because the absorption rate is predictable and the absorption of the drug can be stopped at any time by discontinuing the IV infusion. Its effect on the body usually ceases very quickly after the drug is discontinued; the pregnant woman's plasma, near term, contains a high concentration of the enzyme pitocinase, which breaks down one-half of an IV dose of oxytocin within 2 to 3 minutes (Oxorn, 1980). If the patient is highly sensitive to the drug, the drug's effect can persist for 20 to 30 minutes or for as long as 2 hours after cessation.

Nursing assessment and intervention

Because of the potential deleterious effects if it is inappropriately administered, the drug must be administered carefully. The following protocol should be implemented.

1. Explain the procedure to the patient and her coach.
2. Apply an external fetal monitor or assist the physician with placement of an internal fetal monitor if available. (An internal monitor is best because the strength of the contractions and fetal heart rate variability can be monitored as well as the frequency and duration of the contractions and fetal heart rate.)
3. Determine a baseline for maternal vital signs, fetal heart rate, and uterine activity for 10 to 20 minutes prior to initiation.
4. Prepare the oxytocin solution according to hospital policy and label properly. (Usually 10 U of oxytocin is mixed with 1,000 ml of IV fluid.)
5. Have the patient positioned on her side.
6. Administer the solution by way of a continuous infusion pump to ensure precise control over the amount of medication administered.

7. Piggyback the oxytocin solution into a well functioning infusion line next to the infusion site so that oxytocin can be discounted and restarted as necessary while maintaining an open vein for any emergency.

8. The pump should usually be started at a low setting to deliver 0.5 to 1 mU/min of oxytocin. (If 10 U have been diluted in 1,000 ml, then there are 10,000 mU/1,000 ml or 10 mU/ml).

9. The dose is gradually increased per physician's orders at 15 to 20 minute intervals because it takes that amount of time for the full effect of oxytocin to be seen. (A typical induction order will read: increase from 1 mU/min to 2 mU/min, then to 4 mU/min, and then increase by 4 mU/min until contractions occur, at which time increase by 1 mU/min until a regular pattern is established or the maximum dose of 32 mU/min is reached. A typical augmentation order will read: increase from 0.5 mU/min to 1 mU/min, then to 2 mU/min, and then increase by 2 mU/min until a regular contraction pattern is established or the maximum dose of 32 mU/min is reached.) Most patients will need between 1 and 16 mU/min to augment or induce labor.

10. The goal of oxytocin is to establish a regular contraction pattern of moderate to strong contractions of about 50 mm Hg intrauterine pressure, occurring every 2 to 3 minutes, lasting 45 to 60 seconds, in which the uterus returns to baseline for at least 1 minute between each contraction.

11. Check the patency of the IV frequently so that back-up of the oxytocin solution into the intravenous tubing does not result in a bolus of oxytocin.

12. The fetal heart rate should be continously monitored. The patient's pulse and blood pressure must be assessed every 15 minutes. Periodic vaginal exams should be performed to determine cervical dilatation and fetal descent. To evaluate the progress of labor, cervical dilatation and descent of presenting part should be graphed on a normal labor curve and compared against time in hours.

13. Drug doses, times of increase, maternal vital signs, and fetal heart rate should be charted on a flow sheet and the fetal monitor strip.

14. Reduce oxytocin if contractions occur more often than four every 10 min, last longer than 75 to 90 seconds, or uterine tone fails to return to baseline, around 15 to 20 mm Hg pressure, between contractions for at least 60 seconds.

15. Discontinue oxytocin, administer oxygen, position patient on her side, and notify the attending physician if fetal distress is noted by late or variable deceleration patterns, loss of long- or short-term variability,

tachycardia or bradycardia, or if tetanic contractions occur. Tetanic contractions are strong contractions that (1) occur more often than four every 10 minutes, (2) last 90 seconds or more without a period of relaxation, and (3) have an increased uterine resting tone.

16. The attending physician must be close to the labor and delivery area for the nurse to carry out the induction order.

17. The induction should be discontinued if labor has not started or no progress is made within 2 to 3 hours.

The response to this drug varies between individuals. Therefore a very small amount of the drug is necessary to establish an active labor pattern in some patients; others require a much larger dose. Because there is no way to predict how sensitive a particular patient will be, oxytocin must be administered under very close supervision. Adequate hydration, encouraging the patient to lie on her side, and keeping the bladder empty improve the patient's chances of establishing an effective labor pattern. Once an effective labor pattern has been established and the patient has dilated at least 4 to 5 cm, the oxytocin infusion can often be reduced without changing the strength of the uterine contractions.

Side effects of oxytocin that the nurse should be familiar with are listed below.

1. Excessive uterine stimulation (hypertonus)
2. Water intoxication
3. Hypotension or hypertension
4. Decreased sensitivity to the drug

Uterine contractions increase myometrial pressure, which in turn stops placental blood flow. This usually begins around 30 mm Hg of uterine pressure. The fetus, if healthy, has a good oxygen reserve and can withstand the stress of normal contractions. If the placenta is functioning at maximum prior to the labor contraction, the fetus has a low reserve, or if the contractions are abnormally long and the uterus fails to return to resting tone, the fetus is likely to become hypoxic. Because oxytocin can increase uterine resting tone and frequency, duration, and intensity of contractions, the nurse must be very alert to any abnormal contraction patterns or signs of fetal distress. The internal monitor is most effective in detecting these changes.

Water retention usually occurs after prolonged use of large amounts of oxytocin because oxytocin decreases glomerular filtration rate and renal blood flow and interferes with electrolyte excretion. However, Abdul-Karim and Assali (1961) have documented water retention with a continuous IV infusion of 15 mU/min. The nurse should keep an accurate intake and output on any patient receiving oxytocin and limit fluid intake to approximately 1,000 ml/24 hr. This condition is enhanced if large amounts of electrolyte-free dextrose solution are used to administer the oxytocin (McKenna and Shaw, 1979). Other rare side effects that have been noted due to oxytocin's antidiuretic effect are hyponatremia, congestive heart failure, convulsions, and death (Brenner, 1976).

Hypotension can occur because of the relaxing effect of oxytocin on vascular smooth muscles. In contrast, hypertension might be triggered. These cardiovascular symptoms rarely develop, but the nurse should assess the vital signs frequently; hypotension and hypertension interfere with proper uteroplacental blood flow when they do occur.

A decreased sensitivity to oxytocin can develop if a larger amount of oxytocin is used than needed. This subsequently decreases contractions and causes dysfunctional labor. In these cases, the oxytocin should be stopped and restarted at a later time.

The patient's fear of the pain associated with labor-induced contractions should be determined. Many patients have heard alarming reports about oxytocin. The nurse should inform the patient and her coach that stimulated contractions are usually very similar to normal, active labor contractions. An induced labor usually has a shorter latent phase, but the active and transition phases are not usually altered.

During the actual induction, the patient's level of discomfort should be assessed frequently. The effectiveness of distraction tools should also be determined. If the distraction tools are ineffective for her level of discomfort, the physician should be notified. If the pain is more intense, an analgesic may decrease the pain so that distraction tools are effective and the patient can stay in control. The patient should be allowed a choice in this regard. The nurse should also encourage the patient and her coach by giving them frequent positive reinforcement. This can help alleviate some of the negative feelings associated with a stimulated labor. The response of the patient and her significant other to a labor stimulant should be determined. Many times parents feel as if they have failed when such an intervention is needed. An explanation as to its reason can help to alleviate these feelings.

LABOR STIMULATED WITH PROSTAGLANDINS

Prostaglandins are formed enzymatically from phospholipids and arachidonic acid in most tissues of the body. They act as a local hormone by exerting their action primarily at the site of production. There are 20 known human prostaglandins. Structurally, they are divided into five groups E, F, A, B, and C. Prostaglandin E_2 (PE_2) acts primarily on the myometrium causing contraction of the smooth muscle and the cervix, thus decreasing cervical resistance. Prostaglandin F_{2a} (PF_{2a}) affects the myometrium and the cervix by acting on the ovaries, thereby blocking the release of progesterone and relaxin. Intravenous prostaglandin E_2 and F_{2a} are very effective in stimulating uterine contractions in early pregnancy when oxytocin is ineffective, and they are widely used for medically induced abortions. They have been investigated as labor stimulants and found to be as effective as oxytocin. By intravenous route, they frequently cause side effects such as nausea, vomiting, and diarrhea. Therefore oxytocin may be chosen over IV prostaglandin in patients at term. The two exceptions are patients with renal and cardiac diseases. Prostaglandins are usually preferred for these patients to avoid the antidiuretic effect of oxytocin.

Intravaginal prostaglandins are currently being used as effective labor stimulants. Because the success of induction depends to a great extent on the ripeness of the cervix, intravaginal prostaglandins can have a number of advantages over amniotomy and intravenous oxytocin. PGE_2 is usually the preferred prostaglandin. Neilson and associates (1983) found it to be significantly more effective than PGF_{2a}. Hefni and Lewis (1980) found that 79% of their patients with an unripe cervix could be successfully induced and delivered with PGE_2 suppositories. Of the 21% who did not go into labor within a few hours, all had a ripe cervix within 24 hours and were successfully induced at that time. The patients did not experience the nausea, vomiting, diarrhea, and drug-induced fever common when prostaglandins are administered orally or intravenously. According to Shepherd and Knuppel (1981) intravaginal PGE_2 is as effective as oxytocin in stimulating labor when the cervix is ripe. In patients with an unfavorable cervix, the failed induction rate can be decreased from 42% with oxytocin to 2% with intravaginal PGE_2. The risk of uterine hypertonus is not increased any more than with oxytocin. An added advantage over amniotomy is that the delivery does not have to take place within 24 hours following instillation. Prins and associates (1983) found that labor contractions were usually initiated within a few minutes following insertion.

Nursing assessment and intervention

The patient whose labor is being stimulated with prostaglandins should be monitored as closely as the patient receiving pitocin. Because intravaginal PGE_2 is the most commonly used prostaglandin, the nursing care will focus on this type. The nurse is not responsible for administration, only for assisting the physician with insertion. The nurse's primary role is to assess for such complications as uterine hypertonus and fetal distress. Fetal heart rate and uterine contractions should be monitored continuously, preferably with an internal monitor. The fetal heart rate pattern should be evaluated for deceleration patterns and the rate recorded every 15 minutes. The uterine contraction pattern should be evaluated as to frequency, duration, intensity, and resting tone. This data should be recorded every 15 minutes on the patient's record. Periodic vaginal exams should be done to determine cervical dilatation and fetal descent. To evaluate the progress of labor, cervical dilatation and descent of presenting part should be graphed on a normal labor curve and compared over time in hours. This will facilitate identification of a dysfunctional labor (see Chapter 17).

The patient should be encouraged to lie on either side except during insertion of the suppository or gel. Side lying facilitates effective uterine contractions while preventing the vena cava syndrome.

The patient's level of discomfort should be assessed frequently. The effectiveness of distraction tools should also be determined. If the distraction tools are ineffective for her level of discomfort, the physician should be notified. During active labor an analgesic can be administered as ordered according to the patient's needs. The response of the patient and her significant other to a labor stimulant should be determined. Many times parents feel as if they have failed when such an intervention is needed. An explanation as to its reason can help alleviate these feelings. However, stimulating labor by intravaginal prostaglandin is not usually felt to be as intrusive as IV oxytocin.

The patient should be observed for the development of such side effects as a drug-induced fever, nausea, vomiting, and diarrhea. The temperature should be taken every hour. If an elevation is noted, it should be reported to the physician, and an infection should be ruled out. Prostaglandins can cause the temperature to rise about 2° F (1° C) due to the effect on the hypothalamus. If nausea, vomiting, or diarrhea is persistent, these signs should be reported to the physician because an electrolyte imbalance can develop. This can lead to a dysfunctional labor pattern.

POSTPARTUM INTERVENTION

Following labor induction by an amniotomy, the risk of an infection is greater. The patient's temperature should be taken every 4 hours, the lochia assessed for a foul odor, and the white blood count evaluated. Following prolonged use of oxytocin or intravaginal prostaglandins, the risk of postpartum hemorrhage is also increased. It is usually the result of uterine relaxation and can often be prevented by administering IV oxytocin for the first 2 to 3 hours after delivery. If oxytocin or prostaglandins stimulated the labor to progress abnormally fast, the risk of bleeding as the result of lacerations is greater. Water intoxication is another complication that can result from prolonged use of oxytocin. This may not develop until the postpartum period. A strict intake and output should be kept on all postpartum patients who received oxytocin during labor and for 12 hours or more during the postpartum period. If oxytocin is added to the IV infusion and then administered very rapidly to decrease uterine atony in the early postpartum period, cardiac arrhythmias and hypotension are more likely to develop.

Following any labor stimulant method, the risk of postpartum depression is higher. The nurse should encourage the patient to talk about her labor and delivery experience and express any negative feelings she might have. Then the nurse can help her work through her feelings. If the mother does not work through these feelings, they can negatively affect future childbearing.

S U G G E S T E D   P L A N

Labor stimulation

Potential patient problem	*Outcome criteria*
AROM **A.** Potential fetal distress (hypoxia) related to: Prolapsed cord Increased cephalic pressure	No change in fetal heart rate baseline following AROM No periodic FHR deceleration patterns develop following AROM

EVALUATION

The use of labor stimulants enables many patients to have a vaginal delivery. However, risks are associated with their use. The primary role of the nurse is to monitor closely the labor progress, the uterine contraction pattern, and fetal well-being. Developing complications can then be recognized early so that the labor stimulant can be stopped prior to negative development. A labor stimulant should never be used just to speed up a labor or to initiate a labor for convenience.

O F   N U R S I N G   C A R E

Assessment and intervention

Dx.   Assess the state of the cervix and obtain a Bishop score
Assess FHR prior to and immediately following AROM
Assess color of amniotic fluid
Compare progress of labor to the normal labor curve
Monitor FHR with external or internal monitor
Monitor uterine contractions as to frequency, intensity, duration, and resting tone

Th.   Graph the labor on the Friedman labor curve
If fetal distress develops from a prolapse cord:
   apply and maintain pressure to presenting part
   with other hand push abdomen up
   call for help
   instruct help to:
      Put bed in Trendelenburg position
      Listen for FHR
      Start oxygen by mask at 7 liters/min
      Start intravenous with 18-gauge intracatheter
If fetal distress develops and cord prolapse cannot be determined:
   reposition patient
   administer oxygen by mask at 7 liters/min

Ref.   Notify physician of cord prolapse or signs of fetal distress such as periodic late or variable decelerations, change in baseline, and meconium- or blood-stained amniotic fluid.

Dx., diagnostic; Th., therapeutic; Ed., education; Ref., referral.   *Continued.*

Labor stimulation—cont'd

Potential patient problem	*Outcome criteria*
B. Potential infection related to: AROM	Temperature less than 38° C (100.4° F)

Oxytocin
  A. Potential hypertonic uterus or fetal distress related to:
    Overstimulation with oxytocin

Uterine contractions less than four every 10 min
Uterine contractions that do not last longer than 70 to 90 sec
No rise in resting uterine pressure from 15 to 20 mm Hg
Uterine relaxation for at least 1 min between contractions
Intensity not greater than 80 mm Hg

Assessment and intervention

Dx. Check temperature every 1 hr
Assess odor of amniotic fluid
Th. Keep patient dry and clean as amniotic fluid will continue to leak
Ref. Notify physician if temperature is greater than 38° C (100.4° F)

Dx. Obtain a baseline FHR and uterine activity pattern for 15 to 20 min prior to
starting the induction
Obtain baseline maternal blood pressure and pulse
Monitor uterine contractions and FHR continuously
Assess dosage, rate of flow, blood pressure, pulse, uterine contractions, and
FHR pattern every 15 min after starting induction
Assess intravenous patency every 15 min
Th. Prepare oxytocin solution according to hospital protocol
Piggyback oxytocin solution into a well functioning intravenous line using a
continuous infusion pump
Start IV oxytocin at 0.5 to 1 mU/min
Increase oxytocin rate of flow 1 to 2 mU every 15 to 20 min until adequate
uterine contractility of three contractions in a 10 min period has been established
Monitor with a continuous FHR and uterine contraction monitor
Graph progress of labor on the normal labor curve
Reduce oxytocin if:
uterine contractions last longer than 75 to 90 sec (depending on phase of
labor)
uterine relaxation between contractions is less than 1 min
uterine tone fails to return to baseline of 15 to 20 mm Hg pressure between contractions
mild variable deceleration FHR pattern develops
discontinue oxytocin if the above situations persist after oxytocin reduction
or the following signs of fetal distress develop:
late decelerations
severe variable decelerations
loss of beat to beat variability
sustained fetal bradycardia or tachycardia
Ref. Notify physician if discontinue oxytocin or failure to progress is noted

Continued.

Labor stimulation—cont'd

Potential patient problem	Outcome criteria
B. Anxiety related to: Fear of increased intensity of contractions	Verbalize fears and concerns Participates in decisions affecting care
C. Potential hypotension related to: Relaxing effect of oxytocin on vascular smooth muscle	Blood pressure stable for patient
D. Potential water intoxication related to: Antidiuretic effect of oxytocin	Urinary output greater than 120 ml/4 hr
Intravaginal Prostaglandins **A.** Potential hypertonic uterus or fetal distress related to: Overstimulation with prostaglandins	Less than four uterine contractions every 10 min Uterine contractions that do not last longer than 70 to 90 sec No rise in resting uterine pressure from 15 to 20 mm Hg Uterine relaxation period of at least 1 min between contractions Intensity not greater than 80 mm Hg

Assessment and intervention

Dx. Assess level of anxiety
   Assess knowledge of distraction and relaxation tools
Th. Instruct and support patient and coach with use of distraction and relaxation
    tools as needed
   Administer pain medication during active phase of labor according to pa-
    tient's request and written orders
Ed. Explain procedure and what to expect
Ref. Notify physician if discomfort is greater than patient's tolerance

---

Dx. Check blood pressure every 15 min
   Encourage patient to lay in a lateral recumbent or semi-Fowler's position
   If blood pressure drops below patient's baseline:
    place patient in a modified Trendelenburg position
    increase mainline intravenous infusion
    administer oxygen by mask at 7 liters/min
Ref. Notify physician if blood pressure drops below patient's baseline

---

Dx. Keep an accurate I&O record
Th. Restirct fluids to 1,000 ml/24 hr
Ref. Notify physician if urinary output is less than 120 ml/4 hr

---

Dx. Obtain a baseline FHR and uterine activity pattern for 15 to 20 min prior to
    starting the induction
   Monitor uterine contractions and FHR continuously
Th. Assist with the insertion of the intravaginal prostaglandins
   Graph progress of labor on normal labor curve
Ref. Notify physician if:
    signs of fetal distress develop
    tetanic contractions develop such as:
     greater than four every 10 min
     last longer than 90 sec
     resting time is increased
    failure to progress is noted

Continued.

Labor stimulation—cont'd

Potential patient problem	*Outcome criteria*
B. Anxiety related to: Fear of increased intensity of contractions	Verbalize fears and concerns Participates in decisions affecting care
C. Potential nausea, vomiting, diarrhea, or fever related to: Drug	Signs of nausea, vomiting, diarrhea or fever do not develop

REFERENCES

Abdul-Karim, R., and Assali, N.: Renal function in human pregnancy: Effects of oxytocin on renal hemodynamics and water electrolyte excretion, J. Lab. Clin. Med. **57:**522, 1961.

Bishop, E.H.: Pelvic scoring for elective induction, Obstet. Gynecol. **24:**266, 1964.

Brenner, W.E.: The oxytocics: Actions and clinical indications, Contemp. Obstet. Gynecol. **7**(1):125, 1976.

Elliott, J.P., and Flaherty, J.: The use of breast stimulation to ripen the cervix in term pregnancies, Am. J. Obstet. Gynecol. **145:**553, 1983.

Embrey, M.P., Graham, N.B., and McNeill, M.E.: Induction of labour with a sustained-release prostaglandin E_2 vaginal pessary, Br. Med. J. **281:**901, 1980.

Federal Drug Administration (FDA): Oxytocin injection labeling, Rockville, Md., 1978, Division of Metabolism and Endocrine Drug Products.

Gabbe, S., and others: Umbilical cord compression associated with amniotomy: laboratory observations, Am. J. Obstet. Gynecol. **126:**353, 1976.

Gee, H., and Beazley, J.: Uterine activity plotted on an inductograph as an aid to management of labour, Br. J. Obstet. Gynaecol. **87:**115, 1980.

Gibb, D., and others: Prolonged pregnancy: is induction of labor indicated? a prospective study, Obstet. Gynecol. Surv. **38**(2):87, 1983.

Hefni, M.A., and Lewis, G.A.: Induction of labour with vaginal prostaglandin E_2 pessaries, Br. J. Obstet. and Gynaecol. **87:**199, 1980.

Assessment and intervention

Dx. Assess level of anxiety
Assess knowledge of distraction and relaxation tools
Assess level of discomfort

Th. Instruct and support patient and coach with use of distraction and relaxation tools as needed
Administer pain medication during active phase of labor according to patient's request and written orders

Ed. Explain procedure and what to expect

Ref. Notify physician if discomfort is greater than patient's tolerance

---

Dx. Check temperature every 1 hr
Assess for other signs of an infection
Assess for nausea, vomiting, and diarrhea greater than normal

Th. If nausea or vomiting persists administer antiemetic as ordered

Ref. Notify physician if any of these signs develop

Jeeva, M., and Dommisse, J.: Laminaria tents or vaginal prostaglandins for cervical ripening: a comparative trial, S. African Med. J. **61**:402, 1982.

Liston, W.A., and Campbell, A.J.: Dangers of oxytocin-induced labour to fetuses, Br. Med. J. **3**:606, 1974.

Lumley, J.: Antepartum fetal heart rate tests and induction of labor. In Young, D., editor: Obstetrical intervention and technology in the 1980's, New York, 1983, The Haworth Press, Inc.

McKenna, P., and Shaw, R.W.: Hyponatremic fits in oxytocin-augmented labours, Int. J. Gynaecol. Obstet. **17**:250, 1979.

Neilson, D., and others: A comparison of prostaglandin E_2 gel and prostaglandin F_{2a} gel for preinduction cervical ripening, Am. J. Obstet. Gynecol. **146**:526, 1983.

Norstrom, A.: Influence of prostaglandin E_2 on the biosynthesis of connective tissue constituents in pregnant human cervix, Prostaglandins **23**:361, 1982.

O'Brien, W., and Cefalo, R.: Abnormalities of the active phase: recognition and treatment, Clin. Obstet. Gynecol. **25**:115, 1982.

Oxorn, H.: Human labor and birth, ed. 4, New York, 1980, Appleton-Century-Crofts, Inc.

Petrie, R.: The pharmocology and use of oxytocin, Clin. Perinatol. **8**(1):35, 1981.

Prins, R., and others: Cervical ripening with intravaginal prostaglandins E_2 gel, Obstet. Gynecol. **61**:459, 1983.

Seitchik, J., and Castillo, M.: Oxytocin augmentation of dysfunctional labor: multiparous patients, Am. J. Obstet. Gynecol. **145:**777, 1983.

Shepherd, J., and Knuppel, R.: The role of prostaglandins in ripening the cervix and inducing labor, Clin. Perinatol. **8**(1):49, 1981.

Simkin, P.: Amniotomy. In Young, D., editor: Obstetrical, intervention and technology in the 1980's, New York, 1983, The Haworth Press, Inc.

Weissberg, S., and Spellacy, W.: Membrane stripping to induce labor, J. Reprod. Med. **19**(3):125, 1977.

Wilson, P.D.: A comparison of four methods of ripening the unfavorable cervix, Br. J. Obstet. Gynaecol. **85:**941, 1978.

Index

A

Abdominal breathing, 15
Abdominal ectopic pregnancy, 191
Abdominal pain and abruptio placentae, 227
Abdominal surgery
    and ectopic pregnancy, 196
    postoperative procedures for, 199
Abduction, 15
Abnormal labor patterns, 398-400
Abnormalities
    baseline fetal heart rate, 44, 45
    of baseline variability, 46, 47
ABO incompatibility, 363
Abortion
    complete, 161, 162
        medical management of, 165-167
    early, 157
    elective, and ectopic pregnancy, 197
    habitual, 162
        medical management of, 169-170
    incomplete, 162
        medical management of, 165-167
    inevitable, 161, 162
        medical management of, 165-167
    late, 157-158
    missed, 161, 162
        medical management of, 167-169
    previous, and preterm labor, 311
    septic, 162
        medical management of, 169-170
    spontaneous; see Spontaneous abortion
    threatened, 161, 162
        medical management of, 164-165
    tubal, 189-190
Abruptio placentae
    compared with placenta previa, 244-245
    etiology of, 223-225
    incidence of, 223
    medical diagnosis, 229-230
    nursing care plan, 246-253
    nursing process, 237-243, 254
    physiology, 226-229
    usual medical management, 230-231
Absent variability of baseline fetal heart rate, 46
Accelerations of fetal heart rate, 47, 48, 50-51
Acceptance and grief, 77
Acetyl-CoA, 5
Acetylcholine, 284
Acid-base balance, 137
Acidemia, 139

Actinomycin D and proliferative trophoblastic disease, 213
Active phase of labor, 390
Actual loss, 76
Acute glomerulonephritis, 135
Adaptation, 74-76
    in body functions during pregnancy, 3-9
ADH; see Antidiuretic hormone (ADH)
Adhesions, tubal, and ectopic pregnancy, 188
Adrenal glands, 6
Adrenergic receptors, 318
Afterload, 118
Age
    gestational, and premature rupture of membrane, 351
    maternal
        and Maternal Child Health Care Index, 23
        and postterm pregnancy, 423
Alcohol
    and preterm labor, 324-325
    and spontaneous abortion, 170
Aldomet and renal disease, 146
Aldosterone, 138
Alpha receptors, 318
Ambivalence and grief, 77
Amino acids, 5
    secretion of, 138
Amniocentesis, 61-64
    and diabetic patient, 100
    and hemolytic incompatibility, 370
    and placenta previa, 235
    and polyhydramnios, 94
Amniography and hydatidiform mole, 212
Amnion, 347
Amniotic cavity, 10
Amniotic fluid
    and AROM, 435
    color of, 353
        and hemolytic incompatibility, 373
    normal physiology of, 347-348
    and postterm pregnancy, 421
    test for, 350
Amniotic fluid embolism, 260
Amniotomy, labor stimulated by, 434-435
Amobarbital sodium and convulsions, 288
Ampicillin
    and bacteriuria, 143
    and endometrial infection, 329, 360
Ampullar ectopic pregnancy, 186, 187
Amytal Sodium; see Amobarbital sodium

Analgesics and pregnancy-induced hypertension, 289

Anatomic abnormalities and Hobel scoring system, 25

Anemia
assessment of, 172
and cardiac disease, 121
fetal, and hemolytic incompatibility, 368

Anesthesia
and breech presentation, 408
for cardiac patient, 127
and magnesium sulfate, 324
and renal disease, 147

Aneurysm, dissecting, 119

Anger and grief, 76

Angiotensin II, 270

Angiotensin II test and pregnancy-induced hypertension, 275-276

Ankle circles, 15

ANS; *see* Autonomic nervous system (ANS)

Antepartum assessment
of fetal well-being, 31-67
and interventions, 13-16
maternal, 11-16
physical, and hemolytic incompatibility, 373
and spontaneous abortion, 172-174

Antepartum fetal heart rate monitoring, 52-53

Antepartum fetal surveillance, 52-56

Antepartum intervention
and abruptio placentae, 239-242
for cardiac disease, 123-124
and diabetes, 104-105
and disseminated intravascular coagulopathy, 265
and ectopic pregnancy, 198-199
and hemolytic incompatibility, 374-375
and hydatidiform mole, 214-215
and placenta previa, 239-242
for pregnancy-induced hypertension, 282-284
and premature rupture of membranes, 354-355
and preterm labor, 316-318
and renal disease, 145-146

Antepartum management of diabetes, 97-102

Antepartum monitoring of fetus, 100

Antibacterial substance in amniotic fluid, 348

Antibiotics
and endometrial infection, 329
for intrauterine infection, 352
and renal disease, 143

Antibody screen, 12, 374

Anticipatory grief, 77-79, 82
and diabetes, 94

Antidiuretic hormone (ADH), 6, 137

Antiemetic and spontaneous abortion, 173

Antihypertensive drugs, 143
and renal disease, 146

Antihypertensive therapy, interventions for, 286-287

Antimicrobial drugs and renal disease, 146

Anxiety, 73-74
and cardiac disease, 121
and hemolytic incompatibility, 373
and pregnancy-induced hypertension, 289

Apparent maternal bleeding, 223, 225

Appendicitis compared with ectopic pregnancy, 194

Application
of fetal monitor, 35-39
of Johnson behavioral system model, 27-28
of Orem's model of self-care, 28-29
of Roy adaptation model, 26-27

Apresoline; *see* Hydralazine; Hydralazine hydrochloride

Arm lifts, 15

Arterial pressure, 4

Artifact versus arrhythmia, fetal, 40-41, 42

AROM, 434

Arrest disorders, 396-397, 399, 400

Arrhythmia versus artifact, fetal, 40-41, 42

Assessment
and abruptio placentae, 237-239, 247, 249, 251, 253
antepartum; *see* Antepartum assessment
and cardiac disease, 122-123, 129, 131, 133
and diabetic patient, 103-104, 109, 111, 113, 115
and disseminated intravascular coagulopathy, 263, 264, 265
and dysfunctional labor, 404-407, 411, 413, 415, 417
and ectopic pregnancy, 197-198, 201, 203, 205
and gestational trophoblastic disease, 217, 219
and hemolytic incompatibility, 371-374, 377
and hydatidiform mole, 214
and hypertensive disorders of pregnancy, 293, 295, 297, 299, 301, 303
and labor stimulated by amniotomy, 434-435
and labor stimulated by oxytocin, 436-439
and labor stimulated by prostaglandins, 440-441
and labor stimulation, 443, 445, 447, 449
and placenta previa, 237-239, 247, 249, 251, 253
and postterm pregnancy, 426, 429, 431
and pregnancy-induced hypertension, 279-282
of premature rupture of membranes, 353-354, 357, 359
and preterm labor, 315-316, 329, 331, 333, 335, 337, 339, 341
and psychologic implications of high-risk pregnancy, 79, 81
and renal disease, 144, 149, 151, 153
of self-care of high-risk pregnant woman, 29
and spontaneous abortion, 171-172, 177, 179, 181, 183

Asymptomatic bacteriuria, 141-142

Asymptomatic pyelonephritis, 142
Attachment, 71-73
Augmentation of labor, 432
Auscultation and fetal heart rate, 32
Autonomic nervous system (ANS), 4, 117
Average dilatational curve, 391

B

Back pain and dysfunctional labor, 408
Bacteriuria, 135
  diagnosis of, 141-142
Bandl's ring, 407
Bargaining and grief, 76
Baseline fetal heart rate, 43-47
Bed rest
  and cardiac disease, 120-121, 123
  and pregnancy-induced hypertension, 276, 277, 279, 282
  and premature rupture of membranes, 354-355
  and preterm labor, 312, 316
  and third-trimester bleeding, 240
Bed rest obstetric patient, passive exercises for, 14, 15
Behavioral complications of diabetes, 94-95
Behavioral effects of frustration, 74
Behaviors that result in anxiety, 74
Beta receptors, 318
Beta-sympathomimetics, 125
  and preterm labor, 313
  for suppression of labor, 318-323
Bicarbonate deficit, 141
Bilirubin and hemolytic incompatibility, 368
Biophysical profile, 56, 61
Biopsy, renal, 142
Biparietal diameter (BPD), 351
Birth trauma
  and breech presentation, 388
  and dysfunctional labor, 392
Bladder, full, and labor, 404
Bladder infection, 140
Blastocyte, 9, 158
Bleeding; *see also* Hemorrhage
  third trimester; *see* Abruptio placentae; Placenta previa
  and tubal rupture, 191
  uterine, and hydatidiform mole, 211
  vaginal; *see* Vaginal bleeding
Blood cells, white, 7
Blood flow
  renal, 136
  uterine, and preterm labor, 310
Blood gases, 4
Blood glucose monitoring, antepartum, 98
Blood loss
  and abruptio placentae, 230-231
  and ectopic pregnancy, 192
  estimation of, 238
  and pregnancy-induced hypertension, 290

Blood pressure and renal disease, 144
Blood pressure cuff, 275
Blood pressure measurement, 14
Blood pressure readings
  evaluation of, 273
  and pregnancy-induced hypertension, 275, 283
Blood sugar, assessment of, 12-13
Blood supply to endometrium and placenta previa, 233
Blood type, 12
  fetal, 364-366
Blood urea nitrogen (BUN), 7, 142
Blood volume, 3, 4
  during pregnancy, 33, 116-117, 269
Body fluids, 3
Body functions, adaptations in, during pregnancy, 3-9
Bonding and hemolytic incompatibility, 373-374, 377-378
Booking examination, 56
Boredom
  and pregnancy-induced hypertension, 284
  and preterm labor, 317
BPD; *see* Biparietal diameter (BPD)
Bradycardia, 46
  fetal, 44, 45
Brain, blood supply to, 271
Breast feeding and magnesium, 291
Breasts, changes in, during pregnancy, 9
Breathing and labor, 404
Breech presentation, 388, 389, 402-403
  principles for, 408-409
Brethine; *see* Terbutaline sulfate
Bridging, 15
Brow presentation, 386, 387, 402-403
Buffering substances, 139
BUN; *see* Blood urea nitrogen (BUN)

C

Calcium antagonists and preterm labor, 325
Calcium deficit, 140
Calcium excess, 140
Calcium gluconate, 286
  and magnesium sulfate therapy, 324
Caloric intake
  of diabetic patient, 100
  during pregnancy, 17
Carbohydrate, 5
Carbon dioxide, partial pressure of, 4
Carbonic acid, 137
Cardiac disease and pregnancy, 116-134
  etiology of, 116
  incidence of, 116
  medical diagnosis, 120
  nursing care plan, 128-133
  nursing process, 121-129, 132
  physiology, 116-120
  usual medical management, 120-121

Cardiac output, 3
Cardiac physiology, 116-120
Cardiotachometer, 40
Cardiovascular adaptations, maternal, 3-4, 33
Cardiovascular factors and Hobel scoring system, 24
Catecholamines, 6
Catheter, uterine pressure, 38-39
CBC; *see* Complete blood count (CBC)
Cells of placenta, 233
Central maternal bleeding, 223, 225
Central nervous system (CNS) of fetus, 35
Central venous pressure (CVP), 122, 123
Cephalopelvic disproportion (CPD), 390
Cephalosporin and endometrial infection, 329, 360
Cerclage, 169
Cervical ectopic pregnancy, 191
Cervix, 160
    dilatation of, 166
        and mixed abortion, 168
    incompetent, and habitual abortion, 169
    and labor stimulation, 433
    during pregnancy, 8
    and prolonged latent phase disorder, 395
Cesarean delivery
    and breech presentation, 388, 408
    complications of, 391
    and diabetes, 94
    and dysfunctional labor, 391
    and hemolytic incompatibility, 373
    and placenta previa, 236-237
    and pregnancy-induced hypertension, 289
    and protraction disorders, 395
    and renal disease, 147
    and third-trimester bleeding, 242-243
Chart
    fetal activity, 64
        and diabetic patient, 102
    insulin comparison, 106
Charting of labor, 405, 406
Chemotherapy for proliferative trophoblastic disease, 213-214
Chest pain and beta-sympathomimetics, 321-322
Chloramphenicol, 146-147
Chorioadenoma destruens, 208
Chorioamnionitis, 348-349
    determination of, 351
    and suppression of labor, 321
    symptoms of, 354
Choriocarcinoma, 208
Chorion, 347
Chorion frondosum, 10
Chorionic villi, 189, 210
    types of, 233
Chorionic villi sampling, 63
CHP; *see* Concurrent hypertension and pregnancy (CHP)

Chromosomal disorder
    and habitual abortion, 169
    and spontaneous abortion, 157
Chronic hypertension, 268
    versus pregnancy-induced hypertension, 142-143
Chronic renal disease, 140
Chronic renal impairment, 141
Cigarette smoking; *see* Smoking
Circulation and cardiac disease, 120
Circulatory adaptations, maternal, 33
Circulatory volume and urinary output, 241-242
Classical hydatidiform mole, 210
Classification
    of abruptio placentae, 223, 224, 225, 244
    of cardiac disease, 119
    of hypertensive states of pregnancy, 268
    of obstetric diabetes, 88
    of placenta previa, 231, 232, 244
    of spontaneous abortion, 162
Cleanliness and premature rupture of membranes, 353
Clinistix, 98, 322
Clomid; *see* Clomiphene citrate
Clomiphene citrate, 210
Clonus, 280
Closed-loop insulin pump, 99-100
Clot, blood, 8
    formation of, 257-258, 259
Clot-observation test, 242
Clot-retraction test, 261, 264
CNS; *see* Central nervous system (CNS)
Coagulation, 7-8
Coagulation defects and abruptio placentae, 231
Coagulation factor values, normal, 261
Coagulation process, 257
Coma, 288
Combined maternal bleeding, 223, 225
Complete abortion, 161, 162
    medical management of, 165-167
Complete blood count (CBC), 11-12
Complete breech, 388, 389
Complete hydatidiform mole, 210
Complications
    of abruptio placentae, 245
    of cesarean delivery, 391
    of dysfunctional labor, 406-407
    of placenta previa, 245
    of pregnancy-induced hypertension, 282
    of ritodrine, 320
    of steroid therapy, 326-327
    of terbutaline, 320
Compound presentation, 388, 402-403
Concealed maternal bleeding, 223, 225
Concurrent hypertension and pregnancy (CHP), 267, 268
Conflict and high-risk pregnancy, 73-74
Congenital heart block, fetal, 41

Congenital heart defect, 120
Congenital heart disease, 116
Constipation and premature rupture of membranes, 355
Consumptive coagulopathy, 257
Contraception and cardiac disease, 121-122, 128
Contraction phase of contraction, 384
Contraction stress test (CST), 55-56, 57-60
  in diabetic patient, 102
  and postterm pregnancy, 424
Contractions
  external monitoring of, 37
  initiation of, with nipple stimulation, 57
  intensity of, 405
  and labor stimulated by prostaglandins, 440-441
  normal physiology of, 384
  steps leading to, 309
  stimulation of, with oxytocin, 57
Contractility, 118
Contraindications for labor stimulation, 433
Conventional grief, 76-77
Convulsions
  and nursing responsibilities, 287-288
  prevention of, 284-286
Coping mechanisms, 75
  and hemolytic incompatibility, 372
Corometrics Model 115 fetal monitor, 35
Corometrics tocotransducer, 36
Corometrics ultrasound transducer, 36
Corpus luteum during pregnancy, 9
Cortisol, 6
Cotyledons, 10, 33
Couvelaire uterus, 226
CPD; *see* Cephalopelvic disproportion (CPD)
Crisis, 74-76
Criteria
  for interpretation of contraction stress test, 57, 58-60
  for interpretation of nonstress test, 54, 55
  for labor stimulation, 432-433
  outcome; *see* Outcome criteria
CST; *see* Contraction stress test (CST)
Cuff, blood pressure, 275
Cul-de-sac of Douglas, 192, 193
Culdocentesis, 196
Curettage, 166
  and missed abortion, 167-168
Curl-ups, 15
CVP; *see* Central venous pressure (CVP)
Cyanotic heart disease, 119
Cytotrophoblast, 10

D

Data base for assessment of bleeding, 237-238
Dating of gestation, 425
Death; *see* Mortality

Deceleration phase of labor, 390-391
Decelerations of fetal heart rate, 47, 48-49, 51
Decidua, 10, 159
Decidua basilis, 10, 159
Decidua capsularis, 159
Decidua vera, 159
Decreased variability of baseline fetal heart rate, 46, 47
Deep tendon reflex (DTR) grading, 280, 281
Deformities, fetal, and ectopic pregnancy, 193
Degrees of edema, 280, 281
Dehydration and dysfunctional labor, 404
Delivery
  cesarean; *see* Cesarean delivery
  and premature rupture of membranes, 351-352
  preterm, 347
  vaginal; *see* Vaginal delivery
Demerol; *see* Meperidine hydrochloride
Denial and grief, 76
Depression, 77
  and grief, 77
  postpartum, and labor stimulation, 442
DES; *see* Diethylstilbesterol (DES)
Developmental tasks, 71-73
Dexamethasone, 327
Diabetes and pregnancy, 87-115
  classification of, 88
  etiology of, 87
  incidence of, 87
  medical diagnosis, 96-97
  nursing care plan, 108-115
  nursing process, 103-107
  physiology, 87-96
  signs and symptoms of, 92, 93
  usual medical management, 97-103
Diabetic renal disease, 135
Diagnosis, medical; *see* Medical diagnosis
Diagnostic work-up for ectopic pregnancy, 195
Diastole phase of contraction, 384
Diastolic filling pressure, 118
Diastolic pulmonary artery pressure, 123
Diazepam
  and convulsions, 288
  and spontaneous abortion, 166
DIC; *see* Disseminated intravascular coagulation (DIC)
Diet
  and pregnancy-induced hypertension, 282-283
    high-protein, 276
  and premature rupture of membranes, 353
Diet management of diabetes, 98, 100, 101
Diethylstilbesterol (DES) and preterm labor, 310-311
Diffusion
  facilitated, 10
  simple, 34
Digitalis, 125

Dilatation of cervix, 166
  and missed abortion, 168
Dilatational curve, average, 391
Dipstick readings, 280, 281
Direct monitoring of fetus, 38-39
Diseases
  ectopic pregnancy compared with, 194
  and placental aging, 421
Disequilibrium, 74
Disopyramide phosphate, 126
Dissecting aneurysm, 119
Disseminated intravascular coagulation (DIC),
    167, 257-266
  and abruptio placentae, 228
  and eclampsia, 288
  etiology of, 257
  incidence of, 257
  medical diagnosis, 261
  and missed abortion, 168
  nursing care plan, 262-265
  nursing process, 261, 264-266
  physiology, 257-261
  usual medical management, 261
Distraction tools and oxytocin, 439
Diuresis, postpartum, 289
Diuretics
  and pregnancy-induced hypertension, 277
  and renal disease, 143, 146
Documentation and postterm pregnancy, 426
Double footling breech, 388
Double voided specimen, 98
Drug therapy
  and cardiac disease, 124-126
  for diabetic patient, 105-107
  for hemolytic incompatibility, 375
  and preterm labor, 313
  for renal disease, 146-147
  for stimulation of fetal lung maturity, 326-327
  for suppression of labor, 318-326
Dry method of blood glucose monitoring, 98
DTR grading; *see* Deep tendon reflex (DTR)
    grading
Duration of tubal pregnancy, 191
Dysfunctional labor, 383-418
  etiology of, 383-384
  incidence of, 383
  medical diagnosis, 392
  nursing care plan, 410-417
  nursing process, 401-409
  physiology, 384-392
  usual medical management, 392-401
Dysfunctional labor disorders, 394-400
Dystocia, 383-385

E

Early abortion, 157
Early deceleration of fetal heart rate, 48, 51
ECG monitoring and cardiac patient, 122

Eclampsia, 268, 274
  and disseminated intravascular coagulopathy,
    260
  intervention for, 287-288
  nursing care plan for, 298-303
  signs of, 287
Eclamptic tray, 287
Ectoderm, 11
Ectopic pregnancy, 186-207
  etiology of, 186, 188
  incidence of, 186
  medical diagnosis, 193-196
  nursing care plan, 200-205
  nursing process, 197-201, 206
  physiology, 188-193
  sites of, 186, 187
  usual medical management, 196-197
Edema
  assessment of, 14
  degrees of, 280, 281
  during pregnancy, 270
  and pregnancy-induced hypertension, 273
  pulmonary; *see* Pulmonary edema
Education
  of diabetic patient, 104-105
  and ectopic pregnancy, 206
  and postterm pregnancy, 425
  and pregnancy-induced hypertension, 282-283
  and premature rupture of membranes, 360
  and spontaneous abortion, 175
Educational needs, maternal, 14
Edward's simplified index, 24
Elective abortion and ectopic pregnancy, 197
Elective induction, 432
Electrode, fetal scalp, 38, 39
Electrolyte imbalance, signs of, 140
Emboli, systemic, 119
Embryo, 9-10
Embryoblast, 159, 210
Emotional effects
  of diabetes, 94
  of postterm pregnancy, 422
Emotional support
  and dysfunctional labor, 409
  and premature rupture of membranes, 357
  and spontaneous abortion, 175
Endoderm, 11
Endometrial infection
  postpartum, 328-329
  and premature rupture of membranes, 357,
    360
Endometrium, blood supply to, and placenta
    previa, 233
Entrainment, 72
Epinephrine, 6
Equivocal contraction stress test, 57, 58, 59
Erythrocytes, fetal, 366-367
Escherichia coli, 136
Estriol and labor, 307-308

Estriol determinations, 63-64
  and diabetic patient, 102
Estrogen, 8, 159
  and oxytocin, 436
  during pregnancy, 269
Ethanol and preterm labor, 324-325
Etiology
  of abruptio placentae, 223-224, 244
  of arrest disorders, 399
  of cardiac disease, 116
  of decreased or absent variability, 46
  of diabetes, 87
  of disseminated intravascular coagulopathy,
    257
  of dysfunctional labor, 383-384
  of ectopic pregnancy, 186, 188
  of fetal bradycardia, 44
  of fetal malpresentations, 402
  of fetal tachycardia, 44
  of hemolytic incompatibility, 363
  of hydatidiform mole, 208, 210
  of increased variability, 46
  of placenta previa, 233, 244
  of postterm pregnancy, 419-420
  of precipitous labor, 400
  of pregnancy-induced hypertension, 268-269
  of premature rupture of membranes, 347
  of preterm labor, 306-307
  of prolonged labor phase, 398
  of protraction disorders, 398
  of renal disease, 136
  of spontaneous abortion, 157-158
Evacuation of uterus
  and hydatidiform mole, 212-213
  methods for, 165-166
  and missed abortion, 167-168
  reasons for, 164
Evaluation
  and abruptio placentae, 254
  and cardiac patient, 129, 132
  of diabetic patient, 107
  and disseminated intravascular coagulopathy,
    266
  and dysfunctional labor, 409
  and ectopic pregnancy, 206
  and hemolytic incompatibility, 378
  and hydatidiform mole, 220-221
  and labor stimulation, 443
  and placenta previa, 254
  and postterm pregnancy, 427, 430
  and pregnancy-induced hypertension, 291
  and premature rupture of membranes, 360
  and preterm labor, 342
  and renal disease, 148-149
  and spontaneous abortion, 175
Examination
  pelvic, and postterm pregnancy, 424-425
  vaginal
    and AROM, 435

Examination—cont'd
  vaginal—cont'd
    and dysfunctional labor, 405
    and fetal malpresentations, 403
    and premature rupture of membranes, 350
Exercise(s)
  for diabetic, 100
  passive, for bed rest obstetric patient, 14, 15
  and pregnancy-induced hypertension, 284
  and preterm labor, 317
Expectant management, 236
  and premature rupture of membranes, 350-
    351
  role of nurse in, 239
External cephalic version, 401
External fetal monitoring, 37
External os, 160
Eyes, blood supply to, 271

F
FAC; *see* Fetal activity chart (FAC)
Face presentation, 385-386, 402-403
Facilitated diffusion, 10
Fallopian tube
  ectopic pregnancy in, 186, 187
  normal physiology of, 188-189
False labor, 401, 414
Fatty acids, 5
Faulty metabolism in diabetic, 90
Fear
  and grief, 76
  and postterm pregnancy, 422
Feelings, ambivalent, and grief, 77
Fenoterol, 318
Fertilization, 9
Fetal activity, 14
  and hemolytic incompatibility, 373
  and pregnancy-induced hypertension, 280
Fetal activity chart (FAC), 64
  and diabetic patient, 102
Fetal anemia and hemolytic incompatibility, 368
Fetal blood types, 364-366
Fetal capabilities for withstanding stressors, 34-
    35
Fetal causes of preterm labor, 307
Fetal death
  and disseminated intravascular coagulopathy,
    260
  and ectopic pregnancy, 193
  and spontaneous abortion, 163
Fetal distinction, 72-73
Fetal distress
  and abruptio placentae, 229
  and AROM, 435
  determination of, 353
  and hemolytic incompatibility, 375-377
  and labor stimulation, 434
  nursing interventions for, 41-52
  and premature rupture of membranes, 350

Fetal dystocia, 383-388
  causes of, 383-384
  incidence of, 383
Fetal effects
  of abruptio placentae, 224, 229
  of cardiac disease, 120
  of diabetes, 95-96
  of disseminated intravascular coagulopathy,
    261
  of dysfunctional labor, 391-392
  of ectopic pregnancy, 193
  of gestational trophoblastic disease, 212
  of hemolytic incompatibility, 367-368
  of labor stimulation, 434
  of placenta previa, 235
  of postterm pregnancy, 422-423
  of pregnancy-induced hypertension, 274-275
  of premature rupture of membranes, 349-350
  of preterm labor, 311
  of renal disease, 141
  of spontaneous abortion, 163
Fetal embodiment, 72
Fetal erythrocytes, 366-367
Fetal factors and Hobel scoring system, 25
Fetal heart rate, 14
  and hemolytic incompatibility, 373
  and labor stimulated by prostaglandins, 440
  and pregnancy-induced hypertension, 280
  regulation of, 35
Fetal heart rate (FHR) monitoring, 31-52
  antepartum, 52-53
  application of fetal monitor, 35-40
  arrhythmia versus artifact, 40-41
  basic FHR pattern recognition, 41-52
  and cardiac disease, 120, 122-123
  instrumentation, 40
  nursing interventions for fetal distress, 41-47
  physiologic basis for, 33-35
Fetal heart rate patterns, 47-52
Fetal lung maturity
  determination of, 351
  drug therapy for stimulation of, 326-327
Fetal malpresentations, 401, 402-403
  and vaginal delivery, 407-408
Fetal monitor, application of, 35-39
Fetal monitoring
  and cardiac disease, 124
    during labor, 126
  and dysfunctional labor, 406
  and hemolytic incompatibility, 374
Fetal movement and hydatidiform mole, 211
Fetal outcome of placenta previa and abruptio
    placentae, 245
Fetal scalp electrode, 38, 39
Fetal surveillance, antepartum, 52-56
Fetal well-being
  antepartum and intrapartum assessment of,
    31-67
  and cardiac disease, 124

Fetal well-being tests, 283
Fetopelvic disproportion (FPD), 390
  and arrest disorders, 396-397
  and trial labor, 407
α-Fetoprotein, 63
Fetus, 11
  effects of beta-sympathomimetics on, 323
  viable, 157
FHR monitoring; *see* Fetal heart rate (FHR)
    monitoring
Fibrin breakdown during pregnancy, 8
Fibrinogen and disseminated intravascular coag-
    ulopathy, 168
Fibrinoid material and placenta, 421
Fibrinolysis, 258, 259
Financial loss, 76
Financial strain of diabetes, 94
First trimester, diabetes during, 93
Fluid intake
  and pregnancy-induced hypertension, 278
  and urinary tract infection, 145
Fluid overload, 241
Fluids and renal disease, 144
Follow-up and hydatidiform mole, 213
Footling breech, 388, 389
FPD; *see* Fetopelvic disproportion (FPD)
Frank breech, 388, 389
Fructose, 5
Frustration, 73-74
Fundal height, 14
Fundal measurements and hemolytic incompati-
    bility, 373
Furosemide and cardiac disease, 125

G
Galactose, 5
Gastrointestinal responses to pregnancy, 8
Gastrulation, 11
Genetic evaluation and amniocentesis, 61-62
Genetics and pregnancy-induced hypertension,
    269
Gestation, dating of, 425
Gestational age and premature rupture of mem-
    branes, 351
Gestational diabetes, 88
Gestational hypertension, 268
Gestational trophoblastic disease, 208-222
  etiology of, 208, 210
  incidence of, 208
  medical diagnosis, 212
  nursing care plan, 216-219
  nursing process, 214-218, 220-221
  physiology, 210-212
  usual medical management, 212-214
Glandular developments during pregnancy, 6
Glomerular filtration rate, 7, 269
Glomerulus, 136
Glucocorticoid therapy, 326-327
  and premature rupture of membranes, 352

Glucola-load blood sugar, 12-13
Glucose, 5, 6
  and pregnancy, 86-88, 90
Glucose-6-phosphate, 5
Glucose reflectance meter, 98
Glucose tolerance test, 97
Glucostix, 98
Glyconeogenesis, 90
Goodell sign, 8
Grades of preeclampsia, 273-274
Grading, deep tendon reflex, 280, 281
Granulocytes, 7
Grief and loss, 76-79, 82
Grief work, 76-77

H

Habitual abortion, 162
  medical management of, 169-170
HCG; *see* Human chorionic gonadotropin (HCG)
Heart rate
  fetal; *see* Fetal heart rate
  during pregnancy, 33
Height, fundal, 14
Hematocrit and pregnancy-induced hypertension, 271
Hematologic changes during pregnancy, 7-8
Hemoconcentration, 271
Hemodynamic monitoring during labor and cardiac disease, 127
Hemodynamic pressure readings, 123
Hemodynamic response to labor, 117
Hemoglobin, fetal, 34
Hemoglobin A_1C, 97
Hemolytic incompatibility, 363-379
  etiology of, 363
  incidence of, 363
  medical diagnosis, 368-369
  nursing care plan, 376-377
  nursing process, 371-378
  physiology, 363-368
  usual medical management, 369-371
Hemorrhage; *see also* Bleeding
  and disseminated intravascular coagulopathy, 260
  and dysfunctional labor, 409
  and labor stimulation, 441
  postoperative, and ectopic pregnancy, 199
  postpartum, 243, 254
  and spontaneous abortion, 165, 174
Heparin
  and abruptio placentae, 231
  and cardiac disease, 124-125
  and disseminated intravascular coagulopathy, 168
Hepatic adjustments to pregnancy, 7
Heterozygous blood systems, 364-366
High-protein diet and pregnancy-induced hypertension, 276

High-risk pregnancy, 22; *see also* specific risk factors
  antepartum assessments and interventions, 13-16
  identification of, 22-30
    common scoring systems, 22-26
    nursing models, 26-29
  physiologic considerations in, 1-68
  psychologic adaptations to; *see* Psychologic adaptations to high-risk pregnancy
History
  and antepartum assessment, 13
  and beta-sympathomimetics, 320-321
  and diabetes, 103-104
  and ectopic pregnancy, 197
  and hemolytic incompatibility, 371-372
  and high-risk pregnancy, 22
  and Hobel scoring system, 24
  obstetric
    and Maternal Child Health Care Index, 23
    and postterm pregnancy, 423
  and renal disease, 144
HLA typing, 170
Hobel scoring system, 24-25
Holistic view of nursing, 25-26
Home care
  and premature rupture of membranes, 355
  and third-trimester bleeding, 240
Homozygous blood systems, 364-366
Hope and anticipatory grief, 77
Hormone(s)
  antidiuretic, 137
  and cardiac output, 117
  and labor, 307-308
  produced by placenta, 11
Hospitalization
  and attachment, 72-73
  and pregnancy-induced hypertension, 277-278
Hostility and grief, 77
Human chorionic gonadotropin (HCG), 159
  and ectopic pregnancy, 195
  and fetal death, 163
  and hydatidiform mole, 212, 220-221
  and proliferative trophoblastic disease, 213
Human leukocyte antigen typing, 170
Hydatidiform mole, 208-222
Hydralazine, 286-287
  and renal disease, 146
Hydralazine hydrochloride and pregnancy-induced hypertension, 277
Hydration and preterm labor, 317
Hydrocortisone and vasomotor collapse, 290
Hydrops, 363
Hydrops fetalis, 368
Hyperbilirubinemia and labor stimulation, 434
Hyperemesis gravidarum and hydatidiform mole, 211
Hyperemia gravidarum, 93

Hyperglycemia, 89
  and beta-sympathomimetics, 322
  effect of, on fetus, 95, 96
Hyperplasia, 16
Hyperstimulated uterine activity, 57, 59
Hypertension
  antepartum, 145-146
  and cardiac disease, 123-124
  chronic versus pregnancy-induced, 142-143
  concurrent, and pregnancy, 267, 268
  gestational, 268
  postpartum, 147-148
  pregnancy-induced; *see* Pregnancy-induced hypertension
  signs of, 271
Hypertensive disorders of pregnancy, 267-305
  etiology of, 268-269
  incidence of, 267
  medical diagnosis, 275-276
  nursing care plan, 292-303
  nursing process, 278-291
  physiology, 269-275
  usual medical management, 276-278
Hyperthyroidism and hydatidiform mole, 211
Hypertonic uterine contractions, 384
Hypertonus and oxytocin, 438
Hypertrophy, 16
Hypoglycemia, 90, 91, 92
Hypokalemia and beta-sympathomimetics, 322
Hypotension
  and magnesium sulfate therapy, 324
  and oxytocin, 439
Hypotonic uterine activity, 384
Hypovolemic shock and third-trimester bleeding, 241, 242
Hypoxia and dysfunctional labor, 392
Hypoxic mortality and morbidity, 32
Hysterectomy and ectopic pregnancy, 188

I

Identification of high-risk pregnancy, 22-30
Illness and attachment, 72-73
Immunologic deficit
  and habitual abortion, 170
  and pregnancy-induced hypertension, 268-269
Immunologic factors in spontaneous abortion, 158
Incidence
  of abruptio placentae, 223
  of cardiovascular disease during pregnancy, 116
  of diabetes during pregnancy, 87
  of disseminated intravascular coagulopathy, 257
  of dysfunctional labor, 383
  of ectopic pregnancy, 186
  of fetal malpresentations, 402
  of hemolytic incompatibility, 363
  of hydatidiform mole, 208
  of hypertensive disorders of pregnancy, 267

Incidence—cont'd
  of labor stimulation, 432
  of placenta previa, 231, 233
  of postterm pregnancy, 419
  of premature rupture of membranes, 347
  of preterm labor, 306
  of renal disease in pregnancy, 135-136
  of spontaneous abortion, 157
Incompatibility, hemolytic; *see* Hemolytic incompatibility
Incomplete abortion, 162
  medical management of, 165-167
Incompetent cervix and habitual abortion, 169
Incoordinated uterine contractions, 384
Increased variability of baseline fetal heart rate, 46, 47
Inderal; *see* Propranolol
Indomethacin and preterm labor, 325
Inevitable abortion, 161, 162
  medical management of, 165-167
Infant mortality
  and dysfunctional labor, 391-392
  and preterm labor, 313
Infection
  and abruptio placentae, 254
  and AROM, 435
  bladder, 140
  and diabetes, 94
  and dysfunctional labor, 407, 409
  and ectopic pregnancy, 197
  endometrial
    postpartum, 328-329
    and premature rupture of membranes, 357, 360
  and glucocorticoid, 328-329
  and hydatidiform mole, 215
  and labor stimulation, 441
  and placenta previa, 254
  postoperative, and spontaneous abortion, 174
  and premature rupture of membranes, 347
  and preterm labor, 311
  signs of, 172
  and spontaneous abortion, 165
  urinary tract; *see* Urinary tract infection
Infertility and ectopic pregnancy, 200-201
Initiation of contractions with nipple stimulation, 57
Injections, instructions for, 125
Inlet contraction, 388, 390
Instrumentation for monitoring fetal heart rate, 40
Insulin, 5, 6, 105-106
  abundance of, 91
  lack of, 89
Insulin comparison chart, 106
Insulin-dependent diabetes, 88
Insulin infusion and labor, 102-103
Insulin management, antepartum, 98-99
Insulin pump, antepartum use of, 98, 99-100
Insulin zinc suspension, 106

Intensity of uterine contractions, 405
Intermediate-acting insulin, 106
Internal monitoring of fetus, 38-39
Internal os, 16
Interpretation
  of contraction stress test, 57, 58-60
  of nonstress test, 54, 55
Intervention(s)
  antepartum; *see* Antepartum intervention
  for antihypertensive therapy, 286-287
  for drug therapy for stimulation of fetal lung
    maturity, 326-327
  for eclampsia, 287-288
  intrapartum; see Intrapartum intervention
  for magnesium sulfate therapy, 284-286
  nursing; *see* Nursing interventions
  postpartum; *see* Postpartum intervention
  for self-care of high-risk pregnant woman, 29
Intervillous space, 34-35, 420
Intraamniotic injection of hypotonic saline, 169
Intrapartum assessment
  of fetal well-being, 31-67
  and hemolytic incompatibility, 373
Intrapartum intervention
  and abruptio placentae, 242-243
  and cardiac disease, 126-127
  and diabetes, 107
  and disseminated intravascular coagulopathy,
    265
  and dysfunctional labor, 407-409
  and hemolytic incompatibility, 375-377
  and placenta previa, 242-243
  and pregnancy-induced hypertension, 288-289
  and premature rupture of membranes, 355-
    357
  and preterm labor, 327-328
  and renal disease, 147
Intrapartum management of diabetes, 102-103
Intrauterine infection, 352
Intrauterine transfusion, 370-371, 374
Intravaginal prostaglandins, 440
Intravascular coagulation and fibrinolysis, 257
Intravenous beta-sympathomimetic therapy, 321-
    322
Invasive mole, 208
Iron supplementation, 17
Ischemia, uterine, and pregnancy-induced hyper-
    tension, 269
Isoimmunization, 366-367
Isolation and grief, 76
Isoxuprine hydrochloride, 318
IUD and ectopic pregnancy, 188

J

Johnson behavioral system model, 27-28

K

Kegel exercise, 15
Ketoacidosis and diabetes, 104
Ketodiastix, 98

Ketogenesis, 90
Ketonuria, 98
Kidneys
  blood supply to, 270-271
  function of, 136-137
Kimmelsteil-Wilson disease, 135
Krebs cycle, 5

L

Labor
  augmentation of, 432
  and cardiac disease, 126-127
  charting of, 405, 406
  and diabetes, 93
  dysfunctional; *see* Dysfunctional labor
  and eclampsia, 288
  false, 401, 404
  hemodynamic response to, 117
  and insulin infusion, 102-103
  normal, 390-391
  normal physiology of, 307-309
  precipitous, 397, 400
  preterm; *see* Preterm labor
  and renal disease, 147
  stages of, 405
  suppression of, 312
    drug therapy for, 318-320
    protocol for, 316-318
  trial, 392, 393
    and fetopelvic disproportion, 407
    and third-trimester bleeding, 242, 243
Labor induction and cardiac disease, 127
Labor patterns
  abnormal, 398-400
  normal, 393
Labor stimulation, 432-450
  criteria for, 432-433
  evaluation of, 443
  fetal and neonatal effects, 434
  incidence of, 432
  labor stimulated by amniotomy, 434-435
  labor stimulated by oxytocin, 435-439
  labor stimulated by prostaglandins, 439-441
  maternal effects, 434
  nursing care plan, 442-449
  postpartum intervention, 441-443
Labor stimulants and protraction disorders, 396
Laboratory studies for antepartum maternal as-
    sessment, 11-13
Laboratory tests and pregnancy-induced hyper-
    tension, 280
Lactation and cardiac patient, 129
Lactosuria, 98
Laminaria, 166, 167
  and hydatidiform mole, 213
Laparoscopy, 185-196
Lasix; *see* Furosemide
Late abortion, 157-158
Late deceleration of fetal heart rate, 47, 48, 51
Latent phase of labor, 390

Lecithin, 62, 326
Lecithin/sphingomyelin (L/S) ratio, 62
  in diabetic patient, 100
  and fetal lung maturity, 351
Leg raises, modified, 15
Leg sliding, 15
Lente insulin, 106
Leukocytes, 7
Life-style
  and high-risk pregnancy, 14, 16
  and pregnancy-induced hypertension, 282
Lipids, 5
Liver, blood supply to, 271
Liver enzymes, 7
Logic system in fetal heart rate processing, 40
Loss and grief, 76-79, 82
L/S ratio; *see* Lecithin/sphingomyelin (L/S) ratio
Lung maturity and amniocentesis, 62
Lupus, 135
Luteal defect and habitual abortion, 169-170
Luteal phase, 159
Luteal phase defect and spontaneous abortion, 158
Lysosomes and labor, 308

M

Magnesium, effects of, on neonate, 290-291
Magnesium sulfate
  and cardiac disease, 125
  and precipitous labor, 397
  and pregnancy-induced hypertension, 277
  and preterm labor, 313
  for suppression of labor, 323-324
Magnesium sulfate therapy, intervention for, 284-286
Magnesium toxicity, 286-287, 324
Malnutrition
  and hydatidiform mole, 214
  during pregnancy, 16
Management
  of contraction stress test, 57
  medical; *see* Medical management
  of nonstress test, 54
Marginal maternal bleeding, 223, 225
Marginal placenta previa, 231, 232
Marital status and Maternal Child Health Care Index, 23
Maternal age
  and Maternal Child Health Care Index, 23
  and postterm pregnancy, 423
Maternal assessments, antepartum, 11-16
Maternal causes of preterm labor, 306-307
Maternal Child Health Care Index (MCHC Index), 22-24
Maternal circulatory and cardiovascular adaptations, 33
Maternal effects
  of abruptio placentae, 228-229
  of cardiac disease, 119

Maternal effects—cont'd
  of diabetes, 92-95
  of disseminated intravascular coagulopathy, 261
  of dysfunctional labor, 391
  of ectopic pregnancy, 193, 194
  of gestational trophoblastic disease, 211-212
  of hemolytic incompatibility, 367
  of labor stimulation, 433-434
  of placenta previa, 234-235
  of postterm pregnancy, 422
  of pregnancy-induced hypertension, 274
  of premature rupture of membranes, 349
  of renal disease, 141
  of spontaneous abortion, 162-163
Maternal factors
  in Hobel scoring system, 25
  in postterm pregnancy, 423
Maternal-fetal unit, development of, 9-11
Maternal monitoring and cardiac disease during labor, 126-127
Maternal mortality
  and ectopic pregnancy, 193
  and pregnancy-induced hypertension, 274
  and spontaneous abortion, 162
Maternal outcome of placenta previa and abruptio placentae, 245
Maternal weight gain, 13-14
Maturational crisis, 75
MCHC Index; *see* Maternal Child Health Care Index (MCHC Index)
Meal patterns for diabetic, 101
Measurements, fundal, and hemolytic incompatibility, 373
Mechanism
  of decreased or absent variability, 46
  of early deceleration, 48
  of fetal bradycardia, 44
  of fetal tachycardia, 44
  of increased variability, 46
  of late deceleration, 48
  of nonuniform accelerations, 48
  of prolonged deceleration, 49
  of variable deceleration, 49
Medical diagnosis
  of abruptio placentae, 229-230, 244
  of cardiac disease, 120
  of diabetes, 96-97
  of disseminated intravascular coagulopathy, 261
  of dysfunctional labor, 392
  of ectopic pregnancy, 193, 195-196
  of fetal malpresentations, 403
  of hemolytic incompatibility, 368-369
  of hydatidiform mole, 212
  of placenta previa, 235-236, 244
  of postterm pregnancy, 423-424
  of pregnancy-induced hypertension, 275-276
  of premature rupture of membranes, 350
  of preterm labor, 311

Medical diagnosis—cont'd
  of renal disease, 141-143
  of spontaneous abortion, 163-164
Medical disorders and Maternal Child Health Care Index, 23
Medical management
  of abruptio placentae, 230-231, 245
  of arrest disorders, 399-400
  of cardiac disease, 120-121
  of diabetes, 97-103
  of disseminated intravascular coagulopathy, 261
  of dysfunctional labor, 392-401
  of ectopic pregnancy, 196-197
  of fetal malpresentations, 403
  of gestational trophoblastic disease, 212-214
  of hemolytic incompatibility, 369-371
  of placenta previa, 236-237, 245
  of postterm pregnancy, 424-425
  of precipitous labor, 400
  of pregnancy-induced hypertension, 276-278
    early, 279
  of premature rupture of membranes, 350-352
  of preterm labor, 312-313
  of prolonged labor phase, 398
  of protraction disorders, 398-399
  of renal disease, 143
  of spontaneous abortion, 164-170
Medical workup for threatened abortion, 164
Meiosis, 158
Membrane(s)
  placental, 10
  premature rupture of; *see* Premature rupture of membranes
Mental rest and preterm labor, 316-317
Mentum, 385-386
Meperidine hydrochloride, 317, 324
Mesoderm, 11
Mesotrophoblast, 10
Metabolic acidosis, 141
Metabolic changes during pregnancy, 5-6
Metabolic factors and Hobel scoring system, 24
Metabolism and placenta, 420
Metastasis and hydatidiform mole, 215, 220
Methotrexate, 213
Midpelvis contraction, 390
Migration, placental, 235-236
Mild abruptio placentae, 223, 224
Mild preeclampsia, 273-274
Mineral supplementation, 17
Miscarriage, 157
Missed abortion, 161, 162
  medical management of, 167-169
Mixed maternal bleeding, 223, 225
Models, nursing, 26-29
Moderate abruptio placentae, 223, 224
Modified leg raises, 15
Mole
  hydatidiform, 208-222
  invasive, 208

Monitor
  fetal, application of, 35-39
  for processing fetal heart rate, 40
Monitor paper and artifacts, 41
Monitoring
  blood glucose, antepartum, 98
  fetal
    and dysfunctional labor, 406
    and hemolytic incompatibility, 374
  fetal heart rate; *see* Fetal heart rate (FHR) monitoring
Morbidity
  maternal, and abruptio placentae, 228-229
  neonatal, and hyperglycemia, 96
Morphine, 324
Mortality
  fetal
    and ectopic pregnancy, 193
    and spontaneous abortion, 163
  infant
    and dysfunctional labor, 391-392
    and preterm labor, 313
  maternal
    and ectopic pregnancy, 193
    and pregnancy-induced hypertension, 274
    and spontaneous abortion, 162
  perinatal, 31
    and abruptio placentae, 229
    and placenta previa, 235
    and pregnancy-induced hypertension, 274-275
    and premature rupture of membranes, 349
    and postterm pregnancy, 419
Morula, 9, 158, 210
Mother-infant attachment, 71
Multipara
  normal labor pattern in, 393
  precipitous labor in, 400
  prolonged labor in, 398
  protraction disorders in, 398
Myocardial depression in fetus, 34-55

N

Narcotics and magnesium sulfate, 324
Negative contraction stress test, 57, 58
Neonatal effects
  of abruptio placentae, 229
  of cardiac disease, 120
  of diabetes, 95-96
  of disseminated intravascular coagulopathy, 261
  of dysfunctional labor, 391-392
  of ectopic pregnancy, 193
  of hemolytic incompatibility, 367-368
  of labor stimulation, 434
  of placenta previa, 235
  of postterm pregnancy, 422-423
  of pregnancy-induced hypertension, 274-275
  of premature rupture of membranes, 349-350
  of preterm labor, 311

Neonatal effects—cont'd
  of renal disease, 141
  of spontaneous abortion, 163
Neonatal intensive care unit (NICU), 290
Neonatal side effects of magnesium sulfate, 290-291, 324
Neonate, postmature, 422-423
Nervous system, autonomic, during pregnancy, 117
Neutral protamine hagedorn (NPH) insulin, 106
Nicotine, effects of, 170
NICU; *see* Neonatal intensive care unit (NICU)
Nifedipine, 325
Nipple stimulation
  initiation of contractions with, 57
  and postterm pregnancy, 425
Nitrofurantoin, 147
Nitrogenous waste products
  increased, symptoms of, 140
  antepartum interventions for, 145
  and renal disease, 139
Non-insulin-dependent diabetes, 88
Nongranulocytes, 7
Nonreactive stress test, 54, 55
Nonstress test (NST), 53-55
  in diabetic patient, 102
Nonuniform acceleration of fetal heart rate, 47, 48, 50
Norepinephrine, 6
Normal coagulation factor values, 261
Normal labor, 390-391
  patterns of, 393
Normal physiology
  of amniotic fluid, 347-348
  cardiac, 116-118
  of coagulation, 257-258
  of contractions, 384
  of fallopian tubes, 188-189
  of fetal circulation, 363-366
  of fetal development, 158-160
  and gestational trophoblastic disease, 210
  of labor, 307-309
  of placenta, 420
  and placenta previa, 233
  of pregnancy, 269-270
  of renal system, 136-138
Norpace; *see* Disopyramide phosphate
NPH insulin; *see* Neutral protamine hagedorn (NPH) insulin
NST; *see* Nonstress test (NST)
Nullipara
  normal labor pattern for, 393
  precipitous labor in, 400
  prolonged labor phase in, 398
  protraction disorders in, 398
Nurse, role of
  and amniocentesis, 63
  and expectant management, 239
  and patient history, 22
  and pregnancy-induced hypertension, 282-284

Nursing care plan
  and cardiac patient, 128-133
  and diabetes, 108-115
  and disseminated intravascular coagulopathy, 262-265
  and dysfunctional labor, 410-417
  and ectopic pregnancy, 200-205
  and gestational trophoblastic disease, 216-219
  and hemolytic incompatibility, 376-377
  and hypertensive disorders of pregnancy, 292-303
  and labor stimulation, 442-449
  and postterm pregnancy, 428-431
  and premature rupture of membranes, 356-359
  and preterm labor, 328-341
  and psychologic implications of high-risk pregnancy, 78-81
  and renal disease, 148-153
  and spontaneous abortion, 176-183
Nursing interventions
  and abruptio placentae, 237-243, 247, 249, 251, 253, 254
  antepartum; *see* Antepartum intervention
  and cardiac disease, 129, 131, 133
  for decreased or absent variability, 46
  and diabetes, 107, 109, 111, 113, 115
  and disseminated intravascular coagulopathy, 263, 265
  and dysfunctional labor, 411, 413, 415, 417
  for early deceleration, 48
  and ectopic pregnancy, 201, 203, 205
  for fetal bradycardia, 44
  for fetal distress, 41-52
  for fetal tachycardia, 44
  and gestational trophoblastic disease, 217, 219
  and hemolytic incompatibility, 377
  and hypertensive disorders of pregnancy, 293, 295, 297, 299, 301, 303
  for increased variability, 46
  intrapartum; *see* Intrapartum intervention
  and labor stimulation, 443, 445, 447, 449
    by amniotomy, 434-435
    by oxytocin, 436-439
    by prostaglandins, 440-441
  for late deceleration, 48
  for nonuniform accelerations, 48
  and placenta previa, 237-243, 247, 249, 251, 253, 254
  postpartum; *see* Postpartum intervention
  and postterm pregnancy, 426-427, 429, 431
  and premature rupture of membranes, 357, 359
  and preterm labor, 329, 331, 333, 335, 337, 339, 341
  for prolonged deceleration, 49
  and psychologic implications of high-risk pregnancy, 79, 81
  and renal disease, 149, 151, 153
  and spontaneous abortion, 177, 179, 181, 183

Nursing interventions—cont'd
  for uniform acceleration, 48
  for variable deceleration, 49
Nursing models, 26-29
Nursing process
  and cardiac disease, 121-129, 132
  and diabetic patient, 103-107
  and disseminated intravascular coagulopathy, 261, 264-266
  and dysfunctional labor, 401, 404-409
  and ectopic pregnancy, 197-201, 206
  and hemolytic incompatibility, 371-378
  and hydatidiform mole, 214-215, 220-221
  and postterm pregnancy, 425-427, 430
  and pregnancy-induced hypertension, 278-291
  and premature rupture of membranes, 353-357, 360
  and preterm labor, 313-329, 342
  and renal disease, 144-149
  and spontaneous abortion, 170-175
Nursing responsibilities
  and abruptio placentae and placenta previa, 239-240
  and beta-sympathomimetics, 318-319
  and cardiac patient, 122
  and convulsion, 287-288
  during evaluation of fetus, in Rh isoimmunization mother, 62
  during genetic amniocentesis, 62
  and spontaneous abortion, 173
Nutrient requirements during pregnancy, 16-17
Nutrition
  and ectopic pregnancy, 199
  and Maternal Child Health Care Index, 23
  and pregnancy-induced hypertension, 278
Nutritional adaptation to pregnancy, 16-18
Nutritional deficiency and pregnancy-induced hypertension, 268

O

Obstetric course and postterm pregnancy, 423
Obstetric diabetes, 88
Obstetric disorders and Maternal Child Health Care Index, 23
Obstetric history
  and Maternal Child Health Care Index, 23
  and postterm pregnancy, 423
Occiput presentation, 402-403
  posterior, 385
OCT; *see* Oxytocin challenge test (OCT)
Oliguria, 280
Open-loop insulin pump, 100
Oral antidiabetic agents, 107
Oral tocolytic therapy, 322-323
Orem model of self-care, 28-29
Oscilloscope and artifacts, 41
Outcome of tubal pregnancy, 191
Outcome criteria
  and abruptio placentae, 246, 248, 250, 252
  and cardiac disease, 128, 130, 132

Outcome criteria—cont'd
  and diabetic patient, 108, 110, 112, 114
  and disseminated intravascular coagulopathy, 262, 264
  and dysfunctional labor, 410, 412, 414, 416
  and ectopic pregnancy, 200, 202, 204
  and gestational trophoblastic disease, 216, 218
  and hemolytic incompatibility, 376
  and hypertensive disorders of pregnancy, 292, 294, 296, 298, 300, 302
  and labor stimulation, 442, 444, 446, 448
  and placenta previa, 246, 248, 250, 252
  and postterm pregnancy, 428, 430
  and premature rupture of membranes, 356, 358
  and preterm labor, 328, 330, 332, 334, 336, 338, 340
  and psychologic implications of high-risk pregnancy, 78, 80
  and renal disease, 148, 150, 152
  and spontaneous abortion, 176, 178, 180, 182
Outlet contraction, 390
Outpatient criteria and pregnancy-induced hypertension, 277
Ovaries
  enlargement of, and hydatidiform mole, 211
  during pregnancy, 9
Overstimulation of labor, 433
Ovum, transperitoneal migration of, 188
Oxygen, partial pressure of, 4
Oxygenation and cardiac disease, 120
Oxytocin, 6
  and cardiac disease, 127
  and hydatidiform mole, 215
  labor stimulated by, 435-439
  and pregnancy-induced hypertension, 289
  and premature labor, 308-309, 310
  side effects of, 175
  and spontaneous abortion, 166
  stimulation of contractions with, 57
Oxytocin challenge test (OCT), 55-56, 57-60

P

Pain
  and abruptio placentae, 227
  back, and dysfunctional labor, 408
  and ectopic pregnancy, 192, 197
  and labor stimulation, 433
  and oxytocin, 439
PAP; *see* Pulmonary artery pressure (PAP)
Papanicolaou (Pap) smear, 13
Parity and postterm pregnancy, 423
Paroxysmal atrial tachycardia, fetal, 41
Partial hydatidiform mole, 211
Partial placenta previa, 231, 232
Partial pressure of blood gases, 4
Passive exercises for bed rest obstetric patients, 14, 15
Pathologic edema and pregnancy-induced hypertension, 273

Pathophysiology
  of abruptio placentae, 226
  of cardiac disease, 118
  of diabetes during pregnancy, 90-92
  of disseminated intravascular coagulopathy, 258, 260
  of ectopic pregnancy, 189-191
  of gestational trophoblastic disease, 210-211
  of hemolytic incompatibility, 366-367
  of implantation, 160
  of labor, 384-390
  of placenta previa, 233-234
  of postterm pregnancy, 420-421
  of pregnancy-induced hypertension, 270-271
  of premature rupture of membranes, 348-349
  of preterm labor, 310-311
  of renal disease, 138-140
Patient
  position of, and labor, 404
  psychologic response of, and spontaneous abortion, 172, 173
Patient education on smoking and drinking, 171
Patient problems, potential; *see* Potential patient problems
Patterns, fetal heart rate, 47-52
PCWP; *see* Pulmonary capillary wedge pressure (PCWP)
Pelvic dystocia, 388, 390
  causes of, 384
  incidence of, 383
Pelvic examination and postterm pregnancy, 424-425
Pelvic scoring system, 433
Penicillin and cardiac disease, 121
Perinatal mortality; *see* Mortality, perinatal
Perineal hygiene, 145
Peripheral vascular resistance, 270
PG; *see* Phosphatidyglycerol (PG)
pH, 4-5
Phenobarbital, 276
Phosphatidyglycerol (PG), 62
  and fetal lung maturity, 351
Phospholipase A_2 and labor, 307-308
  preterm, 310
Physical assessment and hemolytic incompatibility, 373-374
Physical discomfort and postterm pregnancy, 422
Physiologic adaptations to pregnancy, 3-21
Physiologic basis for fetal heart rate monitoring, 33-35
Physiologic changes, factors unrelated to, and preterm labor, 310-311
Physiologic considerations of high-risk pregnancy, 1-68
Physiologic edema, 270
  and pregnancy-induced hypertension, 273
Physiology
  of abruptio placentae, 226-229

Physiology—cont'd
  cardiac, 116-120
  of diabetes, 87-96
  of disseminated intravascular coagulopathy, 257-261
  of dysfunctional labor, 384-392
  of ectopic pregnancy, 188-193
  of fetal development, 158-163
  of gestational trophoblastic disease, 210-212
  of hemolytic incompatibility, 363-368
  of placenta previa, 233-235
  of postterm pregnancy, 420-423
  of pregnancy-induced hypertension, 269-275
  of premature rupture of membranes, 347-350
  of preterm labor, 307-311
  of renal disease, 136-141
PIH; *see* Pregnancy-induced hypertension (PIH)
Pitocin, 436
Pituitary gland, 6
Placenta, 10-11
  blood supply to, 270
  cells of, 233
  deterioration of, in postterm pregnancy, 423
  formation of, 210
  and hemolytic incompatibility, 366
  maximum functioning time of, 420-421
  normal physiology of, 420
  organ functions of, 33
  separation of, and disseminated intravascular coagulopathy, 260
  and spontaneous abortion, 165
Placenta previa
  compared with abruptio placentae, 244-245
  etiology of, 233
  incidence of, 231-233
  medical diagnosis, 235-236
  nursing care plan, 246-253
  nursing process, 237-243, 254
  physiology, 233-235
  usual medical management, 236-237
Placental causes of preterm labor, 307
Placental factors and Hobel scoring system, 25
Placental membrane, 10
Placental migration, 235-236
Plasma progesterone, 13
Plasma volume, 3
Plasma volume expanders and pregnancy-induced hypertension, 277-278
Plasma volume increase during pregnancy, 33
Plasmin, 258
Plasminogen, 258
pO_2, fetal, 34
Polycystic kidney disease, 135
Polyhydramnios and diabetes, 93-94
Position of patient and labor, 404
Positive contraction stress test, 57, 60
Postmaturity, 419, 422-423
Postoperative intervention
  and ectopic pregnancy, 199-201

Postoperative intervention—cont'd
and hemolytic incompatibility, 377-378
and hydatidiform mole, 215, 220
and spontaneous abortion, 174-175
Postpartum depression and labor stimulation, 442
Postpartum diabetes, 93
Postpartum diuresis, 289
Postpartum intervention
and abruptio placentae, 243, 254
and cardiac disease, 127-129
and diabetes, 107
and disseminated intravascular coagulopathy, 265
and dysfunctional labor, 409
and labor stimulation, 441-442
and placenta previa, 243, 254
and pregnancy-induced hypertension, 289-291
and premature rupture of membranes, 357, 360
and preterm labor, 328-329, 342
and renal disease, 147-148
Postpartum management of diabetes, 103
Postpartum physical assessment and hemolytic incompatibility, 373-374
Postterm pregnancy, 419-431
etiology of, 419-420
incidence of, 419
medical diagnosis, 423-424
nursing care plan, 428-431
nursing process, 425-427, 430
physiology, 420-423
usual medical management, 424-425
Potassium deficit, 140
Potential loss, 76
Potential patient problems
and abruptio placentae, 246, 248, 250, 252
and cardiac disease, 128, 130, 132
and diabetes, 108, 110, 112, 114
and disseminated intravascular coagulopathy, 262, 264
and dysfunctional labor, 410, 412, 414, 416
and ectopic pregnancy, 200, 202, 204
and gestational trophoblastic disease, 216, 218
and hemolytic incompatibility, 376
and hypertensive disorders of pregnancy, 292, 294, 296, 298, 300, 302
and labor stimulation, 442, 444, 446, 448
and placenta previa, 246, 248, 250, 252
and postterm pregnancy, 428, 430
and premature rupture of membranes, 356, 358
and preterm labor, 328, 330, 332, 334, 336, 338, 340
and psychologic implications of high-risk pregnancy, 78, 80
and renal disease, 148, 150, 152
and spontaneous abortion, 176, 178, 180, 182
Precipitous labor, 397, 400

Preeclampsia, 268
and diabetes, 93
and disseminated intravascular coagulopathy, 260
grades of, 273-274
and hydatidiform mole, 211
nursing care plan for, 292-299
signs of, 273
Pregnancy
blood volume increase in, 33
and cardiac disease; *see* Cardiac disease and pregnancy
cardiovascular adaptations during, 3-4
changes in renal function during, 137-138
diabetes and; *see* Diabetes and pregnancy
ectopic; *see* Ectopic pregnancy
gastrointestinal responses during, 8
glandular developments during, 6
hematologic changes during, 7-8
hepatic adjustments to, 7
high-risk; *see* High-risk pregnancy
hypertensive disorders of; *see* Hypertensive disorders of pregnancy
metabolic changes during, 5-6
nutritional adaptations to, 16-18
plasma volume increase during, 33
postterm; *see* Postterm pregnancy
physiologic adaptations to, 3-21
renal adaptations to, 6-7
and renal disease; *see* Renal disease and pregnancy
reproductive system adaptations during, 8-9
respiratory changes during, 4-5
vaginal bleeding during, 163
validation of, 72
Pregnancy-induced hypertension (PIH), 267, 268
etiology of, 268-269
fetal and neonatal effects, 274-275
incidence of, 267
maternal effects, 274
medical diagnosis, 275-276
medical management of, 276-278
pathophysiology, 270-271, 272
physiology, 269-275
versus chronic hypertension, 142-143
Pregnancy termination
and pregnancy-induced hypertension, 276
and renal disease, 143
Preload, 118
Premature arterial contractions, fetal, 41
Premature rupture of membranes (PROM), 347-362
etiology of, 347
incidence of, 347
medical diagnosis, 350
nursing care plan, 356-359
nursing process, 353-357, 360
physiology, 347-350

Premature rupture of membranes (PROM)—cont'd
usual medical management, 350-352
Premature ventricular contractions, fetal, 41
Prematurity and labor stimulation, 434
Prenatal evaluation and postterm pregnancy, 424
Preoperative protocol and ectopic pregnancy, 198
Pressure readings, hemodynamic, 123
Preterm delivery and premature rupture of membranes, 347
Preterm labor, 306-346
etiology of, 306-307
incidence of, 306
medical diagnosis, 311
nursing care plan, 328-341
nursing process, 313-329, 342
physiology, 307-311
and premature rupture of membranes, 349
and urinary tract infection, 141
usual medical management, 312-313
Prevention
and abruptio placentae, 237
and cardiac disease, 121-122
and diabetes, 103
and disseminated intravascular coagulopathy, 261, 264
and dysfunctional labor, 401, 404
and ectopic pregnancy, 197
and hemolytic incompatibility, 371
and hydatidiform mole, 214
and placenta previa, 237
and postterm pregnancy, 425
and pregnancy-induced hypertension, 278-279
and premature rupture of membranes, 353
and preterm labor, 313-315
and renal disease, 144
and spontaneous abortion, 170-171
Primary abdominal pregnancy, 191
Procedure
for amniocentesis, 62
for contraction stress test, 57
for nonstress test, 54
Process, nursing; *see* Nursing process
Progesterone, 4, 159
and labor, 307-308
prophylactic use of, 314
Proliferative trophoblastic disease, 208, 213-214
and hydatidiform mole, 215, 220
Prolonged deceleration of fetal heart rate, 47, 49, 51
Prolonged labor phase, 398
Prolonged latent phase disorders, 394-395
PROM; *see* Premature rupture of membranes (PROM)
Prophylactic antibiotics, 352
Prophylactic chemotherapy and proliferative trophoblastic disease, 213-214

Propranolol
and cardiac disease, 125-126
and intravenous beta-sympathomimetic therapy, 321
Prostaglandin
and labor, 307-309
labor stimulated with, 439-441
and missed abortion, 168
and preterm labor, 310
and spontaneous abortion, 173-174
Prostaglandin E_2 (PE_2), 439, 440
Prostaglandin F_{2a} (PF_{2a}), 439-440
Prostaglandin inhibitors and preterm labor, 325-326
Protein(s), 5
and pregnancy-induced hypertension, 278
in urine, 139
Protein requirements during pregnancy, 16
Proteinuria
and dipstick readings, 280, 281
and pregnancy-induced hypertension, 273
Prothrombin activator, 258
Protocol
for administration of oxytocin, 436-438
preoperative, and ectopic pregnancy, 198
for suppression of labor, 316-318
Protraction disorders, 395-396, 398-399
Psychologic adaptations to high-risk pregnancy, 71-83
anxiety, frustration, and conflict, 73-74
attachment and developmental tasks, 71-73
crisis, coping, and adaptation, 74-76
loss and grief, 76-79, 82
suggested plan of nursing care, 78-81
Psychologic effects of diabetes, 94
Psychologic impact of postterm pregnancy, 427
Psychologic implications of high-risk pregnancy, nursing care plan for, 78-81
Psychologic needs
and pregnancy-induced hypertension, 290
and premature rupture of membranes, 360
and preterm labor, 342
Psychologic response of patient and spontaneous abortion, 172, 173
Psychologic status and preterm labor, 316
Psychosocial impact of Rh sensitization, 372
Pulmonary artery pressure (PAP), 122, 123
Pulmonary capillary wedge pressure (PCWP), 122, 123
Pulmonary edema, 119
and cardiac disease, 122
and ectopic pregnancy, 199
and magnesium sulfate, 324
signs of, 141
Pulmonary hypertension, 119
Pump, insulin, 98, 99-100
Pyelonephritis, 140
antepartum intervention for, 145
Pyruvate, 5

Q

Quinidine, 126

R

Race and Maternal Child Health Care Index, 23
Radioimmunoassay tests for ectopic pregnancy, 195
Rapid-acting insulin, 106
RDE; *see* Respiratory distress syndrome (RDS)
Reactive nonstress test, 54, 55
Referral
    antepartum, and hemolytic incompatibility, 375
    of diabetic patient, 105
Regulation of fetal heart rate, 35
Relaxation phase of contraction, 384
Renal adaptations to pregnancy, 6-7, 137-138
Renal biopsy, 142
Renal blood flow, 6-7, 136
Renal calculi, 135
Renal disease and pregnancy, 135-153
    etiology of, 136
    incidence of, 135-136
    medical diagnosis, 141-143
    nursing care plan, 148-153
    nursing process, 144-149
    physiology, 136-141
    usual medical management, 143
Renal factors and Hobel scoring system, 24
Renal failure, postpartum, 254
Renal function, marginal, antepartum intervention for, 145
Renal function studies, 142
Renal transplant, pregnancy following, 135-136
Renal ultrasound, 143
Renin-angiotensin system, 138
Reproductive system adaptations during pregnancy, 8-9
Respiratory changes during pregnancy, 4-5
Respiratory distress syndrome (RDS), 326
    and premature rupture of membranes, 349
    and preterm infant, 311
Rest
    and dysfunctional labor, 409
    and pregnancy-induced hypertension, 279
Rh, 12
Rh incompatibility, 363
Rh immune globulin, 374, 375
Rh isoimmunization
    and amniocentesis, 62
    and ectopic pregnancy, 199
    and hydatidiform mole, 215
Rheumatic fever and cardiovascular disease, 116
Right angle retractors and breech presentation, 408-409
Rigidity, uterine, and abruptio placentae, 226-227
Ripe cervix, 433
Risk, maternal, and cardiac disease, 124

Risk factors for diabetics, 96-97
Ritodrine, 125
    and external cephalic version, 401
    and preterm labor, 313
    for suppression of labor, 318-323
Role transition, 73
Rollover test and pregnancy-induced hypertension, 275
Roy adaptation model, 26-27
Rubella screen, 12
Rupture
    of membranes; *see* Premature rupture of membranes
    tubal, 190-191
    uterine, and dysfunctional labor, 407

S

Salbutamol, 318
Salpingectomy, 196
Salpingitis compared with ectopic pregnancy, 194
Salpingo-oophorectomy, 196
Salpingotomy, 196
    for infertility, 200-201
Scoring systems
    for high-risk pregnancy, 22-26
    pelvic, 433
Scotoma, 280
Screening
    for diabetes, 97
    and hemolytic incompatibility, 368-369, 371, 374
    for pregnancy-induced hypertension, 275
Second trimester, diabetes in, 93
Secondary abdominal pregnancy, 191
Sedatives
    and magnesium sulfate, 324
    and pregnancy-induced hypertension, 276
    and preterm labor, 317
    and prolonged latent phase disorder, 394-395
Seizure; *see* Convulsion
Selective transfer, 34
Self, loss of, 76
Sensitive period, 71
Sensitivity, decreased, to oxytocin, 439
Sensitization, 366, 368-369
Septic abortion, 162
    medical management of, 169-170
Septicemia and premature rupture of membranes, 349
Serial human chorionic gonadotropin titers and hydatidiform mole, 212
Serum creatinine, 142
Serum creatinine levels, 7
Serum magnesium levels, 285
Severe abruptio placentae, 223, 224
Severe preeclampsia, 274
Shelf life of insulin, 106

Shock
  and abruptio placentae, 227-228
  and disseminated intravascular coagulopathy,
    260
  and ectopic pregnancy, 198
  hypovolemic, and third-trimester bleeding,
    241, 242
Shoulder pain and ectopic pregnancy, 197
Shoulder presentation, 386, 387, 402-403
Side effects
  of ethanol, 325
  of hydralazine, 287
  of isoxsuprine, 318
  of magnesium sulfate, 324
  of oxytocin, 438-439
  of prostaglandin, 441
  of Rh immune globulin, 375
  of ritodrine, 320
  of terbutaline, 320
Significance
  of decreased or absent variability, 46
  of early deceleration, 48
  of fetal bradycardia, 44
  of fetal tachycardia, 44
  of increased variability, 46
  of late deceleration, 48
  of nonuniform accelerations, 48
  of prolonged deceleration, 49
  of uniform accelerations, 48
  of variable deceleration, 49
Signs and symptoms
  of abruptio placentae, 224, 226-228, 244
  of cardiac disease, 118-119
  of chorioamnionitis, 354
  of diabetes, 92, 93
  of disseminated intravascular coagulopathy,
    260-261
  of dysfunctional labor, 390-391
  of eclampsia, 287
  of ectopic pregnancy, 191-193
  of hemolytic incompatibility, 367
  of hydatidiform mole, 211
  of placenta previa, 234, 244
  of postmaturity, 422-423
  of postterm pregnancy, 421
  of preeclampsia, 273
  of pregnancy-induced hypertension, 271, 273-
    274, 283
  of premature rupture of membranes, 349
  of preterm labor, 315
  of renal disease, 140-141
  of spontaneous abortion, 160-162
Simple diffusion, 34
Single footling breech, 388, 389
Sinusoidal pattern of fetal heart rate, 368, 369
Sites of ectopic pregnancy, 186, 187
Situational crisis, 75
Smoking
  and abruptio placentae, 224

Smoking—cont'd
  and premature rupture of membranes, 353
  and pregnancy-induced hypertension, 279,
    283
  and preterm labor, 314
  and spontaneous abortion, 170-171
Socioeconomic status and preterm labor, 310,
    313-314
Sodium and renal disease, 138-139
Sodium chloride and vasomotor collapse, 290
Sodium depletion during pregnancy, 269
Sodium excess, signs of, 140
Sodium intake
  and cardiac disease, 121
  during pregnancy, 17
  and pregnancy-induced hypertension, 276
Sodium retention, 271
Somogyi effect, 92
Speculum examination and placenta previa, 235
Split dose insulin, 99
Spontaneous abortion, 157-185
  and cardiac disease, 120
  classification of, 162
  with ectopic pregnancy, 194
  etiology of, 157-158
  incidence of, 157
  medical diagnosis, 163-164
  nursing care plan, 176-183
  nursing process, 170-175
  physiology, 158-163
  usual medical management, 164-170
Staphylococcal bacteria, 136
Steroid therapy for stimulation of fetal lung ma-
    turity, 326-327
Stimulation
  of fetal lung maturity, 326-327
  labor; *see* Labor stimulation
Streptococcal bacteria, 136
Stress test, 55-56, 57-60
Stressors, fetal capability for withstanding, 34-35
Stroke volume, 118
Studies, renal function, 142
Subsequent abortion, risk of, and spontaneous
    abortion, 162-163
Substrates for cellular metabolism, 5
Suction curettage and missed abortion, 168
Sugar in urine, 138
Sulfonamides, 147
Sulphonylureas, 107
Superimposed preeclampsia and eclampsia, 268
Supplementation during pregnancy, 17
Suppression of labor, 312
  drug therapy for, 318-326
  protocol for, 316-318
Surgery
  abdominal, postoperative procedures for, 199
  preparation for, and hydatidiform mole, 214-
    215
Suspicious contraction stress test, 57, 58

Sympathomimetic drugs, 318
Sympathomimetic tocolytic drugs, 318
Symptoms; *see* Signs and symptoms
Synchrony, 72-73
Syncytial trophoblast, 10
Syncytiotrophoblast, 420
Syntocinon, 436
Systemic diseases and spontaneous abortion, 158
Systemic emboli, 119
Systemic vascular resistance, 118
Systole phase of contraction, 384
Systolic pulmonary artery pressure, 123

T

Tachycardia, 46
    fetal, 44, 45
Tactile interactions, mother-infant, 71
Tasks, developmental, 71-73
Temperature and infection, 172
Tenderness, uterine, and abruptio placentae, 227
Terbutaline, 125
    and external cephalic version, 401
    and precipitous labor, 397
    for suppression of labor, 318-323
Terbutaline sulfate and preterm labor, 313
Test(s)
    contraction stress, 55-56, 57-60
    for diabetes, 96
    nonstress, 53-55
Testape, 98, 322
Tetracycline, 146
Therapeutic induction, 432
Therapy, drug; *see* Drug therapy
Thiazides, 125
Third trimester, diabetes in, 93
Third trimester bleeding; *see* Abruptio placenta;
        Placenta previa
Threatened abortion, 161, 162
    medical management of, 164-165
Thyroid gland, 6
Tocolytic agents
    and cardiac disease, 125
    and preterm labor, 317-318
Tocotransducer, 37, 40
Total placenta previa, 231, 232
Toxemia, 267
Toxicity, magnesium, 286-287, 324
Transfer
    through placenta, 420
    selective, 34
Transfusion, intrauterine, 370-371, 374
Transition, role, 73
Transition phase of labor, 390-391
Transperitoneal migration of ovum, 188
Transplant, renal, 135-136
Trauma
    birth
        and breech presentation, 388
        and dysfunctional labor, 392

Trauma—cont'd
    and preterm labor, 315
Tray, eclamptic, 287
Treatment; *see* Medical management
Trial labor, 392, 393
    and fetopelvic disproportion, 407
    and third-trimester bleeding, 242, 243
Trimester manifestations and consequences of di-
        abetes, 93
Trimesters, growth of fetus by, 11
Trophoblast, 9, 158-159, 210
Tubal abortion, 189-190
Tubal adhesions and ectopic pregnancy, 188
Tubal ectopic pregnancy, 189-191
Tubal rupture, 190-191
Tubules, 137
    inflammation of, 138

U

Ultrasound
    and abruptio placentae, 230
    and cardiac disease, 120
    and diabetic patient, 100
    and ectopic pregnancy, 195
    and external cephalic version, 401
    and fetal monitoring, 56, 61
    and gestational age, 351
    and hydatidiform mole, 212
    and placenta previa, 235
    and postterm pregnancy, 424
    renal, 143
    and vaginal bleeding, 163
Ultrasound transducer, 37
Uniform accelerations of fetal heart rate, 47, 48,
        50
Unsatisfactory contraction stress test, 57, 59
UPI; *see* Uteroplacental insufficiency (UPI)
Uric acid, 142
Urinalysis, 12, 144
Urinary creatinine clearance, 142
Urinary output
    and cardiac disease, 122
    and circulatory volume, 241-242
Urinary pregnancy tests and ectopic pregnancy,
        195
Urinary protein, 142
Urinary tract infection, 136, 138
    antepartum intervention for, 145
    postpartum intervention for, 147
    and preterm labor, 141
Urine testing, antepartum, 98
Uterine abnormalities and preterm labor, 310-
        311
Uterine bleeding and hydatidiform mole, 211
Uterine blood flow, 4
    and preterm labor, 310
Uterine causes of preterm labor, 307
Uterine contractions; *see* Contractions

Uterine disorders
  and habitual abortion, 169
  and spontaneous abortion, 158
Uterine dystocia, 383, 384
Uterine ischemia, 269
Uterine pressure catheter, 38-39
Uterine rigidity and abruptio placentae, 226-227
Uterine rupture and dysfunctional labor, 407
Uterine scarring and placenta previa, 233
Uterine tenderness and abruptio placentae, 227
Uteroplacental-fetal exchange, 33-34
Uteroplacental insufficiency (UPI), 53
Uterus
  blood supply to, 270
  effect of oxytocin on, 438
  enlarged, and hydatidiform mole, 211
  evacuation of
    and hydatidiform mole, 212-213
    methods for, 165-166
    and missed abortion, 167-168
    reasons for, 164
  during pregnancy, 8

V

Vacuum aspiration, 165-166
  and missed abortion, 167-168
Vagina during pregnancy, 8
Vaginal bacterial flora and premature rupture of
    membranes, 348
Vaginal bleeding
  and abruptio placentae, 227
  assessment of, 171-172
  causes of, 163
  and ectopic pregnancy, 192, 197-198
  and placenta previa, 234
  and spontaneous abortion, 160
Vaginal delivery
  and abruptio placentae, 230, 231, 240-241
  and arrest disorders, 397
  and breech presentation, 388, 408
  and cardiac disease, 121
  and eclampsia, 288
  and malpresentations, 407-408
  and placenta previa, 237, 240-241
  and pregnancy-induced hypertension, 289
Vaginal examination
  and AROM, 435
  digital, and premature rupture of membranes,
    350
  and dysfunctional labor, 405

Vaginal examination—cont'd
  and fetal malpresentations, 403
Vaginitis and diabetes, 94
Validation of pregnancy, 72
Valium; *see* Diazepam
Variability of fetal heart rate, 46-47
Variable deceleration of fetal heart rate, 47, 49,
    51
Vascular deterioration and diabetes, 92-93
Vasodilan; *see* Isoxsuprine hydrocholoride
Vasomotor collapse and pregnancy-induced hy-
    pertension, 290
VDRL, 12
Verbal interactions, mother-infant, 72
Vesicles, grapelike, and hydatidiform mole, 211
Viable fetus, 157
Villi, 10
Viruses and spontaneous abortion, 158
Visual interactions, mother-infant, 72
Vital signs and pregnancy-induced hypertension,
    279-280
Vitamin supplementation, 17
Vitamins, water-soluble, in urine, 138
Volume, stroke, 118
Vulva during pregnancy, 8

W

Warfarin, 124
Warning signs of postterm pregnancy, 426
Water intoxication and labor stimulation, 441-
    442
Water retention, 271
  and oxytocin, 438-439
Water-soluble vitamins in urine, 138
Weight gain, maternal, 13-14, 18
  and renal disease, 144
White blood cell count (WBC) and infection,
    172
White blood cells, 7

X

X-ray pelvimetry, 392

Y

Yolk sac, 10
Yutopar; *see* Ritodrine

Z

Zinc deficiency during pregnancy, 17
Zygote, 158, 210